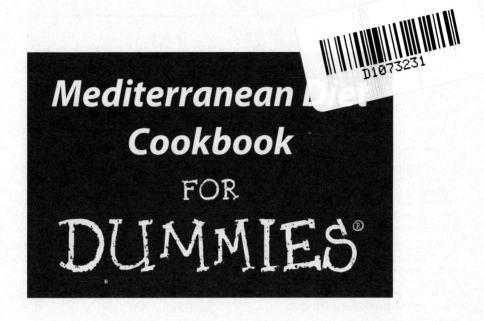

Mediterranean Diet Cookbook

FOR

DUMMIES®

by Meri Raffetto, RD, LDN
and Wendy Jo Peterson, MS, RD

WILEY

John Wiley & Sons, Inc.

Mediterranean Diet Cookbook For Dummies®

Published by
John Wiley & Sons, Inc.
111 River St.
Hoboken, NJ 07030-5774
www.wiley.com

10

WILEY

About the Authors

Meri Raffetto is a registered dietitian and recognized professional in the area of nutrition and wellness. Meri is the founder of Real Living Nutrition Services® (www.reallivingnutrition.com), providing one of the few interactive online weight-loss and wellness programs where people can work with a dietitian to get advice, support, and coaching to reach their goals. She also develops custom online corporate wellness programs for small to large companies. Meri is a freelance writer and the author of *The Glycemic Index Diet For Dummies* and coauthor of *The Glycemic Index Cookbook For Dummies* (both published by John Wiley & Sons, Inc.).

She is a wife and a mother of triplets and loves every crazy minute! She has a passion for great food and enjoys getting outside as much as possible for camping, swimming, and hiking with her family.

Wendy Jo Peterson, MS, RD, is a registered dietitian with a master's degree in nutritional sciences from San Diego State University. Wendy Jo specializes in culinary arts, public speaking, sports nutrition, and nutrition for musicians. She is the owner of the San Diego–based private practice Edible Nutrition® (www.EdibleNutrition.com), which includes nutrition counseling, corporate wellness consulting and speaking, and culinary nutrition. When she's not in San Diego, you can find her on the road working as the Roadie Nutritionist® (FuelinRoadie.com) with traveling musicians. Wendy Jo has a love of food and nutrition and shares her knowledge as an adjunct professor at San Diego Mesa Community College.

She is a proud military wife and a mother of the four-legged variety. If she's not in the kitchen, you may be able to find her in the surf, on the rocks, or in the mountains, but two things will be certain: She'll be eating well and listening to good music!

Dedication

Inspiration for this book came from those closest to us — friends and family — who continue to celebrate food in respect to their unique cultures. We dedicate this book to all the mothers, fathers, and grandparents who keep their family food traditions alive for the next generation. You inspired us not only to write but also to continue with our own traditions and the joy of celebrating delicious food. Thank you for your dedication and love of food and family.

Authors' Acknowledgments

To start, we want to thank Matt Wagner from Fresh Books and our acquisitions editor, Erin Calligan Mooney. Thank you for always being such a pleasure to work with and for your flexibility and creative solutions to make this book happen. Our project editor, Chad Sievers, was wonderful to work with, and we greatly appreciate his time and support in making this book organized and fun to read, not to mention his going the extra mile to help us balance work life and family life.

A big thank you to Megan Knoll for her dedication in helping us find the perfect wording, especially when using traditional recipes that are sometimes complex, and to our technical reviewer and nutritional analyst, Rachel Nix, for ensuring the information in the book was accurate and offering helpful suggestions to enhance the book. Emily Nolan, thank you for testing all these recipes to ensure that they're easy to follow and turn out the way we hoped they would: delicious!

Writing a cookbook and developing recipes is always a fun experience with so many people involved in different ways. Wendy Jo would specifically like to thank her amazing husband for taste-testing every recipe and supporting her even from afar; her parents, Bob and Nancy, for inspiring and setting the foundation of cooking; her best friend, Kathie, and her mother, Maria, for providing her Italian love and a guiding hand in the recipes; Teresa and Anita for shedding light on the Middle Eastern influence within Mediterranean food; Leslie for sharing family favorites; Becky and Micki for helping her make food to feed an army; and her interns, Bryana, Merri, Marty, and Nicole, for helping with the research and development of the recipes.

Meri would specifically like to thank her husband, Mark, for his never-ending support; her sisters, Marla and Rosemarie, for always being there to share ideas; and her parents, Joe and Iolanda, for modeling the southern Italian culture in her American upbringing. Lastly a special thank you to her grandmother, Linda, for being her greatest inspiration and writing muse while working on this book. Thank you!

Publisher's Acknowledgments

We're proud of this book; please send us your comments at http://dummies.custhelp.com. For other comments, please contact our Customer Care Department within the U.S. at 877-762-2974, outside the U.S. at 317-572-3993, or fax 317-572-4002.

Some of the people who helped bring this book to market include the following:

Acquisitions, Editorial, and Vertical Websites

Senior Project Editor: Chad R. Sievers

Acquisitions Editor: Erin Calligan Mooney

Copy Editor: Megan Knoll

Assistant Editor: David Lutton

Editorial Program Coordinator: Joe Niesen

Technical Editor: Rachel Nix

Recipe Tester: Emily Nolan

Editorial Manager: Michelle Hacker

Editorial Assistant: Rachelle Amick

Art Coordinator: Alicia B. South

Cover Photos: T.J. Hine Photography

Cartoons: Rich Tennant (www.the5thwave.com)

Composition Services

Project Coordinator: Nikki Gee

Layout and Graphics: Carl Byers, Joyce Haughey, Corrie Socolovitch, Christin Swinford

Proofreaders: Dwight Ramsey, Nancy L. Reinhardt

Indexer: Sharon Shock

Illustrator: Liz Kurtzman

Photographer: T.J. Hine Photography

Food Stylist: Lisa Bishop

Publishing and Editorial for Consumer Dummies

    Kathleen Nebenhaus, Vice President and Executive Publisher

    David Palmer, Associate Publisher

    Kristin Ferguson-Wagstaffe, Product Development Director

Publishing for Technology Dummies

    Andy Cummings, Vice President and Publisher

Composition Services

    Debbie Stailey, Director of Composition Services

Contents at a Glance

Recipes at a Glance

Table of Contents

Introduction

*I*magine the Mediterranean Sea, where the water and the land are big parts of life. Picture people eating fresh foods and relaxing with friends and family. That image is the essence of the traditional Mediterranean diet. In other words, the Mediterranean diet is part of certain lifestyle habits, including diet, physical activity, stress management, and fun, used in various regions of the Mediterranean coast. Research has shown that people who live in these areas have less heart disease and better longevity. Throughout this book, you uncover more about the details of these habits and how they affect your health and well-being. You can dive in and use all these concepts as a way of life or adopt a few of the strategies that work for you.

No matter what inspired you to pick up *Mediterranean Diet Cookbook For Dummies*, we know that changing habits isn't always easy. These particular life strategies can be challenging because they all focus on one main trend — slowing down — that's at odds with many people's busy lifestyles. Our goal in this book is to show you that implementing a Mediterranean diet and lifestyle can be simple and flavorful. You don't have to follow a strict dietary plan or omit any foods; in fact, the Mediterranean diet is more about adding than taking away. This book is here to help you make small changes so you can find more balance in your life.

About This Book

If you're curious about using the Mediterranean style of cooking in your life, *Mediterranean Diet Cookbook For Dummies* is the perfect book for you. In the following pages, you can find historical information about the region, the balance of foods the people there eat, the health benefits of this style of eating, and more than 160 recipes full of delicious flavor. You also find some cooking tips and meal-planning tools to help make your transition simple.

You can use this book as a resource, and you don't have to read it from cover to cover. Instead, you can find that perfect recipe you've been looking for or head straight to the chapter on meal planning (that'd be Chapter 4) to get examples of how to pull meals together easily. You find everything you need to begin making changes toward a Mediterranean style of life.

Conventions Used in This Book

Like all cookbooks, we recommend that you read all the way through each recipe before you start making it. That way, you can account for any necessary refrigeration time, marinating time, and so on and for any special tools, such as a stick blender, that the recipe may require.

Here are a few other guidelines to keep in mind about the recipes in this book:

- All butter is unsalted unless otherwise stated. Margarine isn't a suitable substitute for butter.
- All eggs are large.
- All milk is lowfat unless otherwise specified.
- All onions are yellow unless otherwise specified.
- All pepper is freshly ground black pepper unless otherwise specified.
- All salt is kosher.
- All dry ingredient measurements are level.
- All temperatures are Fahrenheit (see the appendix to convert Fahrenheit temperatures to Celsius).
- All lemon and lime juice is freshly squeezed.
- All sugar is white granulated sugar unless otherwise noted.
- All flour is all-purpose white flour unless otherwise noted.
- When a recipe says to steam a vegetable, the amount of water you need to use in your pot or steamer depends on your steaming method, so we don't include the water in the ingredients list. As a general rule, if you're using a basket in a pot, the water level should be just below the basket.

Although most of the recipes in this book require relatively few ingredients, we include a few classics that have longer ingredient lists; a culinary tour of the Mediterranean just wouldn't be complete without these dishes. Don't be intimidated by the longer lists of ingredients. They may look overwhelming, but the recipes themselves are still pretty simple.

Finally, we include the following basic conventions throughout the rest of the book:

- For the purposes of this book, a Mediterranean lifestyle and dietary pattern focuses on the traditional habits seen at least 50 years ago in Crete, Greece, Spain, southern Italy, and Morocco.
- We use **boldface** to highlight keywords and the specific action steps in numbered lists.

✔ We use *italic* to define or emphasize a word or phrase.

☼ We use this little tomato icon to highlight the vegetarian recipes in this book.

✔ Websites appear in `monofont`; we haven't added any extra spaces or punctuation in them, so type exactly what you see in the text.

What You're Not to Read

You're probably very busy with everyday life and may only have time to read the essential information in this book to help you make the transition to the Mediterranean diet. If so, go ahead and skip the following bits of information:

✔ **Sidebars:** Like all *For Dummies* books, this book has gray-shaded boxes called *sidebars* that contain interesting but supplementary information. Sidebars often have anecdotes or some nitty-gritty information that isn't vital to your understanding of the topic at hand. We won't hold you accountable for this info — promise!

✔ **Text marked with the Technical Stuff icon:** The text marked with the little Technical Stuff icon in the margin usually is notable but nonessential information about the Mediterranean or medical stuff. Check out the section "Icons Used in This Book" for more detail about how we use icons.

Foolish Assumptions

When writing this book, we made the following few assumptions about you, our dear reader:

✔ You're looking for meal-planning tips that will help you succeed with your health and weight-loss goals.

✔ You want to incorporate these recipes into your lifestyle.

✔ You have an understanding of cooking basics. In other words, you know your way around a kitchen and know how to use a knife without cutting your finger. If you need to brush up on your cooking skills, check out *Cooking Basics For Dummies*, 4th Edition, by Bryan Miller, Marie Rama, and Eve Adamson (John Wiley & Sons, Inc) before you get rolling.

✔ You're used to the standard American way of eating and wonder whether anything called a "diet" can be yummy and satisfying.

✔ You aren't afraid to embrace a lifestyle that goes against the grain of what many around you may be doing.

✔ You're looking for ways to get more vitamins, minerals, and antioxidants into your diet.

✔ You're genuinely willing to make changes and stick to them until they become habits.

How This Book Is Organized

We've set up this book to make it easy to navigate. The book is divided into five parts to help you incorporate the benefits of a Mediterranean-style diet into your life with recipes, helpful pointers, and more. Consider it your map of the Mediterranean (diet). Here's how it breaks down:

Part I: Exploring the Mediterranean Lifestyle

The Mediterranean lifestyle is a way of life encompassing a unique set of dietary habits, physical activity, stress management, and fun. Research shows that following a Mediterranean diet has a strong correlation to heart health and longevity. *Our* research shows that it's a delicious and enjoyable way to live life.

This part discusses the main principles behind the Mediterranean diet and lifestyle. It delves into the health benefits, such as heart health, a reduced risk of cancer, and weight loss, that you can achieve by incorporating these same habits into your own life.

Part II: Creating a Healthy Lifestyle with Mediterranean Cooking

Understanding the main principles of the Mediterranean lifestyle is the first step, but how do you make them work in everyday life, especially when you live a fast-paced lifestyle and can't realistically slow down as much as you want? In this part, we show you how to make small changes so that you can easily make a Mediterranean lifestyle work for you. This part is full of meal planning strategies, sample meal plans, cooking tips, guidelines for stocking your kitchen, and grocery shopping ideas to help you adopt the Mediterranean way of life.

Part III: Starters and Sides

Mediterranean cooking is all about exploring your senses through delicious foods. The chapters in this part show you how to make some amazing breakfast dishes, classic appetizers and sauces, and delicious vegetable and grain sides that prove how much flavor is possible with healthy cooking. And don't forget salads, soups, and stews! These recipes are perfect for everyday cooking or to share with friends.

Part IV: Main Entrees and Desserts

Whether you're in the mood for seafood, meat, or pasta, you can find a wonderful collection of entrees for any occasion in Part IV. The chapters in this part celebrate some of the timeless classics of Mediterranean cooking along with tasty meals you can serve up in minutes.

Don't worry; we wouldn't leave you without desserts! This part also includes an assortment of dessert recipes perfect for large celebrations or weekly treats. With these recipes, you can easily satisfy your sweet tooth and still stick to a healthy diet plan.

Part V: The Part of Tens

In this part, we provide ten healthy lifestyle tips often practiced on the Mediterranean coast, along with easy ways to incorporate more plant-based foods in your diet. We also debunk some of the misconceptions floating around about the Mediterranean lifestyle. (Hint: You can't really consume all the cheese, pasta, and wine you want.)

The appendix contains some great hands-on information to help you implement some of the cooking strategies found in this book. It provides simple conversion tables to make switching from ounces to grams (and other metric measurements) simple.

Icons Used in This Book

The icons in this book are like bookmarks, pointing out information that we think is especially important. Here are the icons we use and the kind of information they point out:

Even if you forget everything else in this book, remember the paragraphs marked with this icon. They help you make good choices and stay on track with your health goals.

The information marked with this icon is interesting to know, but it goes beyond what's essential for your basic understanding. If you're the type of person who likes to know more about any particular topic, you'll enjoy these tidbits. If not, feel free to skip 'em.

This helpful icon marks important information that can save you time and energy, so make sure you don't overlook it.

Watch out for this icon; it warns you about potential problems and common pitfalls of implementing a Mediterranean diet into your lifestyle.

Where to Go from Here

Where to go from here depends on your immediate needs. Ready to start cooking and want to make some fabulous seafood tonight? Head over to Chapter 18. Interested in finding out more about the health benefits of the Mediterranean diet? Sit back and read Chapter 2. If you're not sure where you want to begin, peruse the table of contents, pick out the topics that mean the most to you, and start there. *Mediterranean Diet Cookbook For Dummies* contains a wide variety of recipes, so we encourage you try as many as you can at your own pace. We hope that you end up with lots of smudge marks on this book because you use it so lovingly and frequently in your kitchen.

Part I
Exploring the Mediterranean Lifestyle

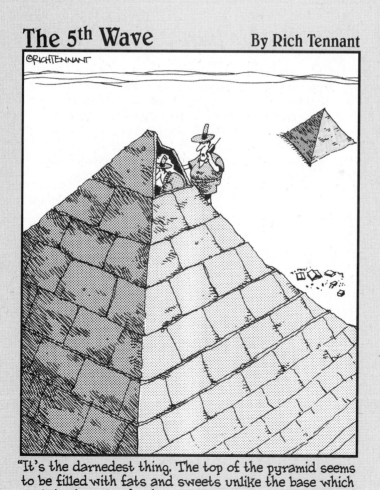

The 5th Wave   By Rich Tennant

"It's the darnedest thing. The top of the pyramid seems to be filled with fats and sweets unlike the base which contained mostly fresh vegetables, grains, and legumes."

In this part . . .

Research indicates that certain regions of the Mediterranean coast show an interesting connection among their people's lifestyle habits (unique dietary patterns, physical activity, stress management, and a contagious love for life), a reduced risk of heart disease and cancer, and improved longevity. This part focuses on these healthy Mediterranean lifestyle principles and how they can help with disease prevention, weight management, and overall wellness.

Chapter 1

Introducing the Mediterranean Diet

*W*hen you picture the Mediterranean diet, you may imagine the sea lapping up on a beach near a quaint village whose residents are lounging and eating fresh grapes and olives. That picture is a good start. The Mediterranean diet is a way of life — one where you eat lots of fresh food and slow down. More technically, *the Mediterranean diet* is a modern set of guidelines inspired by traditional diet patterns of southern Italy, the Greek island of Crete, and other parts of Greece. The lifestyle was first researched in the 1960s, and in 2010, the United Nations Educational, Scientific and Cultural Organization (UNESCO) officially recognized this diet pattern to be part of the cultural heritage of Italy, Greece, Spain, and Morocco. A more rural lifestyle is a common thread among all these regions.

Research shows that following a traditional Mediterranean diet significantly reduces the risk of heart disease and cancer. The key word here is *traditional*. The Mediterranean region is changing, with faster-paced lifestyles and more modern conveniences. These changes bring with them an increased prevalence of heart disease and cancer.

For the purposes of this book, when you think of a Mediterranean lifestyle and dietary patterns, the focus is on the traditional habits seen at least 50 years ago in the regions we note here. For instance, if you visited northern Italy in a recent trip, you may not have experienced any of the dietary patterns we promote in this book. So no, that huge portion of butter-laden pasta you had doesn't qualify for this diet.

Although diet is a big component of the health benefits experienced in the Mediterranean, all the lifestyle patterns combined, including physical activity and relaxation, may provide insight into the health benefits found in this region. This chapter serves as your jumping-off point into the Mediterranean diet and breaks down the Mediterranean dietary patterns and lifestyle choices that you can use as strategies for your own healthy lifestyle.

Identifying the Flavors of the Mediterranean Coast

The Mediterranean Sea is actually part of the Atlantic Ocean; a total of 21 countries have a coastline on the Mediterranean. However, only a few truly epitomize the Mediterranean diet and lifestyle that we discuss in this book. Having a decent understanding of these countries and their cooking styles can help you have a better appreciation for this way of life.

The recipes in this book are inspired by Mediterranean cooking — specifically, the areas of southern Italy, Greece, Morocco, and Spain. Although you may see some of the same ingredients in many recipes, the flavors used in different countries or regions create entirely different dishes. For example, if you've eaten both Italian and Greek meatballs, you know that the two varieties sure don't taste the same. Table 1-1 lists some of the countries in the Mediterranean that are part of this lifestyle and the associated flavors and cooking styles commonly used in those areas.

Table 1-1	Common Mediterranean Flavors by Region	
Region	*Commonly Used Ingredients*	*Overall Cuisine Flavor*
Southern Italy	Anchovies, balsamic vinegar, basil, bay leaf, capers, garlic, mozzarella cheese, olive oil, oregano, parsley, peppers, pine nuts, mushrooms, prosciutto, rosemary, sage, thyme, tomatoes	Italian food is rich and savory, with strongly flavored ingredients. Look for tomato-based sauces and even an occasional kick of spicy heat.
Greece	Basil, cucumbers, dill, fennel, feta cheese, garlic, honey, lemon, mint, olive oil, oregano, yogurt	Greek cooking runs the gamut from tangy with citrus accents to savory. Ingredients such as feta cheese add a strong, bold flavor, while yogurt helps provide a creamy texture and soft flavor.

Region	Commonly Used Ingredients	Overall Cuisine Flavor
Morocco	Cinnamon, cumin, dried fruits, ginger, lemon, mint, paprika, parsley, pepper, saffron, turmeric	Moroccan cooking uses exotic flavors that encompass both sweet and savory, often in one dish. The food has strong flavors but isn't necessarily spicy.
Spain	Almonds, anchovies, cheeses (from goats, cows, and sheep), garlic, ham, honey, olive oil, onions, oregano, nuts, paprika, rosemary, saffron, thyme	Regardless of what part of Spain you're in, you can always count on garlic and olive oil setting the stage for a flavorful dish. Spanish dishes are often inspired by Arabic and Roman cuisine with emphasis on fresh seafood. You often find combinations of savory and sweet flavors, such as a seafood stew using sweet paprika.

Discovering Where the Food Comes From

Although you may be used to cruising to the grocery store and buying whatever you need, folks on the Mediterranean coast 50 years ago didn't roll that way. Instead, they depended on what was farmed and fished locally, making culinary specialties by using everything on hand. Those habits may be fading, but they're still the cornerstone of the Mediterranean diet, and you can still embrace them by incorporating fresh foods into your meals even if you don't live near the Mediterranean.

The following sections highlight where people in the Mediterranean get their food and why these strategies are so important.

Focusing on farming

In addition to creating travel-worthy beaches, a moderate climate of wet winters and hot summers makes many of the areas along the Mediterranean ideal for agriculture. As a result, people living in the Mediterranean area can grow their own food in gardens and small farms, and many do so. A few areas have this type of climate (similar to the climate of southern coastal California), which makes growing specialized foods like olives and fig trees easier, thus providing ingredients for some of the signature recipes from this region.

Many people in the Mediterranean also abundantly use fresh herbs, spices, onions, and garlic to provide big flavor to their cooking. Table 1-2 is a partial list of common foods grown on the Mediterranean coast; it can give you a glimpse of what fresh ingredients the recipes in Part III and IV use.

Table 1-2	Foods Commonly Grown in the Mediterranean
Category	*Ingredient*
Legumes	Chickpeas
	Lentils
	Peas
Fruits	Olives
	Mandarin oranges
	Figs
	Grapes
	Lemons
	Persimmons
	Pomegranates
Grains	Barley
	Corn
	Rice
	Wheat
Herbs	Rosemary
	Oregano
	Sage
	Parsley
	Basil
	Dill
	Thyme
	Mint
	Fennel
Nuts	Almonds
	Hazelnuts
	Pine nuts
	Walnuts
Vegetables	Asparagus
	Broccoli

Category	Ingredient
	Cabbage
	Green beans
	Garlic
	Onions
	Eggplant
	Tomatoes
	Broccoli rabe
	Artichokes

Eating seasonally

As a side effect of eating what they grow locally (see the preceding section), folks in the Mediterranean also eat seasonally; after all, you can't eat what you can't grow. Eating in-season food makes an impact for the following reasons:

- ✔ **Seasonal abundance makes you cook more creatively.** If you have an abundant amount of, say, green beans, you want to utilize them in any way possible. Finding different, tasty ways to prepare green beans as a side dish or as part of an entree requires more of a thought process, and more care goes into the food itself.

- ✔ **You eat an increased variety of produce throughout the year.** On one hand, you may eat a lot of one food while it's in season, but when that season's over, you'll switch to other foods associated with the new time of year. Relying on produce available year-round at the grocery store means you can easily get stuck in a rut of eating the same standbys throughout the year.

More variety in produce means more variety of health-promoting nutrients that help you prevent disease. Although eating a few different types of fruits and vegetables throughout the year is better than nothing, getting a wide variety is the ultimate goal for good health.

We know that eating seasonally isn't feasible for many people in certain climates. Don't worry! We cover how you can adopt more of these ideas in Chapter 5.

Fishing the Mediterranean Sea

People in the Mediterranean area rely on the nearby sea as a food source. Fish appear in many common traditional recipes, providing an abundance of healthy omega-3 fatty acids. You can add seafood to a few weekly meals and reap the same benefits. The least expensive seafood in the Mediterranean region includes sardines, anchovies, mackerel, squid, and octopus. Mid-priced fish and shellfish include tuna, trout, clams, and mussels. For a pricey, special-occasion meal, options include lobster and red mullet.

During the 1960s, before the area was over-fished, a variety of seafood was available in the Mediterranean. Unfortunately, fish stocks today are significantly low in the Mediterranean due to overfishing, and many important species, such as tuna, are threatened.

Eating and Living the Mediterranean Way

The Mediterranean diet includes a specific balance of foods that's high in vitamins, minerals, and antioxidants and contains the perfect balance of fatty acids. Alas, you can't just eat your way to Mediterranean health. Living a healthy lifestyle means you have to look at all aspects of your life. Along with the food plan is a way of life that includes regular physical activity and time for rest, community, and fun; for the folks on the Mediterranean coast, this combination seems to have created that ever-elusive life balance.

To tie all the Mediterranean diet and lifestyle concepts together, Oldways Preservation and Exchange Trust came up with the Mediterranean Food Guide Pyramid based on the dietary traditions of Crete, other parts of Greece, and southern Italy around 1960, when chronic diseases such as heart disease and cancer were low. As you can see in Figure 1-1, the focus is on eating a diet rich in vegetables, fruits, whole grains, legumes, and seafood; eating less meat; and choosing healthy fats such as olive oil. Note also the importance of fun activities, time shared with family and friends, and a passion for life. The following sections examine each aspect so that you can find it, too.

Focusing on healthy fats

Although Mediterranean residents don't consume a lowfat diet, their dietary pattern is considered heart-healthy. How can that be? Not all fats are created equal. People in the Mediterranean consume more of the healthier types of fats (monounsaturated fats and polyunsaturated omega-3 fatty acids) and less of the omega-6 polyunsaturated fatty acids and saturated fats other cultures tend to overload on. Instead of focusing on total fat intake, these folks maintain a healthier ratio of these different groups of fats than you see in the United States; they consume about 35 percent of their total daily calories from fat, but less than 8 percent of their calories come from saturated fats. According to the National Health and Nutrition Examination Survey, the average intake of saturated fats in the United States is 11 percent of daily calories. You can find out more about the details of this fat ratio in Chapter 2.

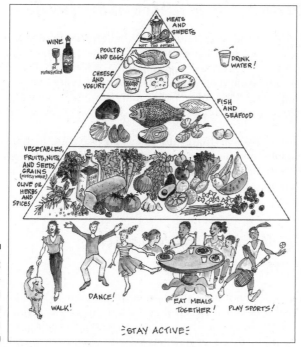

Figure 1-1:
The Mediterranean Food Guide Pyramid.

To start rebalancing your fat ratio, limit your use of fats such as butter and lard in cooking and use more olive oils or avocadoes for spreads.

Don't say "cheese": Using dairy in moderation

You may think of the Mediterranean as a cheese-eater's heaven, but the truth is that the Mediterranean areas we focus on don't consume an abundance of cheese. Dairy is consumed on a daily basis in the Mediterranean diet, and cheese (along with yogurt) is a common source of calcium; however, moderation is the key (isn't it always?).

Incorporate two to three servings of dairy products daily. One serving may include an eight-ounce glass of milk, eight ounces of yogurt, or an ounce of cheese. Stick with the lowfat versions of milk and yogurt to help lower your saturated fat intake; because you're eating so little of it, you can go with regular cheese if you want.

Eating primarily plant-based foods

One of the most important concepts of the Mediterranean diet pattern is consuming tons of plant foods such as fruits, veggies, legumes, and whole grains. People in the Mediterranean commonly eat five to ten servings of fruits and vegetables each day, which often means having two to three vegetable servings with each meal. Other daily staples include legumes such as beans, lentils, and peas, and whole grains such as bulgur wheat or barley.

Foods in these categories are naturally low in calories and high in nutrients, which makes weight- and health-management easy. Begin by finding ways to incorporate more unprocessed plant foods in your diet on a daily basis; Chapter 21 can help.

Punching up the flavor with fresh herbs and spices

Fresh herbs and spices not only add tremendous flavor to food but also have many hidden health benefits, which we cover in Chapter 6. If you already use ample herbs and spices in your own cooking, you're on the right track. If not, this book can help you discover new flavors and simple ways to add more of these plants into your diet.

Enjoying seafood weekly

Seafood is a weekly staple in the Mediterranean diet, and with good reason. Not only is it a local product (see the earlier section "Fishing the Mediterranean Sea"), but it's also a great source of those coveted omega-3 fatty acids. If you live near a coast, you have a great opportunity to find fresh fish in your local stores and restaurants. If you're landlocked, don't discount lakes and rivers for fresh fish.

Check out www.montereybayaquarium.org/cr/seafoodwatch.aspx for a list of recommended fish in your region. This guide is a great tool to help you choose local fish with low contaminants and also to protect against overfishing.

Don't like fish? You can get omega-3 fatty acids in other ways, such as with fish oil supplements or by eating lots of fresh herbs, walnuts, and flaxseeds. Even if you don't like fish, we still encourage you to try some of the seafood recipes in Chapter 18 to see whether we can change your mind!

Limiting red meat

Red meat used to be a luxury item in rural parts of the Mediterranean, so folks there ate it less frequently. Even though it's now more accessible to the average Joe, the serving limits have stuck over the years.

Beef is only served once or twice a month in the Mediterranean rather than several times a week like in many U.S. kitchens. And when it does hit the table, it's usually as a small (two- to three-ounce) side dish rather than an eight-plus-ounce entree. This habit helps ensure a reasonable intake of saturated fats and omega-6 fatty acids. (See the earlier section "Focusing on healthy fats" for info on balancing fat intake.)

Don't panic at the idea of cutting your meat portion so drastically. You can easily replace some of that meat with lentils or beans to add plant-based protein to your meals, or add more vegetable servings to help fill the plate. Also keep in mind that Mediterranean beef recipes are so full of flavor that a small serving becomes more satisfying. (You can see this difference for yourself by trying out the recipes in Chapter 19.)

Having a nice glass of vino

Wine lovers, rejoice! Drinking a glass of wine with dinner is certainly a common practice in the Mediterranean regions. Red wine has special nutrients that are shown to be heart-healthy; however, moderation is so important. Enjoying some red wine a couple times a week is certainly a good plan for heart health, although you want to check with your doctor to ensure its okay for you. Check out Chapter 2 for specifics on the benefits of red wine.

Getting a good dose of daily activity

Historically, the people in the rural Mediterranean got plenty of daily activity through work, getting where they needed to go on foot, and having fun. Although you may rely heavily on your car and think this lifestyle isn't realistic for you, you can still find ways to incorporate both aerobic exercise (which gets your heart rate up) and strength-training exercises regularly.

Now that's a long weekend!

If you don't believe that slowing down can really do that much for your health, consider this study. Researchers from the University of Rochester found that from Friday night until Sunday, study participants, even those with high income or exciting work lives, were in better moods, showed greater enjoyment in life, and had fewer aches and pains.

Having unscheduled time on the weekends provided individuals with opportunities to bond with others, explore interests, and relax. Hey, wait; those are some of the main tenets of the Mediterranean lifestyle! And if just a couple of days of downtime can make a difference, think about the effects of making this type of time a priority throughout the week.

Walking encompasses both aerobic and strength training and helps relieve stress. If you live close to markets or restaurants, challenge yourself to walk to them rather than drive, or simply focus on taking a walk each day to unwind.

Taking time for the day's biggest meal

Even though the Mediterranean residents of days gone by were hard workers, often doing a significant amount of manual labor, they always made time for their largest meal of the day. Traditionally, this meal was lunch, where people sat down as a family and enjoyed a large meal full of vegetables, legumes, fruits, and seafood or meat. Taking time for meal and family was a priority; you didn't see people eating in five minutes at the countertop.

In many cultures, having this large relaxing meal at lunchtime is difficult because of work schedules. However, you can adapt this strategy into your life by focusing on supper. Prioritizing some time to unwind and relax from a busy work day provides other benefits for your family. According to a Columbia University survey, teenagers who eat with their families at least five days a week have better grades in school and are less prone to substance abuse.

Although taking time for a large, relaxing meal sounds like one of those optional strategies you can skip, keep in mind that even small lifestyle choices can make a very big impact on overall health. Family dinners can help you clear your head from work and provide enjoyment through good food and conversation. If you're go, go, go all day at work, prioritizing family meal time can be priceless for your daily stress management.

Fighting stress with daily rituals

Many principles of the Mediterranean lifestyle revolve around family, community, and fun. It's so easy to get caught up in a busy, hectic life and put these small experiences on the back burner because they don't appear to be that important. However, these little rituals throughout the day add up for a big impact on stress management. Stress impacts your health in so many ways, from increasing your risk of high blood pressure and heart disease to promoting weight gain, so managing it is key. Here are two examples of daily routines that illustrate how little experiences sprinkled throughout the day can provide more stress relief:

1. **Using Mediterranean lifestyle strategies**

✔ Wake up and have a light breakfast

✔ Workday begins (stress inducer)

✔ Lunch break with a light walk (stress reliever)

✔ End work day

✔ Home for sit-down dinner with family (stress reliever)

✔ Clean-up and evening tasks, such as kids' homework

✔ Reading or journaling (stress reliever)

✔ Bedtime (stress reliever)

In this example, the person has opportunities to let go of a little stress multiple times during the day. Now take a look at an example far too many people get trapped in:

2. **Using fast-paced lifestyle strategies**

✔ Wake up and skip breakfast (stress inducer)

✔ Workday begins (stress inducer)

✔ Lunch break, eating quickly in ten minutes at the desk (neutral — doesn't induce stress or reduce it)

✔ Work late (stress inducer)

✔ Rush through the drive-through to pick up a meal for family, eating in five minutes at the countertop (neutral)

✔ Clean-up and evening tasks, such as kids' homework

✔ Television (may be a stress inducer or reliever)

✔ Bedtime (stress reliever)

The first example has one big stress inducer (work) and four stress relievers sprinkled throughout the day. The second example has three to four stress inducers and only one or two stress relievers. That stress builds up in your body, setting you up for an increased risk of disease and possible weight gain. Taking the time for those small experiences during the day, such as a family dinner or a walk, make a big difference. And remember that the activities here are just examples. You can find stress relievers that work for you, such as knitting, yoga, tea time, painting, meditation, exercise, or conversation with a dear friend. Refer to Chapter 3 for more help.

Enjoying time with friends and family

Community spirit is a large part of the Mediterranean culture and is something that's disappearing in American culture. Getting together on a regular basis with friends and family is an important priority for providing a sense of strong community and fun. The fun and laughter that come with friendly get-togethers are vital for stress management. Without these little joyful experiences, stress can tip to an unhealthy balance.

To put this strategy into practice, invite some of your close family and friends over each week, perhaps for dinner. It can be as casual as you like. The important thing is to add this type of fun and enjoyment to your life more often.

Having a strong passion for life

The Mediterranean coast is full of sunshine, good food, and beautiful surroundings, so the people who live there naturally tend to have a strong passion for life, family, friends, nature, and food. Choosing to have a strong passion and love of life is associated with more happiness and fulfillment and less stress.

What are you passionate about? Perhaps you love the arts, or maybe nature is your thing. Whatever your passions are, make sure to find a way to make them a part of your life.

Chapter 2

Discovering the Health Benefits of the Mediterranean Diet

The Mediterranean diet has long been touted for providing health benefits, such as reducing coronary artery disease and decreasing the risk of some cancers. Including fresh vegetables and fruits, legumes, and healthy fats into your diet can help improve your health in many ways. And in addition to the health benefits, you're eating foods with full flavor. Thinking of bland or boring Greek or Italian food isn't easy.

This chapter highlights why this diet is full of health benefits (focusing on heart disease, cancer, diabetes, and anti-aging) by looking at some of the main nutrients found in Mediterranean eating.

As you read this chapter, note that a healthy diet, exercise, and stress management can significantly reduce your risk of certain diseases, but nothing can bring a guarantee. Genetic components also play a role with chronic diseases. However, if you have family history of heart disease, diabetes, or cancer, incorporating these lifestyle and diet changes into your daily life can help you decrease those risks.

Highlighting the Main Nutrients of the Mediterranean Diet

A plant-based diet such as the Mediterranean diet offers a plethora of nutrients that can help your body stay healthy. These plant foods are loaded with vitamins, minerals, antioxidants, phytochemicals, and healthy fats. The following sections highlight some of these key nutrients found in the foods associated with the Mediterranean coast.

These nutrients don't just benefit humans; the plant itself needs them so that it can grow and protect itself from the elements, bacteria, and other damage. Without nutrients, the plant can't grow or protect itself from oxidative damage or bacteria.

Fighting free radicals with antioxidants

Antioxidants are a key component of many plant foods that help slow down the process of oxidation (when your body's cells burn oxygen). This slowing decreases the amount of *free radicals,* or unstable molecules, that cause damage to your cells, tissues, and DNA. Antioxidants are a crucial part of your diet because you can't avoid oxidation all together. Consider the many contaminants, such as car exhaust, sunlight, unhealthy foods, and air pollution, that you're exposed to during a typical day. These types of exposures can cause free radicals to gain speed in your body, damaging everything in their path and leaving you at greater risk of chronic conditions like heart disease and cancer.

Think about slicing an apple. Before you know it, the exposed flesh turns from white to brown. This browning occurs because of oxidation. But adding orange juice or lemon juice to the apple right after you slice it keeps it whiter longer because the antioxidant vitamin C in the juice protects the flesh.

Eating a diet high in antioxidants such as vitamin C, vitamin E, and beta-carotene means better protection for your body and overall health (no, the benefits of antioxidants aren't just for apples). The ATTICA study in the September 2005 issue of the *American Journal of Clinical Nutrition* measured the total antioxidant capacity of men and women in Greece. It found that the participants who followed a traditional Mediterranean diet had an 11 percent higher antioxidant capacity than those who didn't adhere to a traditional diet. The findings also showed that the participants who followed the traditional diet the most had 19 percent lower oxidized LDL (bad cholesterol) concentrations showing a benefit in reducing heart disease.

You don't have to look far or even cook that much to get antioxidants into your diet. You can find plenty of antioxidants in fruits and vegetables. If you're only eating one to three servings of fruits and vegetables per day, you need to increase your intake to take advantage of the produce's antioxidants. We challenge you to increase your intake of fresh fruits and vegetables to five to eight servings daily! Table 2-1 shows some common foods, including lots of fruits and veggies, that are rich in certain antioxidants.

Table 2-1	Antioxidant-Rich Foods
Antioxidant	*Foods*
Vitamin C	Asparagus
	Broccoli
	Cantaloupe
	Cauliflower
	Grapefruit
	Green and red bell peppers
	Guava
	Lemons
	Oranges
	Pineapple
	Strawberries
	Spinach, kale, and collard greens
	Tangerines
	Tomatoes
Vitamin E	Mustard greens, Swiss chard, spinach, and turnip and collard greens
	Almonds
	Peanuts
	Sunflower seeds
Beta carotene	Broccoli
	Cantaloupe
	Carrots
	Cilantro
	Kale, spinach, and turnip and collard greens
	Romaine lettuce

To supplement or not to supplement? That's still the question

Although you've likely heard the news that antioxidants found in foods promote good health, scientists are still researching whether taking supplements such as beta carotene, vitamin C, vitamin E, or other antioxidant blends can replace eating the real thing.

Research has provided a great deal of information about many individual nutrients and their impacts on health, but researchers still don't have the answers to many questions, such as how much of a supplement is enough and whether supplemented antioxidants have the same effect working on their own as the natural ones do working with accompanying nutrients. For instance, many fruits are high in vitamin C, so you may think that you can get the same vitamin C effects from taking a supplement if you don't eat a lot of fruit. However, the vitamin C in an orange may work with the phytochemicals in the orange to more significantly affect your

health than the vitamin C supplement does by itself. Even supplements made from fruits and vegetables may not contain the other nutrients.

Another supplement concern is that taking high doses of antioxidants may actually cause the antioxidants to work as pro-oxidants that promote rather than neutralize oxidation. And in some cases, you actually want free radicals to attack harmful cells such as bacteria and cancer cells. High doses of antioxidant supplements may interfere with this natural process.

The bottom line is that eating whole foods is still your best bet to combat diseases and live your healthiest life. As we note throughout the book, folks in the Mediterranean eat scads of produce, and this type of food intake is one of the reasons you see more longevity in people who live in this region.

Understanding phytochemicals

Besides vitamins and minerals, plants also contain phytochemicals. Don't be scared by the big word. *Phytochemicals* are simply healthy chemicals that offer your body healthful benefits. As we say repeatedly throughout this book, a plant-based diet high in fruits, vegetables, and legumes can provide you with an increased amount and variety of phytochemicals, helping to promote heart health and working to prevent certain cancers.

Research in this area is relatively new and is uncovering a whole side of previously unknown health benefits. To date, certain phytochemicals have been shown to work as antioxidants (see the previous section), contain anti-inflammatory properties, and promote heart health.

Phytochemicals provide the pigment to your fruits and vegetables, so you can literally know which class of phytochemicals you're consuming simply by noting the color you're eating. Table 2-2 shows a few specific health benefits found in each color.

Table 2-2	Potential Health Benefits of Foods by Color	
Color	*Health Benefits*	*Foods*
Blue/purple	A lower risk of some cancers; improved memory; and healthy aging	Blueberries, eggplants, purple grapes, and plums
Green	A lower risk of some cancers; healthy vision; and strong bones and teeth	Broccoli, green peppers, honeydew melon, kiwi, salad greens, and spinach
Red	A lower risk of heart disease and of some cancers, and improved memory function	Pink watermelon, red bell peppers, and strawberries
White	A lower risk of heart disease and of some cancers	Bananas, garlic, and onions
Yellow/orange	A lower risk of heart disease and of some cancers; healthy vision; and a stronger immune system	Carrots, oranges, yellow and orange bell peppers, and yellow watermelon

Vitamin D: Getting a little of the sunshine vitamin

Your body gets vitamin D, otherwise known as the sunshine vitamin, both from food sources and from exposure to sunlight. You want to make sure you get the appropriate amount of vitamin D; people in the Mediterranean may be healthier because they have strong levels of the vitamin.

The scientific community has been buzzing in the last ten years about the health benefits of vitamin D. Research shows this vitamin can help

- Protect against osteoporosis
- Reduce the risk of coronary artery disease
- Decrease the risk of certain cancers
- Lower the risk of infectious diseases such as the common flu

One theory suggests that the people of the Mediterranean coast are healthier because they're exposed to more sunlight — specifically, the ultraviolet B rays that are responsible for producing vitamin D — because of their location near the equator and because they're outside more often walking, gardening, working, or enjoying family and friends.

To produce vitamin D, you want exposure to sunlight for 15 minutes each day with no sunscreen (sunscreen blocks up to 90 percent of vitamin D production). Of course, unprotected sun exposure increases the risk of skin cancer, so you have to weigh the good with the bad. Note that many people don't make enough vitamin D from the sun, including those who have darker skin tones, are overweight, are older, or live in northern climates.

In addition to the sun, you can get vitamin D from a few foods, such as fish, fortified cereals, and fortified milk. Food sources are limited, so you mostly need to depend on sun exposure to get the proper amounts.

Researchers agree that people's vitamin D levels need to increase, although the level of increase is still up for debate. In 2010, the Institute of Medicine released a report recommending the following daily intake of vitamin D:

- ✔ People ages 1 to 70 should take 600 IU (international units) a day.
- ✔ People over the age of 70 should take 800 IU (international units) a day.

You can easily get your vitamin D levels checked with a simple blood test at your annual physical. Just let your primary care provider know if you have concerns about your level. Many people need to add a supplement to ensure they're getting the daily dose they need, but don't try to guess how much you need; taking too much vitamin D can have harmful consequences. Check out *Vitamin D For Dummies* by Alan L. Rubin, MD, (John Wiley & Sons, Inc.) for more information.

Choosing healthy fats

The Mediterranean diet is lower in omega-6 polyunsaturated fats (or *fatty acids*) and saturated fats than most people's diets are; it's also higher in healthy fats, such as monounsaturated fats and omega-3 polyunsaturated fats. (For reference, you find monounsaturated fats in foods such as olive oil, avocadoes, and certain nuts. Polyunsaturated fatty acids are in corn, safflower, soybean, sesame, and sunflower oils and seafood. Saturated fatty acids appear in animal-based foods such as meat, poultry, butter, and dairy products, as well as in coconut and palm oils.) The higher percentage of monounsaturated fats found in the Mediterranean diet is associated with

- ✔ A lower risk of heart disease
- ✔ Lower cholesterol levels
- ✔ Decreased inflammation in the body
- ✔ Better insulin function and blood sugar control

Omega-3 fatty acids are one of the big contributors to the health benefits of the Mediterranean diet, and many people don't get enough of them. Research shows that omega-3s help reduce inflammation, which is specifically important for those with inflammatory diseases such as arthritis, cardiovascular disease, or inflammatory bowel disease. These fats are also shown to be helpful for immune system function, behavioral issues such as attention deficit (hyperactivity) disorder, mood disorders such as depression, and prevention of Alzheimer's disease.

Omega-6 fatty acids occur abundantly in the diet through sources such as grains, nuts, and legumes as well as sunflower, safflower, sesame, and corn oils. Animal protein is also high in a specific omega-6 fatty acid called *arachidonic* acid. Omega-6 fats lower cholesterol, help keep the blood from clotting, and support skin health. Both omega-3 and omega-6 fats are considered *essential,* which means your body doesn't make them and needs to get them from your diet.

The big trouble begins when omega-3s aren't balanced appropriately with omega-6s. Although your omega-6 intake should be higher than your omega-3 intake, a diet too high in omega-6 fatty acids and too low in omega-3 fatty acids can promote conditions of chronic inflammation, including atherosclerosis, arthritis, and inflammatory bowel disease. Preliminary research also shows a possible connection to obesity, depression, dyslexia, and hyperactivity. This out-of-balance fat intake is very common in the American diet (with a ratio of 20 omega-6s to 1 omega-3) and less common in a Mediterranean style diet. Experts say the ratio to shoot for is about 4 parts omega-6 and 1 part omega-3.

Rebalance your diet by incorporating more sources of omega-3s, such as fresh herbs, canola oil, walnuts, flaxseeds, and cold-water fish (such as salmon, herring, and sturgeon), into your meals. You can also find products (such as eggs) fortified with omega 3s. Limit other sources of animal proteins (such as beef, poultry, unfortified eggs, and pork) by reducing your portion sizes to two to three ounces.

You can also repair the balance by replacing your cooking oils with olive oil, which is high in a third fat called omega-9 fatty acids. Your body can make omega-9s on its own, but adding more of them to your diet can help you lower your omega-6 intake.

Boosting your fiber intake

"Eat more fiber." You've probably seen this message in advertisements and the media. You can get all the fiber you need by eating the Mediterranean way, focusing on fruits, vegetables, whole grains, and legumes.

Fiber is what you may call the "roughage" found in plants. Your body doesn't digest fiber like it does nutrients; fiber goes through your gastrointestinal tract intact. This process has a bigger impact on health than you may think; it's very important roles include the following:

✔ Helps maintain a healthy gastrointestinal tract by decreasing constipation and reducing your risk of *diverticulosis,* or small pouches that form in your colon.

✔ Lowers total cholesterol and bad cholesterol levels, helping to keep your heart healthy. This is the role played by the soluble fiber found in foods such as oat bran, beans, and flaxseeds.

✔ Slows the absorption of sugars you consume from carbohydrate foods, which helps keep blood sugar stable. This function is important for those who have insulin resistance diseases, such as diabetes or PCOS, and helps people manage their weights more effectively.

✔ Acts as a natural appetite suppressant, helping you to feel full and satisfied after a meal. No need to buy those diet pills that are supposed to suppress your appetite. Save your money and try eating more fresh produce, beans, and whole grains with every meal.

Understanding the Importance of Wine

Drinking more red wine, like many people in the Mediterranean coast do, may be one reason you're excited about switching to a Mediterranean diet. Red wine has certain properties that research has shown are beneficial for heart health. If you drink alcohol in moderation, add a little red wine in place of other alcoholic beverages. (If you're not a fan of red wine, drinking grape juice made from Concord grapes and eating purple grapes also provide similar heart-health benefits.)

The cardio protection red wine provides is attributed to the antioxidants from *flavonoids* found in the skin of the grapes. The flavonoids reduce your risk of heart disease by lowering bad cholesterol, increasing good cholesterol, and reducing blood clotting. A specific flavonoid called *reservatol* may have additional benefits, including inhibiting tumor development in certain cancers, but that research is still in early stages.

Although red wine can indeed be part of a healthy lifestyle, a fine line determines what amount is considered healthy. The recommended daily intake is one 4-ounce glass for women and one to two 4-ounce glasses for men. Excessive drinking can become unhealthy and is linked to high blood pressure, cardiovascular conditions, and extra calories.

You also need to be in good health to enjoy this perk of the Mediterranean diet. If you have high blood pressure, high triglycerides, pancreatitis, liver disease, or congestive heart failure, drinking even moderate amounts of alcohol may worsen your condition. Also, if you take aspirin regularly for heart health, you want to slow down on the drinking. Talk to your health care provider to see what's right for you.

Looking at the Mediterranean Diet's Effect on Heart Disease

The Mediterranean diet is most noticed in the scientific community for its effect on heart health. Heart disease is the number one cause of death in the United States, even though a few lifestyle changes make it easily preventable. Genetics still play a strong role, of course, but making small changes to your diet and exercising make a big difference.

The first research focused on the Mediterranean diet started with a scientist named Ancel Keys and the Seven Countries Study. This study found that southern Europe had far fewer coronary deaths than northern Europe and the United States did, even when factoring in age, smoking, blood pressure, and physical activity. These results made researchers look more closely at the differences in dietary habits. This study is still important today because more people in the Mediterranean regions studied no longer eat in their traditional way, and those regions show higher occurrences of heart disease.

Recent research continues to show a correlation between a traditional Mediterranean diet and lower incidence of heart disease. According to a 2008 study published in the *British Medical Journal,* research showed a 9-percent decrease in deaths from coronary artery disease. A 2011 review of several studies covering 535,000 people that was published in the *Journal of the American College of Cardiology* reported that a traditional Mediterranean diet is associated with lower blood pressure, blood sugar, and triglyceride levels.

Many more studies have shown the heart health protection of a diet high in fruits, vegetables, legumes, wine, and seafood, which supports the idea that the Mediterranean diet is a healthy lifestyle. We're sure you'll continue to see more and more research on this topic in the future.

Fighting Cancer

Another area research on the Mediterranean diet has focused on is the diet's effects on preventing and managing cancer. Specific staples of the diet have been shown to provide cancer-preventing and cancer-fighting benefits:

- **Plant foods:** A diet high in plant foods such as fruits, vegetables, legumes, and nuts may provide cancer protection. The high amounts of phytochemicals in these foods provide unique properties that can help inhibit or slow tumor growth or simply protect your cells. Head to the earlier section "Understanding phytochemicals" for details on these powerhouses.

- ✔ **Meat:** Beginning in 1976, researchers from the Harvard School of Public Health followed 88,000 healthy women and found that the risk of colon cancer was 2.5 times higher in women who ate beef, pork, or lamb daily compared with those who ate those meats once a month or less. They also found that the risk of getting colon cancer was directly correlated to the amount of meat eaten.

- ✔ **Olive oil:** A study of 26,000 Greek people published in the *British Journal of Cancer* showed that using more olive oil cut cancer risk by 9 percent.

In addition to these ingredient-specific studies, the diet as a whole has some promising research. A 2008 study review published in the *British Medical Journal* showed that following a traditional Mediterranean diet reduced the risk of dying from cancer by 9 percent. That same year, the *American Journal of Clinical Nutrition* published a study that showed that among post menopausal women, those who followed a traditional Mediterranean diet were 22 percent less likely to develop breast cancer. Although more research is needed in this area, you can enjoy a Mediterranean diet and know that you're helping increase your odds against cancer.

Battling Diabetes

The foods in a Mediterranean diet make perfect sense for a person with type 2 diabetes because the food choices lean toward being low-glycemic. The *glycemic index* is a measurement given to carbohydrate-containing foods that shows how quickly they turn into blood sugar. High-glycemic foods create a quick, high blood sugar spike, while low-glycemic foods offer a slow blood sugar rise. A diet that provides this slow rise in blood sugar is best for diabetics, who can't manage a large influx of sugar normally. Most vegetables, fruits, whole grains, and legumes (hallmarks of the Mediterranean diet) provide a much slower blood sugar response compared to white bread, white pasta, or sugary snacks. A 2009 study from the Second University of Naples in Italy published in the *Annals of Internal Medicine*, found that diabetics who followed a Mediterranean diet instead of a lowfat diet had better glycemic control and were less likely to need diabetes medication.

The portion sizes in the Mediterranean diet can also make a significant difference for a diabetic. Starchy foods such as the whole grains found in cereals and breads can also make blood sugar rise if a person consumes too much of them, but the portion sizes associated with a Mediterranean pattern of eating are much lower and help keep total carbohydrate intake during the meal in check.

Getting the facts about sulfites in wine

Sulfites are used as preservatives in many food products and also occur naturally in foods. Many people have sensitivities and allergies to sulfites, causing asthma-like symptoms, hives, and swelling. The headache that commonly results from drinking wine may be due to sulfite sensitivity, but it's more likely a question of overindulgence, dehydration, or lack of food in your stomach while drinking. If your headaches aren't consistent when you drink wine, you can't blame the sulfites (sorry). The best way to determine whether you have an allergy is to get yourself tested by an allergist, especially if you already suffer from asthma.

Sadly, you won't have much luck finding a sulfite-free wine; grape skins themselves are high in sulfites, and more are added in winemaking to give your wine a long shelf life. Without added sulfites, you get vinegar in a few months. Despite popular belief, European wines don't have fewer sulfites; in some cases, they have more!

But the benefits don't stop at those who already have diabetes; this diet pattern may help you reduce your risk of getting the disease. The SUN cohort study from the University of Navarro, Spain, which involved more than 13,000 participants with no history of diabetes, showed that those participants who followed a Mediterranean style diet were less likely to develop type 2 diabetes. What's more interesting about this study is that participants who had high risk factors for type 2 diabetes (including older age, family history of diabetes, and a history of smoking) and followed the diet pattern strictly had an 83 percent relative reduction for developing the disease.

Aging Gracefully: Anti-Aging Tips from the Mediterranean

A Mediterranean lifestyle can also help you feel and look your best. A diet high in nutrients, moderate activity, and lots of laughter with friends lets you enjoy the benefits of health! Here are some of the ways you can age gracefully with a Mediterranean lifestyle.

 ✔ **Increased longevity:** The NIH-AARP Diet and Health Study published in the *Archives of Internal Medicine* in 2007 found that people who closely adhered to a Mediterranean-style diet were 12 to 20 percent less likely to die from cancer and all causes.

Coffee's health benefits: Full of beans?

The art of drinking coffee was invented by the Italians and has held a strong tradition in many cultures. Coffee is a complex nutrition topic because it's a natural, plant-based food containing healthy antioxidants, which may be to thank for the lower rates of type 2 diabetes, Parkinson's disease, and dementia in coffee drinkers. However, the caffeine in coffee may increase blood pressure (though you can drink decaf to avoid this problem), and coffee in general may increase homocysteine levels, which is a risk factor for heart disease, regardless of the caffeine content. More research is needed to provide any definitive recommendations for or against caffeine and coffee, but enjoying it in moderation is likely the key.

Enjoying *espresso*, a form of concentrated coffee, is a tradition on the Mediterranean coast, but folks there tend to look at espresso as a morning drink only and often drink just one to two ounces of espresso a day (a stark contrast to many coffee-shop regulars in the United States). One ounce of espresso contains around 75 milligrams of caffeine, compared to 135 milligrams in one cup of coffee.

If you don't drink coffee, there is certainly no reason for you to start. If you're a coffee lover, enjoy your coffee, but try to limit yourself to one to two 8-ounce cups of coffee or one to two 1-ounce shots of espresso each day.

- **Wrinkle reduction:** Now we know we've got your attention! A study published in the *Journal of the American College of Nutrition* in 2001 found that people who consumed a diet high in fruits, vegetables, nuts, legumes, and fish had less skin wrinkling. Of course, this arena needs far more research, but try the theory out at home to see your own results. Sure beats plastic surgery, right?

- **Smoother skin:** Eating a diet high in vitamin C foods, such as oranges, strawberries, and broccoli, plays an important role in the production of collagen, the skin's support structure. Head to Table 2-1 earlier in the chapter for more vitamin C-rich foods.

- **Bone density maintenance:** Moderate weight-bearing exercise such as walking or lifting weights can maintain good bone density, keeping your bones strong and helping you avoid bone fractures later in life.

- **Tension taming:** A good laugh reduces tension and stress in the body, leaving your muscles relaxed for up to 45 minutes. Stress can lead to depression, anxiety, high blood pressure, and heart disease, all of which contribute to aging and a reduced quality of life.

- **Inflammation reduction:** Inflammation can affect your heart health, joints, and skin. Eating a diet high in anti-inflammatory foods such as cold-water fish, walnuts, flaxseeds, and fresh herbs can help keep you feeling your best.

- **Lowered Alzheimer's risk:** A 2006 study at Columbia University Medical Center showed that participants who followed a Mediterranean-style diet had 40 percent lower risk of Alzheimer's disease than those who didn't.

Chapter 3

Losing Weight with the Mediterranean Diet

In This Chapter

▶ Changing your habits

▶ Managing (not counting) your calorie intake

▶ Understanding your appetite and craving mechanisms

▶ Getting the biggest bang for your metabolic rate

*W*eight loss is an important issue for many people (and perhaps you) in the world today. You may be looking for a way to lose some weight and think that the Mediterranean diet is the way to go. Choosing a Mediterranean diet isn't going to be a traditional "diet" or a quick fix. Rather, it's a series of healthy lifestyle choices that can get you to your weight loss goal while you eat delicious, flavorful foods and get out and enjoy life. Sounds much better than counting calories and depriving yourself, right?

With that description in mind, you need to focus on a few must-haves with the Mediterranean lifestyle in order to lose weight successfully. You have to pay attention to lifestyle changes, manage your calorie intake through balancing food choices and controlling portions, and increase your physical activity. This chapter covers all these details so that you can reach your weight loss goals with ease.

Focusing on Lifestyle Changes

The focus of the Mediterranean diet is on your entire lifestyle. Paying attention to lifestyle changes, such as changing your portion sizes and exercising regularly, is the only way to see long-term results. Weight-loss diets come and go, and most can help you lose the weight, but they aren't something you can live with long term. The Mediterranean diet helps you pay attention to your individual lifestyle, including the types of foods you eat, the portion sizes you consume, your physical activities, and your overall way of life. You can incorporate these changes into your daily life and create long-term habits that bring you not only weight loss but also sustained weight loss.

Evaluating your life and deciding what types of changes will work for you long term is crucial. You want to incorporate changes you're excited to make; if you feel like you *have* to make them, you may struggle to motivate yourself and find that you keep pushing the changes off for another day. Making changes that work for you sets the stage so that you can keep the weight off long term.

The following sections focus on the main lifestyle changes you can make by integrating the Mediterranean diet into your daily life. These changes first and foremost include setting a goal to quit diets and then a goal to slow down and make time for yourself. After you commit to focusing on lifestyle changes, remember to start small with baby steps.

Although the Mediterranean diet is technically a diet, that's not the kind of diet we're talking about getting away from in this section. When we refer to quitting diets, we're talking about the quick-fix, non-lifestyle types of diets where you eat nothing but grass clippings for two weeks just to lose pounds quickly.

Setting goals

Making goals provides a road map of where you are so that you're less likely to get lost in the details of lifestyle changes. In order for your goals to be attainable, they must be realistic, practical, and measureable:

- ✔ **Realistic goals:** Make sure your goals are realistic ones that you can successfully achieve. For example, if you have 50 pounds to lose, don't set a goal to lose all the weight in two months. This unrealistic timeline may make you frustrated and inclined to give up if you don't hit that mark.

- ✔ **Practical goals:** What's "practical" depends entirely on your lifestyle. If your day is scheduled around traveling from place to place, setting a goal of eating lunch at home may not be practical. Instead, you can make a goal to bring a healthy lunch or have a deli sandwich and salad instead of buzzing through a fast-food joint for a grease-bomb combo (hold the tomato).

- ✔ **Measurable goals:** You won't know whether you're meeting your goals if you can't measure them. Specific goals, such as eating three servings of vegetables per day, are a lot easier to measure your success for than general goals such as "eat healthy."

Ditching diets

Quitting diets once and for all is the first step to weight-loss success. Chronic dieting ends up doing more harm than good. If you've lost weight and regained it many times, you may have noticed how easy it is to gain. Each time you lose and gain weight, you may be lowering your *metabolic rate* (how many calories your body burns at rest), making gaining weight easier and easier; any time you consume more calories than you burn, you gain weight. The biggest issue with traditional dieting is that it almost always provides a short-term solution.

Omitting foods, counting calories, and eating very low numbers of calories aren't habits most people can live with long term. Although you may lose weight quickly with these kinds of methods, you're likely to gain it back (plus possibly even more weight) after you stop the diet, leaving you in a never-ending battle with weight loss that affects your self-esteem and motivation.

Dieting also messes with your head. Research shows that when people restrict and omit foods, they tend to focus more on those foods, which leads to an unhealthy relationship. For example, when you say you aren't going to eat any sugar, you're more likely to dwell on chocolate, ice cream, and other forbidden goodies until you snap and end up eating more of the items than you should. Then you say, "I'll get back on track next week," and the cycle continues and continues.

Assuming you have no health issues that require you to omit certain foods, research shows that enjoying a small piece of, say, chocolate and then moving on is far better for you than omitting sugar all together. You don't become consumed with the chocolate and are less likely to overeat it. Finding the balance of eating healthy foods most of the time and allowing yourself treats once in awhile is the key to mastering weight loss.

Making time in a fast-paced lifestyle

A fast-paced lifestyle is part of reality today, but it also contradicts one of the premises of a Mediterranean lifestyle. When incorporating the Mediterranean diet into your lifestyle, your first goal is to try to slow down. Look at all you have on your (figurative) plate and see whether you can start to say "no" to some things so you can free up time for yourself.

Overbooking yourself with work, kids, and other tasks is easy. Before you know it, you have no time for health and wellness, leading to overwhelm and fatigue. Children, family, certain occupations, and other obligations may make slowing down more difficult. However, you still can do a few things to make adopting the Mediterranean lifestyle easier. Keep the following tips in mind:

- **Have a plan for your weekly grocery shopping and meal planning.** Doing so can save you time and help you to follow through with your food goals. See Chapter 4 for more details on how to make this idea work for you.

- **Pre-make meals and meal components to have at the ready.** Use batch cooking (see Chapter 6) to make meals ahead of time for later in the week or for freezing. Chop up a bunch of fresh veggies and prepare some simple grains like rice, quinoa, or barley at the beginning of the week to have on hand throughout the week so you can cut down your cooking time after your busy day.

- **Follow the great Mediterranean strategy of using fresh, raw produce with your meals.** Sometimes cooking all meal components takes up too much time. Add unadorned veggies such as sliced tomatoes and cucumbers or carrot sticks to your plate. Focus on easy-to-prepare meals for every day and use the more labor-intensive cooking for special occasions.

- **Embrace the convenience of the produce aisle.** Make use of pre-washed, pre-cut vegetables you can find at your local grocery store, such as salad mixes, baby carrots, grape tomatoes, and celery sticks.

- **Keep your kitchen well stocked.** That way, you always have Mediterranean foods such as olive oil and beans on hand for throwing together whatever meal strikes your fancy. Head to Chapter 5 for a complete pantry, refrigerator, and freezer list.

- **Schedule time for physical activity.** In today's world, you may say you're going to go walking, but before you know it, it's bedtime. To combat this kind of failed intention, find 20 to 30 minutes for walking or doing other kinds of exercise four to five times week and pencil it into your schedule. Make sure you stick to your schedule. For example, do you watch mindless TV for an hour each evening? If so, reduce your TV time and go walking for 30 minutes. Do you take an hour lunch at work? Go outside and walk for 20 to 30 minutes before you eat.

Creating small changes that stick

Before you begin your weight-loss journey, you want to take baby steps and start small with a few changes at a time. Look at small goals you can integrate into your daily life and do it.

For example, perhaps you start by making sure you have a fruit or vegetable with every meal while decreasing your portions of meats and starch. Add a scheduled daily walk to that goal, and you have a great starting point for incorporating changes. Master these few things, and you'll likely lose a few pounds from your new, lower calorie intake and increase in calorie-burning exercise. A little success is a great way to make changes become habits. Then you're on to the next two goals.

Trying to jump into all the new changes at once can be overwhelming and seem impossible, making you quit before you get a chance to really get rolling. Change can be hard, and your habitual mind will keep calling you back to your old habits. Tackling some small, achievable goals and having a few victories is far easier to keep you motivated for the long haul. Even a few small changes each week can lead to weight loss.

Considering Calories without Counting Them

Calories are one of the most important concepts of weight loss. Basically, *calories* are the amount of energy in the foods you eat and the amount of energy your body uses for daily activities. Your body constantly needs energy or fuel not only for daily activities such as cooking, cleaning, and exercising but also for basic biological functions (like, you know, breathing). Everyone has a different metabolic rate that determines how quickly he or she burns calories and depends on factors such as age, genetics, gender, and physical fitness level.

At the end of the day, you can't lose weight if you eat more calories than you burn through daily activity and exercise. To lose weight, you have to create a calorie deficit, but you can do so without actually knowing how many calories you burn. All you have to do is make small changes to your lifestyle, such as reducing portion sizes and exercising more, to reduce your calorie intake.

Counting the calorie level of each and every food and drink you consume all day — commonly known as *counting calories* — isn't much fun at all. As a gauge for cutting the number of calories you consume, it's a no-win situation. Counting calories each and every day isn't something you want to do long term because it takes time and can end up being a daunting task.

Without having some idea of your calorie intake level, however, you'll be in the dark about how much you're eating. That's where the Mediterranean diet comes into play. Instead of counting calories, you think about the kinds of foods you eat and the portion sizes of those foods. By adding more low-calorie fruits and vegetables to your diet and decreasing the portion size of higher-calorie foods like meats and grains, you can decrease your calorie level naturally. When you master this new way of eating, you can ensure you're eating the appropriate number of calories without having to account for every single one.

The following sections show you how to eat at an appropriate calorie level by properly balancing your plate's food make-up, controlling portions, and expending energy through fun activities.

Eating more to lose weight

Unlike many weight-loss diets, a Mediterranean style of eating lets you have more food on your plate while still taking in fewer calories. "How does *that* work?" you wonder. Well, you get to eat far more low-calorie vegetables and fewer high-calorie meats and grains. As an added bonus, these lower-calorie foods also help you feel more satisfied with your meal instead of feeling deprived.

In the United States, a traditional plate of food has a large piece of meat, a large serving of grains or potatoes, and a tiny amount of vegetable. By simply switching up your plate to include small portions of meat and grain, two to three vegetables, and perhaps a serving of legumes, you can easily save calories (in some cases, hundreds of them). For example, one 6-ounce chicken breast is around 276 calories. Decrease the serving size to 3 ounces, and the count drops to 138 calories. That one change saves 138 calories. A serving of vegetables (½ cup cooked or 1 cup raw) is only 25 calories. By the time you put two to three of those servings on your plate, you've spent about 75 calories and don't have space for much else. You can see how simply changing the balance of the foods you eat makes a huge difference in your calorie intake.

Taking portion size into account

Paying attention to portion sizes is a far better way to decrease your calorie intake than counting calories. Portion sizes in the Mediterranean are different than they are in the United States, which is one reason folks in the Mediterranean region tend to manage their weights more effectively. Although the U.S. serving-size guidelines are appropriate, few Americans actually follow them.

Part of the problem is that the portion sizes in restaurants have become gigantic — big enough to feed three adults in some circumstances. Even the plate sizes are huge! And food manufacturers are following this trend as well.

Consider these few examples of how commercial portion sizes have gotten out of control:

- In the 1970s, a typical fountain drink from a restaurant or convenience store was 12 ounces, with no free refills. Today the typical small size is 20 ounces, and cups go all the way up to 100 ounces, often with as many free refills as your bladder can handle. A 12-ounce soda pop is around 140 calories, so imagine what the count for 44 ounces is.

- Bagels used to weigh 2 to 3 ounces and now weigh 4 to 7 ounces. A 4-ounce bagel is around 300 calories.

- Deli bread has gotten bigger so that people feel like they're getting more for their money. And of course, more bread requires more filling, adding even more calories. Going to a deli for a sandwich on jumbo-sized bread basically amounts to eating a sandwich and a half on regular bread at home.

The more you see these types of portion sizes, the more normal they seem.

On the Mediterranean coast, people actually eat portion sizes of meats and grains closer to what the recommended serving sizes are in the United States: 2 to 3 ounces of meat as a side dish (recommended U.S. serving: 3 ounces) and about ½ cup of grains/pasta as a side dish (recommended U.S. serving: the same). Unfortunately, the average American is eating closer to 8 ounces of meat and 1½ to 2 cups of grains at any given meal. Table 3-1 is a serving guide that can help you create smaller, appropriate portions and thus a lower-calorie plate; after you get the hang of it, eating the right portion size will be second nature, and you'll just know how much to put on your plate by eyeballing it.

Table 3-1	Serving Size Guide
Food	*Serving Size*
Grains	1 slice bread
	½ an English muffin, hamburger bun, or bagel
	⅓ cup rice
	½ cup cooked cereal, pasta, or other cooked grain
	¾ cup cold cereal
	One 6-inch tortilla
Other starchy carbohydrates	½ cup beans or lentils (these also contain protein)
Fruit	1 medium piece of fruit
	½ cup canned or sliced fruit
	6 ounces (¾ cup) 100% fruit juice

(continued)

Table 3-1 *(continued)*

Food	Serving Size
Vegetables	1 cup raw
	½ cup cooked
	6 ounces (¾ cup) 100% vegetable juice
Dairy	8 ounces of milk or yogurt
	⅓ cup cottage cheese
	1 ounce cheese
Protein	½ cup beans (beans are also high in carbs)
	2–4 ounces beef, poultry, pork, or fish (size of a deck of cards)
	1 ounce cheese
	1 egg
	1 ounce nuts
	1 tablespoon nut spreads (such as peanut butter, almond butter, and so on)
Fats	⅛ of an avocado (2 tablespoons)
	1 teaspoon oil, butter, margarine, or mayonnaise
	2 teaspoon whipped butter
	8 olives
	1 tablespoon regular salad dressing
	2 tablespoons lowfat salad dressing

Here's an example of what a Mediterranean style meal may look like using these serving sizes.

- 2 ounces of grilled lemon chicken
- ⅔ cup of wild rice, black bean, and fresh herb mixture
- 2 cups mixed green salad with sliced tomatoes and radishes with 1 tablespoon vinaigrette salad dressing
- ½ cup grilled zucchini

This large meal contains several vegetable servings, and the estimated calorie level is about 500 calories. Compare that to an 8-ounce chicken breast with 2 cups of rice and a small vegetable; that calorie level is about 680 calories. This sample Mediterranean meal isn't too bad when you consider that you get to eat a greater variety of food, a good balance of protein between the chicken and black beans, and loads of fiber from the beans and veggies to help you feel full and satisfied. It also contains a good dose of healthy fats from the salad dressing and any oil used while grilling the zucchini.

Watching your fat calories

The Mediterranean diet also allows you to keep track of the calories you get from fat. Although people on the Mediterranean coast eat slightly more fat than is recommended in the United States (35 percent of their calories come from fat, versus the U.S. recommendation of 30 percent), they consume different types of fat, such as the healthy fats from olive oil. Flip to Chapter 2 for more on the types of fat you consume on a Mediterranean diet.

No matter what type of fat you eat, it still has 9 calories per gram. Make sure you're careful about not using too much fat with your meals. Otherwise, you can end up gaining weight from excessive fat calories. The recipes in this book help you use the right amount of fat your body needs.

To help you gauge how much fat to use in your cooking, measure your added fats, such as salad dressing or drizzles of olive oil, for a few days so that you get the idea of what the appropriate portion size looks like on your food. You want to use about one tablespoon of salad dressing and one teaspoon for oil drizzles added to vegetables or breads. You don't need to measure forever, and you don't need to be exact. Just get comfortable with the portion, and pretty soon you'll be able to eye what a teaspoon of oil looks like.

Increasing activity you love

Exercise is an important component to weight loss and health, especially with the Mediterranean diet. You have to use up some of your calorie intake as energy, or those calories will store as fat. Exercise allows you to not only burn calories but also strengthen your heart, manage stress, and increase your energy level.

Starting an exercise program may be challenging for you — maybe the thought of going to a busy gym and running on a treadmill sounds more painful than a double root canal. Never fear; look to the Mediterranean. On the Mediterranean coast, the main focus on exercise is walking, working, and enjoyable activities instead of formalized exercise programs. That is, people walk to run errands; lift and carry groceries home; work in the yard; and enjoy fun activities like bike riding or swimming. With modern conveniences, people in the United States and Canada typically don't move and exercise as part of daily life much anymore. They typically sit in front of a computer or behind a desk, which is why exercise programs are more popular. Those programs are great, but if you don't enjoy it, you may not stick with it for long.

If starting an exercise program sounds difficult for you, find activities that you actually enjoy doing and look for ways to get out every day for a walk. The American College of Sports Medicine and the American Heart Association recommend getting 30 minutes of moderate exercise (you get your heart rate up but can still have a conversation) a day, five days a week for those who are 18 to 65 years old, as well as adding two days a week of strength-training exercises like lifting weights.

Suppressing Your Appetite Effortlessly

Eating a Mediterranean style diet is not only great for your health but can also work as a natural appetite suppressant to help manage your weight. When you eat the right balance of plant-based foods and healthy fats, your body works in a natural way to feel satisfied. Because you're full, you're not tempted (at least, not by your stomach) to snack on high-calorie junk food a short while after your last meal. The following sections highlight the three main reasons a Mediterranean diet helps to control your appetite.

Loading up on fiber

Fiber, found in fruits, vegetables, whole grains, and legumes, provides bulk and slows down digestion to help you feel full for a longer period of time. With the Mediterranean diet, you consume much more fiber-rich food with each meal and snack, which can make you feel satisfied all day. The average American diet contains little fiber and often doesn't include fibrous foods with each meal; this lack of fiber can actually stimulate your appetite even shortly after you've eaten.

These high-fiber foods also make you chew a little longer, helping you to slow down at mealtime. Your brain takes 20 minutes to register that you're full, which is longer than many people spend eating a meal. As a result, your brain may give you the okay to keep eating because it doesn't realize yet that you've actually eaten enough to be full. Chewing more helps you to slow down and reach that 20-minute mark.

Turning on your fullness hormones

The Mediterranean diet is naturally high in *low-glycemic foods,* those carbohydrate-containing foods that illicit a lower blood sugar spike. Low-glycemic foods may just help kick on your fullness response. Appetite is controlled by an intricate dance of hormones that trigger the feelings of hunger and fullness.

When you're eating, your body releases two separate hormones that play a role in regulating your appetite and letting you know you're full. Those hormones are

- ✔ **Leptin:** This hormone releases a process telling you it's time to stop eating — you're comfortably full.

- ✔ **GLP-1:** This hormone tells your body, "Hey, I'm not messing around. You need to stop eating pronto because the food is making you uncomfortably full." It brings things to a halt by telling your stomach to stop moving anything along to your intestines until they've broken down what's already there. You know how after you eat a huge meal like Thanksgiving dinner, all you can do is lie on the couch in sweatpants? That's your GLP-1 kicking in.

    In 2009, researchers from King's College in London took a close look at GLP-1 in respect to a low-glycemic diet. Volunteers who ate a low-glycemic breakfast ended up with 20 percent higher levels of GLP-1 in their blood compared to those who ate a high-glycemic breakfast. More research is needed, but as you start eating the Mediterranean way, you can take note of whether you feel a larger degree of fullness after your meals than you have in the past.

To help you pay attention to your body, start by filling your plate with appropriate portion sizes of food (see the serving size guide in Table 3-1). Eat slowly, spending at least 20 minutes with your meal. Keep checking in with your stomach and pay attention to whether it feels hungry, neutral, or full. You'll be surprised that a relatively small amount of food will make you feel comfortably full. At this point, you want to stop eating.

Feeling biologically full and psychologically satisfied with your meal are two very different things that are often hard to distinguish. Biological fullness occurs in your stomach, where you feel hungry, neutral, or comfortably full. Feeling psychologically satisfied is in your brain; you want to eat more because it tastes so good!

Overindulging once in awhile because something is so tasty is completely normal, but when you consistently ignore your fullness cues and eat until you're psychologically satisfied, you consume too many calories far too often. If you fall into this trap, tell yourself you can have more of the food later in the day or even tomorrow. Heck, you can even make this meal again and again so that you can enjoy it every week.

Note: One of the first signs of dehydration is hunger, so when you feel hungry even though you just ate a short time ago, grab a glass of water, wait 15 minutes, and see how you feel.

Controlling Food Cravings

Food cravings occur for many reasons, whether they're physiological, psychological, or a combination of both. For instance, having a stressful day at work may lead to food cravings. Perhaps you end up skipping a meal (putting more stress on your body) and start craving some particular candy that was your go-to feel-better solution growing up. At this point, eating that candy is easy, even if you have an apple sitting in your drawer.

Unfortunately, no one-size-fits-all-answer exists to deal with food cravings, but you can do a few things to manage them more effectively. The following strategies are natural byproducts of a Mediterranean style of living.

Avoiding blood sugar spikes

Keeping your blood sugar stable throughout the day is a good strategy to help manage food cravings. Eating high-glycemic foods causes a high blood sugar spike and then a crash, leaving you with symptoms of low blood sugar that include hunger and irritability, which can lead down the path to food cravings. Waiting too long to eat between meals and snacks can also elicit those low blood sugar symptoms. The combination of feeling both very hungry and edgy can often set you up to make the wrong food choices.

To avoid this trap, do as they do on the Mediterranean coast, including the following:

- ✔ **Make sure you don't skip meals or wait longer than 5 hours to eat.** Eat a meal or snack every 3 to 5 hours. Eat when you are hungry instead of waiting until you have extreme hunger.

- ✔ **Eat protein-rich foods and a bit of fat.** Include foods such as fish, beans, nuts, or eggs with a fat with each meal to help slow down your digestion

- ✔ **Eat high-fiber, fruits, vegetables, grains, and legumes with each meal and snack.** You don't have to eat these foods all at once, but including some combination of them at meals and incorporating a fruit, veggie, or whole grain with your snacks is a good idea.

Managing your stress hormones

Stress occurs for many different reasons, and unfortunately, it's a prevalent part of everyday life for many people. You may have a demanding job and small children to care for. Perhaps the lack of time to stick to a proper diet and exercise plan is stressful. Luckily, the Mediterranean lifestyle can help you handle your stress and find a little bit of relaxation.

Stress releases hormones that trigger the "fight or flight" response (where your body gears up its energy levels for a big event like fighting or fleeing) and kick on your hunger hormones. Biologically, this concept makes sense. How are you supposed to fight like a warrior or run to the hills with no fuel? The body is working as it's supposed to. The increase in stress is what's leading to more hunger and food cravings.

You can tackle stress-induced cravings a few different ways:

- ✔ **Try to limit or prevent stressful situations in your life.** Some things you can't help, like work-related stress, but you can certainly prevent stress in other ways, like saying "no" more often if you have too much going on or avoiding unnecessary confrontations by letting the small stuff in life go.

- ✔ **Manage stress levels.** This step is a priority in traditional Mediterranean life. You can accomplish it by exercising, getting enough sleep, drinking water, practicing deep breathing, meditating, and relaxing. For example, if you are getting ready for a stressful meeting, take a few moments to do some deep breathing. Simply take a deep breath, hold it for a few seconds, and let the air out. Keep repeating for as long as you can. Even a few minutes can help.

- ✔ **When you're feeling a craving, go for a low-glycemic snack and include some omega-3 fatty acids.** A good snack is some tuna fish spread on whole-grain crackers. This combination can help you get the fuel your body is craving but also help your central nervous system calm down. Eating high-glycemic foods in this situation can keep you in a state of blood sugar spikes, making the craving cycle worse.

- ✔ **Know when to give in a little.** If you're really craving sugar, are in a truly edgy state, and couldn't care less about what you *should* eat, eat the omega-3 and low-glycemic snack and then have a small piece of the sugar you're craving. The healthy snack will do its work biologically, and the small sugar hit will help you avoid feeling deprived to the point where you want to eat the whole package.

These tips may require changing your coping habits. Your brain may be used to going for comfort food when you're stressed, so you need to go through a period of retraining your brain to try some new coping skills, such as having a cup of tea and journaling for a few minutes to help come down from the stressful day.

Mastering the Art of Mindful Eating

A traditional Mediterranean style of eating engages regularly in mindful eating, something that many have completely lost track of. With *mindful eating,* you can manage your weight by paying attention to your internal body cues. Yes, your own body has a very sophisticated weight management system built in that include hormones that tell you when you should eat and when to stop (see the earlier section "Suppressing Your Appetite Effortlessly" for details). The problem is that too many people often ignore that reflex. The following sections highlight how to refocus on these internal cues and become completely satisfied with what you're eating.

Slowing down

Slowing down is a theme in the Mediterranean lifestyle that even goes for meals. A good goal is to spend at least 20 to 30 minutes eating your larger meals. As we note earlier in the chapter, this time frame gives your biological system time to let you know when you're full. Plus, it allows you to sit and enjoy your food. Use these tips to help you slow down at meal time:

- ✔ Set your fork down between bites to begin retraining yourself how to slow down while you eat.

- ✔ Take a deep breath and count to ten before each bite. Don't worry, you don't have to do this forever, just until you've learned how to pace yourself.

- ✔ Have great table discussions with your family and friends. Ask a question about everyone's day or talk about current events.

- ✔ Take some time to be grateful for what you have.

- ✔ Make meal time a television-, computer-, and phone-free zone to avoid mindless eating.

Enjoying food to its fullest

When you eat, take time to enjoy every aspect of your food. When you think about Italians, Greeks, Spaniards, and other Mediterranean people, you think about cultures who love their food. They don't wolf down their food in a few minutes. They sit around their dining tables and enjoy every aspect of the food. This enjoyment of food helps them to manage their weights by feeling psychologically satisfied with what they're eating, which leaves less chance for overeating.

Incorporate the following mealtime tips to help you enjoy eating to the fullest:

- ✔ **Take a deep breath.** Before you dig into any food, smell the flavors coming from it. You've spent time creating these dishes, so let your nose enjoy them as well.

- ✔ **Act like the natives.** Put yourself in the shoes of an Italian or Greek when you're eating a meal and rave over every bite. That's how you want to enjoy your food.

- ✔ **Taste each and every flavor.** During each bite, let the food sit in your mouth. Chew it slowly and take pleasure in the freshness and the many tastes that roll across your taste buds. By slowing down and really tasting the flavors, you'll be more satisfied than you would be eating it quickly.

  Additionally, serving lots of food in small portion sizes helps you enjoy each flavor. Adding several vegetables, sliced tomatoes, olives, salads, and protein to a meal helps you to enjoy all the different flavors and temperatures. Don't underestimate the power of food satisfaction. Not being satisfied with what your eating can lead to overeating relatively easily.

You can do the chocolate kiss test at home to see for yourself how luxuriating in your food makes you eat less. Take a chocolate kiss and wolf it down quickly. How did it taste? Would you be able to report to someone about the texture and flavor? Wouldn't it be easy to pop another couple in your mouth considering how quickly that went? Now, try again, and let the candy melt in your mouth for as long as you can. No chewing; just slowly melt it. You can see how you're more satisfied with the flavor and need less food to get you to that psychological satisfaction level.

Maximizing Your Metabolic Rate

As we note in the earlier section "Ditching diets," your metabolic rate is how many calories you burn at rest. You don't have control over some of the factors that influence this rate, but you can take some steps to kick your metabolic rate into full gear.

Some people have moved away from these strategies in the United States and Canada as life has gotten more fast-paced and more convenient. You can model the Mediterranean lifestyle and incorporate some of these strategies in your daily living; try to include at least two to three of these strategies regularly:

- ✔ **Build lean muscle mass.** Muscle burns 90 percent more calories than fat does, so the more muscle you have, the more calories you burn each day. You can build more muscle by lifting weights, using resistance bands, walking, and performing other forms of strength-training exercises.

✔ **Increase your heart rate.** Regular aerobic exercise not only gets your heart rate up but also raises your metabolism during the activity and for several hours afterwards. Aerobic exercise includes any activity that gets your heart rate up, such as walking, biking, dancing, jogging, swimming, or aerobics classes.

✔ **Take the extra stairs.** Any time you increase your heart rate, even for two minutes, you give your metabolic rate a small boost. So doing little things all day like taking the stairs, dancing to your favorite song, or walking farther in the parking lot provides little rises in your metabolic rate over the course of a day. Those little individual rises add up to help you with weight loss and wellness. As you move through your day, think of ways you can increase these little bursts of energy.

✔ **Enjoy some resistant starches.** Research shows a connection between metabolism and certain starch-resistant foods that can increase the body's efficiency at burning stored fat. *Resistant starch* refers to a type of fiber that opposes digestion. Unlike other types of fiber, resistant starch ferments in the large intestine, which creates beneficial fatty acids, including one called *butyrate*.

This particular fatty acid has been shown to help the body burn more stored fat. You can find resistant starches in bananas, yams, pearl barley, and corn — all pieces of a Mediterranean-style diet. The only trick is to eat these foods cold or at room temperature for their best effect, and remember that they're not a miracle cure.

Part II
Creating a Healthy Lifestyle with Mediterranean Cooking

The 5th Wave   By Rich Tennant

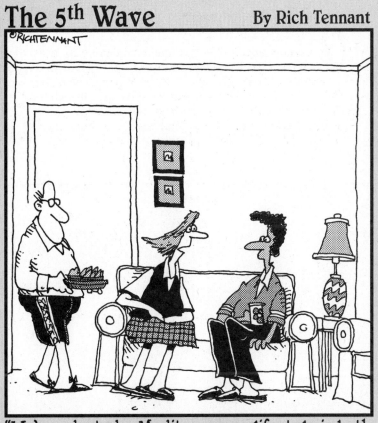

"We've adopted a Mediterranean lifestyle in both diet and exercise. Brian and I bullfight three nights a week."

In this part . . .

Understanding the healthy Mediterranean principles and incorporating them into your daily life are two very different things. Changing habits can be challenging and often overwhelming; sometimes even knowing where to begin is difficult. The chapters in this part show you the practical steps of meal planning, grocery shopping, stocking your kitchen, and cooking so that you can get your new, balanced lifestyle off on the right foot.

Chapter 4

Planning Your Mediterranean Meals

. . . .

In This Chapter

▶ Building your meals with the Mediterranean mindset

▶ Getting started with a week's worth of sample meals

▶ Searching out the best recipes for kids

▶ Celebrating the holidays with unique recipe and gift ideas

. . . .

*W*hat differentiates the eating habits of people living on the Mediterranean coast and other cultures is actually quite subtle. These small differences include eating smaller portion sizes and regulating how often certain foods are consumed. The changes may be small, but they make a significant difference for weight management, health, and well-being. As dietitians, we know you may have trouble believing that such small shifts can really make that big an impact, but we want to emphasize in this chapter how much they really do.

This chapter dives into meal planning to show you some small changes based on the Mediterranean lifestyle that have big effects on the amounts of calories and nutrients you consume. We also give you a seasonal sample menu along with some valuable lifestyle ideas to get you into the Mediterranean spirit.

Grasping the Importance of Meal Planning

Meal planning provides you a road map for the week of what you're going to eat, when you'll prepare those meals, and what foods you need to have handy in your kitchen to do so. By taking the steps to do some planning, changing to a Mediterranean diet is much easier and less stressful.

Meal planning on some level is important for several reasons:

- ✔ It ensures that you're efficient with your time and have everything you need on hand from the grocery store and markets. This preparedness also helps keep you on track with your Mediterranean lifestyle because you always have the fixings for fresh meals at your fingertips.

- ✔ It makes cooking easier during the week because you already know what you're making instead of trying to think of what you can cook with the chicken and cauliflower you bought.

- ✔ It saves you money by decreasing food waste. Do you ever buy broccoli and then wonder what to do with it as it starts yellowing in your refrigerator? Waste.

If you have a pit in your stomach right now and are ready to skip this section, hold on! Meal planning needs to (and can) work into your lifestyle. Here are a few different approaches; hopefully, you find one that works for you:

- ✔ **The detailed meal plan:** This plan is for those who love details and planning. Sit down and write out a plan for breakfast, lunch, and dinner for each day of the week. (You may want to include snacks as well.) You can make each day's foods interchangeable, but this planning method at least makes sure you have a plan and can go on your way this week with everything organized. The "Showing the Way with Sample Meals and Lifestyle Plans" section later in this chapter provides a sample week to help you get started.

- ✔ **The rotating two-week meal plan:** If you like details and convenience, this setup is perfect for you. Spend some time making up a two-week meal plan, complete with shopping list, and you've done all the work you need. So it may be that you have Dilled Eggs every other Monday for breakfast and Tortellini with Vegetables and Pesto every other Sunday for dinner. You still get plenty of variety with a two-week meal plan, but you may need to change it up every couple of months to make seasonal menus.

- ✔ **The fast meal plan:** If you're like author, Meri, you don't want to waste time on making a meal plan for each and every meal for the week. In that case, think about your habits and plan accordingly. For example, Meri knows she regularly eats a few different items for breakfast, such as poached eggs or granola and yogurt, and often eats leftovers or sandwiches along with fruit for lunch. (Call her a creature of habit.) So she focuses only on planning dinners and the few staples she needs for breakfast and lunch. She also doesn't plan a meal every night because her family almost always uses leftovers as another meal. Making a menu plan for four to five nights a week works out just fine for her situation. If you go this route, just don't forget your breakfast and lunch staples.

✔ **The super-fast meal plan:** Perhaps you need something even speedier than the fast menu plan. Instead of planning four or five dinners a week, focus on two to three and plan some convenience meals, such as entree salads you can throw together or canned or homemade, frozen soups.

Changing the Way You Fill Your Plate

Folks on the Mediterranean coast eat many of the same foods that people elsewhere do; they just eat smaller portions and incorporate plenty of vegetables. For example, they may eat pizza, but they eat less pizza; go easy on the sauce, cheese, and other toppings; and add a salad and possibly other side vegetables. In this section, we highlight some of the Mediterranean eating habits you can adopt when you're meal planning. These small changes make all the difference in health and flavor.

Focusing on plant-based foods

People of the Mediterranean region are used to using what they have on hand, and the Mediterranean climate makes for abundant amounts of fresh fruits and vegetables. As a result, people in the Mediterranean eat a lot of plant-based foods (five to nine daily servings of fruits and vegetables) and depend less on prepackaged convenience foods. (To compare, Americans eat about three servings of fruits and vegetables a day on average.). Additionally, beans and lentils commonly take the place of meat for fulfilling some protein needs. (See the later section "Finding the right balance with protein" for information on changing your protein mindset.)

To get more plant-based foods on your plate, work to get one to two fruits and/or veggies (in a rainbow of colors) into each meal, and use beans or lentils as your protein several times a week. Meats and starchy carbohydrates become your side dishes. Think about all the fresh flavors of the Mediterranean and try putting some items together. Here are some ideas to get you started:

✔ **Soup and sandwich:** The standby of grilled cheese sandwich and tomato soup is appropriate for lunch or dinner. Why stop at just the tomato soup, though? We say add as many veggies as you love; throw some fresh basil and tomato onto to your sandwich and include a side salad along with your meal.

- ✔ **Sandwiches:** Pump up your favorite sandwich with tomatoes or cucumbers. If you don't like them in a sandwich, toss them with a little oil and vinegar for a side dish. Add a fruit for a complete meal.

- ✔ **Salads, salads, salads:** We recommend always having salad greens on hand because they can make a quick side dish or a whole meal. Add as many veggies and fruits as you can find and top with a protein, such as nuts, beans, hard-boiled egg, or leftover chicken or fish. Add a roll or slice of toast, and you have a quick, light meal for a busy evening.

- ✔ **Rice and beans:** Top brown rice with your favorite beans (try black or pinto), chopped fresh tomatoes, bell peppers, and whatever else you love. Sprinkle with some goat cheese or feta cheese, and you have delicious fast food with lots of fresh produce! For extra flavor, add some fresh herbs such as cilantro or basil.

- ✔ **Scrambled eggs:** Eggs with a slice of toast can work for any meal of the day. Sauté vegetables such as onions, zucchini, bell peppers, tomatoes, and spinach, and add them to your eggs. Top with a little salsa for some kick!

- ✔ **Frozen meals:** Some frozen meals are better than others, so try to find some with lower sodium and fat contents and stick to basic foods. Even if your meal contains vegetables, add more as a side dish or to the entree; it's as easy as tossing some grape tomatoes and cucumbers onto your plate.

- ✔ **Leftovers:** Don't underestimate your leftovers. Think outside the box on how to utilize them the next day. Maybe you just have some cooked barley leftover? Combine it with some beans and veggies. Grilled chicken leftover? Slice it up and add it to a salad. Grilled vegetables left over? Put them in a tortilla with beans and cheese. You can make some quick, creative lunches and dinners from leftovers. Just yesterday, Meri gussied up leftover beans and rice with fresh heirloom tomatoes, a little goat cheese, olives, and avocado — yum!

You may also find that you have time to make a quick entree such as grilled chicken but no time to cook vegetables. Don't worry! You can add all kinds of fresh vegetables in a simple way with no extra cooking. Start with some of these ideas:

- ✔ Slice fresh tomatoes and drizzle with lemon juice and olive oil or toss with goat cheese or feta.

- ✔ Slice fresh tomatoes and cucumbers and toss with a little olive oil and vinegar.

- ✔ Cut up some cucumbers and radishes to serve alongside your meal.

- ✔ Add a tossed salad with oil and vinegar.

✔ Serve frozen (thawed) or canned artichoke hearts along with your meal. Try mixing them with sun-dried tomatoes packed in oil (drained) and fresh basil.

✔ Cut up your favorite raw veggies, such as carrots, cauliflower, and broccoli, and serve with hummus.

Making good use of healthy fats

The good news: Eating Mediterranean cooking doesn't mean you have to go on a lowfat diet. You just focus on different the types of fats, tipping the balance toward healthy monounsaturated fat sources such as olive oil, canola oil, olives, nuts, and avocadoes and away from saturated fats such as animal fats. Using monounsaturated fats is often associated with better heart health. Eating a good amount of dietary fat also helps to keep you feeling full for a longer period of time.

Here are some tips to add healthy fats in place of not-so-healthy fats in your diet.

✔ Use olive oil or canola oil rather than vegetable oils or butter when sautéing meats and vegetables.

✔ Use salad dressings with an olive oil or canola oil base rather than those with a base of cream or other vegetable oils.

✔ When making a grilled sandwich, brush your bread with olive oil rather than butter.

✔ Dip your bread in extra-virgin olive oil and a little balsamic vinegar instead of using butter.

✔ Spread avocado, pesto, or hummus on your sandwiches and use less/no mayonnaise.

Finding the right balance with protein

Many people automatically consider protein foods such as beef, poultry, pork, and fish as an entree. However, meat is typically a side dish in the Mediterranean diet; when meat does serve as the main dish, it's in a smaller portion size than you're probably used to.

The goal is to eat less animal protein and more plant-based protein. Instead of having an 8-ounce steak, you may choose to have a 3- or 4-ounce portion but also have a lentil salad or sprinkle some nuts on a salad to reincorporate some of that lost protein.

Thinking of meat as anything but an entree may be difficult. I know many people are meat lovers, and you may be just about ready to put this book on the shelf because you think you have to give up your favorite foods. Wait! You don't have to become vegetarian to live a Mediterranean lifestyle. Incorporating this lifestyle is more about eating less and adding more variety to your plate than about depriving yourself completely.

If you feel like this lifestyle isn't for you, consider going halfway. Eating your normal portions of meat two to three days a week and going a more Mediterranean route on the other days may work better for you. If you aren't willing to give up your regular portion of steak, look for other places in the meal where you can incorporate Mediterranean concepts. Start with what you're comfortable with; even a partial change in your habits can make a big difference in your overall health.

Looking at a Mediterranean meal makeover

Everyone loves a good makeover story, so in this section, we use the information from the preceding sections to give a meal a Mediterranean renovation. We want to show you how powerful small changes can be and also emphasize that you don't have to give up foods you love. You also get to add more food to your plate at the end of the day. Who can argue with that?

Before: A typical steak-and-potatoes meal

8-ounce rib-eye steak

Whole baked potato with sour cream and butter

½ cup steamed broccoli

Estimated calories: 1,049; Saturated fat: 22 grams; Monounsaturated fat: 15.8 grams

After: A Mediterranean-style steak-and-potatoes meal

3-ounce rib-eye steak

¾ cup Garlic and Lemon Roasted Potatoes (Chapter 12)

½ cup steamed broccoli

Grilled Fennel (Chapter 12)

Estimated calories: 575; Saturated fat 5 grams; Monounsaturated fat 26 grams

The results: As you can see, simply decreasing the amount of steak, changing the (saturated fat) loaded baked potato to the roasted Garlic and Lemon

Potatoes (which use olive oil), and adding more vegetables changed the entire make-up of this meal. The made-over meal has nearly half the calories, significantly lower levels of saturated fats, and much higher levels of healthy monounsaturated fats. Plus, the Grilled Fennel adds vitamins, minerals, and phytochemicals.

Showing the Way with Sample Meals and Lifestyle Plans

You may not be sure exactly where to start with your new Mediterranean diet, but no worries. In this section, we give you a sample menu to get your brain working on possible pairings and meal plans. Staying true to all that is Mediterranean, we include seasonal cooking, exercise, rest, and time with friends and family. The enjoyment of coming together in a community is an important piece of the Mediterranean lifestyle puzzle. Make sure you designate a few nights a week with extended family and/or friends.

Make sure not to follow this sample plan like a weekly diet, because you may get bored or discouraged. Instead, use it as an example of how you can begin making changes to your own lifestyle.

The menus in this section are based on the summer season, with daily calorie counts between 1,600 to 2,200 calories. Everyone has a different calorie level for optimal health, so use your own internal calorie counting system: your fullness level. If you're still hungry after any meal, try going back for seconds or even thirds of your veggie side dishes. This strategy is a great way to fill your appetite and add healthy nutrients without adding too many calories.

Always stop eating when your stomach is comfortably full, which may happen with more or less food than we provide in the sample menus, depending on your sex, genetic makeup, age, and activity level. Keep in mind that people who aren't on a strict diet don't eat the exact same number of calories each day. You may find you eat less on a busy day and more when you're having a gathering. The goal is to always eat when you're hungry and stop when you're full. Make sure to spend at least 20 minutes at meal time to allow yourself to feel that full sensation in your stomach.

In order to make these menus functional, we did make dinner the main meal (rather than lunch, which is typically the main Mediterranean meal) because we know cooking a large meal for lunch can be hard for those working during the day. Breakfast remains light and is followed up with a snack, true to the Mediterranean way of eating. We've also incorporated some leftovers and convenience foods to make the menu plan more like the real world; no one (including folks in the Mediterranean) cooks every meal from scratch every day.

Sunday: Day of relaxation

Sunday is a great day to get some downtime and rest. Sleep, read a book, or watch a game. Put on some sauce and smell the delicious aroma as you lounge. In the afternoon, take some time for activity and go for a walk. Walking (even short walks) is a great daily habit for exercise and stress management.

Breakfast

Farina Farina (Chapter 7)

1 cup coffee or tea (optional)

Snack

6 ounces lowfat Greek yogurt with ⅓ cup blueberries

Lunch

½ a turkey sandwich with lettuce, tomato, provolone cheese, and avocado

½ cup Black Beans with Tomatoes and Feta (Chapter 14)

1 cup tomato soup (the Tomato Basil Soup recipe in Chapter 11 or store-bought)

1 orange

Snack

¼ cup Hummus with 8 Toasted Pita Chips (Chapter 8)

Dinner

1 cup penne pasta with Meat Sauce (Chapter 9) — freeze any leftover sauce for future use

½ cup steamed broccoli

1 cup Tomato, Cucumber, and Basil Salad (Chapter 10)

Monday: Grilling to start off your work week

Monday is a return to the grind for many people, so it's a good day to ease into the week after a relaxing weekend. Take time today for a walk during your lunch break. The fresh air and change of scenery will help you revitalize your day. Tonight is grill night, which means little time spent on cooking, so get outside this evening and go for a bike ride or throw a ball or Frisbee around with the kids (or anyone else).

Breakfast

1 cup cooked oatmeal with 1 sliced banana and 2 teaspoons honey

1 cup lowfat milk

1 cup coffee or tea (optional)

Snack

¼ cup Hummus with 8 Toasted Pita Chips (leftover from Sunday)

Lunch

1 serving Roasted Vegetables with Feta Cheese Pita (Chapter 16)

6 ounces lowfat Greek yogurt

Snack

16 grapes

Dinner

1 serving Grilled Tuna with Braised Fennel (Chapter 18)

¾ cup Couscous with Tomatoes and Cucumbers (Chapter 13) — make extra

1 cup Lemon Asparagus with Parmesan (Chapter 12)

Tuesday: Making it quick!

Although a large part of the Mediterranean lifestyle is slowing down, we also know a few days of the week are always busy. Even on a busy day, prioritize a time for a brisk morning or evening walk. Get up a little earlier to sit on your front porch and enjoy a cup of coffee or tea. The walk and relaxation time combined may take just one hour out of your day, but prioritizing you-time is worth it for your health!

Breakfast

1 cup Greek Yogurt and Fruit Bowls (Chapter 7)

1 cup coffee or tea (optional)

Snack

1 ounce Toasted Almonds (Chapter 8)

1 tangerine

Lunch

1 chicken sandwich on whole-grain bread with tomatoes, lettuce, mozzarella, and Pesto (Chapter 9 or store-bought)

1 cup vegetable soup (canned)

Snack

¼ cup assorted olives with 1 ounce feta cheese

Dinner

1 serving Chicken in Paprika Sauce (Chapter 17)

¾ cup leftover Couscous with Tomatoes and Cucumbers (leftover from Monday)

½ cup sautéed bell peppers

½ cup Sautéed Broccoli Rabe (Chapter 12)

Wednesday: Making easy, delicious meals

Using some of the leftovers from earlier in the week makes this cooking day go smoothly. You can even whip up your salad dressings in the morning and have them ready to go for lunch and dinner. You can complete this dinner in 45 minutes, so plan some downtime to enjoy the evening. Make sure to get some fresh air by going for a walk or even just setting your table up outside.

Breakfast

1 Lemon Scone (Chapter 7)

1 cup coffee or tea (optional)

Snack

1 serving Goat Cheese with Honey and Fruit (Chapter 8)

Lunch

Smoked Salmon and Arugula Salad (Chapter 10)

8 Toasted Pita Chips (leftover from Monday)

Snack

1 ounce Toasted Almonds (leftover from Tuesday)

1 tangerine

Dinner

¾ cup Pork Sausage with White Beans and Tomatoes (Chapter 19)

½ cup steamed broccoli and cauliflower

1 cup Italian Bread Salad (Chapter 10)

Thursday: Winding down the work week

Now that you're approaching the end of the work week, you can enjoy your friends and family. Have a family game night or movie night with friends. Revel in the company of those who are closest to you.

Breakfast

1 Dilled Egg (Chapter 7)

1 to 2 slices of whole-grain toast with 2 teaspoons butter

1 cup coffee or tea (optional)

Snack

6 ounces of lowfat Greek yogurt with ½ cup fresh strawberries

Lunch

1 cup assorted steamed vegetables (broccoli, cauliflower, carrots, and so on; can be leftover from Wednesday)

½ cup Chickpea Salad (Chapter 10)

Snack

¼ cup Hummus (leftover from Sunday) with 5 raw baby carrots

Dinner

1 cup Moroccan Chicken with Tomatoes and Zucchini (Chapter 17)

¾ cup cooked brown rice

2 cups Greek Salad (Chapter 10)

Snack

1 Classic Biscotti (Chapter 20)

Friday: Pizza night

The work week is done, and now you can kick up your feet and start your weekend. Making pizza is a fun activity for all ages. Create a family night where everyone can prepare his or her own individual flatbread pizzas. Don't forget to go for a walk today.

Breakfast

> 1 Classic Biscotti (leftover from Thursday)
>
> 1 banana
>
> 1 cup coffee or tea (optional)

Snack

> 6 ounces of lowfat Greek yogurt with ⅓ cup fresh berries

Lunch

> 2 cups tossed green salad with kidney beans, walnuts, tomatoes, and cucumbers and 1 tablespoon of vinegar-and-oil-based salad dressing
>
> ¾ cup Tabbouleh (Chapter 13)

Snack

> ¼ cup assorted olives

Dinner

> 1 slice Chicken and Arugula Pizza (Chapter 16) or your own favorite pizza — make extra
>
> 1 cup Mediterranean-Style Fruit Salad (Chapter 10)
>
> ½ cup Warm Fava Beans with Feta (Chapter 14)

Saturday: Party all day and night

Saturday is a great day to do some fun activities. All exercise doesn't need to be formal; instead, focus on fun. Get an early start in the morning and go for a hike, take a bike ride, or go for a swim. Do something active that you love. Get home for a quickie leftover lunch and get the stage ready for a fun evening with friends and family. *Note:* You may have to double or triple your dinner recipes depending on how many guests you have. And the serving sizes for the party reflect what you'll eat; we're not suggesting you make only eight pita chips to go around!

Breakfast

1 cup cooked oatmeal with 1 sliced banana and 2 teaspoons of honey

1 cup coffee or tea (optional)

Snack (hopefully while you're out and about!)

1 granola bar

1 apple

Lunch

1 slice of pizza (leftover from Friday)

1 cup Mediterranean-Style Fruit Salad (leftover from Friday)

Snack (appetizers for guests)

¼ cup Roasted Eggplant Dip (Baba Gannoujh) (Chapter 8)

8 Toasted Pita Chips (Chapter 8; you probably won't have enough leftover from Sunday to serve to the entire party)

1 ounce assorted olives and nuts

Dinner

1 cup Paella (Chapter 18)

½ cup saffron rice (store-bought)

½ cup Roasted Broccoli and Tomatoes (Chapter 12)

Snack

1 slice Ricotta Cake (Chapter 20)

Finding Kid-Friendly Recipes

All children have different tastes. Some can handle a lot of spice, and others like foods to be bland. You may have picky eaters on your hands who shudder at the idea of lentils or feta, or adventurous eaters who think lima beans are the best food ever (like Meri's do). This book provides a ton of recipes, so you're sure to find some kid-friendly ones.

Another way to encourage kids to try new things is to involve them in the planning, shopping, and cooking processes. The tykes will be more excited to try new things if those things are their creations.

We encourage you to try many different recipes with your kids because you never know what they may like. Here are a few recipes we think your kids will enjoy to get you started:

Chapter 7

Egg Panini

Greek Yogurt and Fruit Bowls

Orange Ricotta Pancakes

Chapter 8

Toasted Pita Chips

Mini Spanakopita

Chapter 9

All sauce recipes

Chapter 10

All the fruit salad recipes

Chapter 11

Tomato Basil Soup

Pasta Fagioli

Minestrone

Chicken Stew with Chickpeas and Plum Tomatoes

Chapter 12

Roasted Vegetables with Béchamel Sauce

Garlic and Lemon Roasted Potatoes

Rice-Stuffed Tomatoes

Chapter 13

Golden Pilaf

Basic Polenta

Chapter 14

Lentil Loaf

Black Beans with Tomatoes and Feta

Falafel

Chapter 15

Tortellini with Vegetables and Pesto

Vegetarian Lasagne

Spaghetti and Meatballs

Chapter 16

Margherita Pizza

Oven-Fried Fish Sandwich with Fresh Spring Mix

Chapter 17

Chicken Cacciatore

Spanish Kabobs

Chicken Wrapped in Phyllo

Chapter 18

Baked Salmon with Fresh Vegetables

Chapter 19

Mediterranean Beef Kabobs

Roasted Pork Loin with Apricots

Chapter 20

All dessert recipes (of course!)

Cooking Up Creative Ideas for the Holidays

The holidays are a great time for family traditions, and many of those customs include the types of foods that you serve for parties or give away as gifts. Taking the time to cook as part of your celebration is fun and special, and it adds a personal touch that everyone appreciates. This section gives you some great ideas to incorporate Mediterranean cooking into your holiday parties and special gifts to give to your neighbors, friends, and family.

Preparing unique foods for gatherings

The holidays bring a time of family gatherings and parties with colleagues and friends. This book includes some favorite celebration recipes from the Mediterranean that are sure to wow your guests. If you're looking for something different to serve at your get-together, try some of the following options:

- **Starters:** Any of the appetizers in Chapter 8 are great choices, but a few, such as the grape leaves recipes and the Italian Bruschetta, offer beautiful presentations and are very tasty.

- **Sides:** Any of the vegetables, legumes, and grain recipes (Chapters 12, 13, and 14, respectively) are party-worthy, and many are simple to prepare. Serving many different recipes gives your guests lots of variety.

- **Entrees:** Pastitsio (Chapter 19) is common at large Greek celebrations, and it's delicious (even if you aren't Greek). You can't go wrong with this traditional meal, especially if you're serving a large group. The lasagne recipes in Chapter 15 are also great meals for a large bunch. If you're having a smaller gathering, the Spaghetti and Clams (Chapter 15) and Greek Meatballs with Red Pepper and Tomato Puree (Chapter 19) are great finds.

- **Desserts:** You can go so many ways with the desserts in Chapter 20. Make a variety of cookies to offer with coffee, or focus on creating a larger presentation such as the Ricotta Cake or Walnut Baklava.

When it comes to celebrations, making a large variety of dishes is the way to go, but make sure you don't commit to a ton of difficult recipes; include some easy recipes so you aren't overwhelmed. Get some helpers, too. Preparing items such as desserts a day before whenever possible is always a good head start. Now you can enjoy a great feast with your next holiday gathering!

Making tasty treats for friends and family

Crafting homemade treats for friends and family is a great and inexpensive way to give special, unique gifts during the holidays (or anytime). What's even better is giving treats you make from this book!

Giving homemade treats may be a family tradition, like it was in Meri's. Growing up, her mother and grandmother spent a full day making special Italian pastries and fudge for the holidays. They'd place their homemade treats on decorative plates to give to neighbors and close friends, with plenty leftover for visitors. If you're looking for some great gift ideas, here are a few suggestions to get you started (all these recipes appear in Chapter 20):

- ✔ Spend a day making assorted cookies, such as Pucker Up Lemon Polenta Cookies and Orange Cardamom Cookies. Give them away to neighbors and friends and make enough for visitors.

- ✔ Make some biscotti and put them in decorative tins with a bag of gourmet coffee. This beautiful gift is a tasty treat and a wonderful starter for holiday mornings.

- ✔ Bake the Ricotta Cake and give it to special friends or close family. This recipe is a great gift to offer to bring to a dinner party.

- ✔ Spend the day preparing Walnut Baklava and give the results out as gifts. Always amazing!

Chapter 5

Going to the Market and Stocking Your Kitchen

. . . .

. . . .

*L*iving the Mediterranean lifestyle involves making a few changes in the way you grocery shop and stock your pantry. Don't worry; making these changes doesn't have to mean cleaning out your cupboards for days on end or spending lots of money. To help you incorporate these changes, we want you to focus on what you can add to your grocery list so that your kitchen is stocked with the staples and fresh foods you need handy to truly live the Mediterranean lifestyle. Imagine walking into your kitchen to a bowl of fresh fruit on the counter, next to a bowl bursting full of ripe tomatoes. And making the delicious recipes in this book is much easier when you have everything you need at your fingertips.

The first steps to revamping your kitchen are finding the best stores and markets to meet your needs, venturing into a little meal planning, heading to the store to get your kitchen stocked, and having the kitchen appliances and utensils to make the transition easier. You can find all the information you need to get started with your new Mediterranean lifestyle in this chapter.

Knowing Where to Shop

Most North Americans shop for food by simply going to the nearest grocery store. Even on the Mediterranean diet, the grocery store is still where you get most of your staples, but this section challenges you to explore different places in your community as well to get the freshest foods you can find. You may discover some ethnic stores in your community or even locate a new area of your local grocery store. This section discusses some great shopping experiences to get you into the Mediterranean spirit.

Shopping local, no matter where you live

One of the big differences between the North American lifestyle and that of the Mediterranean is where people shop for food. Many people in the Mediterranean, whether they live in large cities or small towns, depend more on local markets, butchers, bakers, and produce stands (though the big-box stores you're used to are popping up more and more in the Mediterranean). This dependence allows them to have fresher foods.

In North America, people often shop in big grocery stores whether they live in large cities or small towns. The conveniences of a big grocery store make life easy, but you often forego the benefit of seasonally fresh foods. Much of the produce found in grocery stores is shipped in from other states and even other countries. The longer the transport time, the more nutrients are lost.

Living in a big city does have some advantages if you want to shop someplace besides a large grocery store. A big city gives you opportunities to shop in specialty stores such as local bakeries and butchers. Take some time to explore your city. Head to the later section "Discovering other hidden food spots" for more on digging up these gems.

Although rural areas may not have the convenience of many different specialty markets, these regions do have their own positives for getting into the swing of Mediterranean cooking. For one, they may have more local produce stands where you can get fresh, locally grown fruits and vegetables. You may even have room to grow your own garden, which is the best way to get truly fresh produce.

If you don't have a lot of options or time and only can shop in your local grocery store, take some time to really explore your produce section. More and more grocery stores are carrying locally grown foods. It's usually not a very large section, but it's a great way to get some fresh, seasonal, local foods and still keep the convenience of your grocery shopping!

Taking advantage of local farmers' markets

Local farmers' markets are a wonderful resource to get fresh, seasonal food for any community. Picking out produce at the grocery store is convenient, but it isn't terribly exciting. Strolling outside through the aisles of the farmers' market is a more enriching experience and helps get your creative juices flowing with what recipes you can make with these fresh foods (some which may have been picked that morning). The additional benefits of shopping at the farmers' market include the following:

- ✔ The foods are local and therefore fresh, seasonal, and more nutrient-rich because of decreased storage and shipping time.
- ✔ You slow down and enjoy the process of selecting your foods.
- ✔ The market provides an outlet to get outside and take a leisurely stroll, which is part of living the Mediterranean lifestyle.
- ✔ You get an experience more similar to the way people in the Mediterranean shop.
- ✔ Buying local is a great way to give back to your community.

If you've never been, take some time to explore your farmers' market and enjoy the sights, smells, and sounds. Check out www.localharvest.com for a map and listing of farmers' markets in your area.

Getting involved with your local CSA

Love vegetables? Buying a share of a Community Supported Agriculture (CSA) is a great way to incorporate fresh, seasonal produce into your diet. With a CSA, you pay an upfront fee to a local farm and receive a box full of fresh produce each week in return. Going with a CSA is as close to having your own garden as you can get without having to get dirt under your fingernails, and it's a great way to get into the Mediterranean style of living. Plus, you support your local farmers.

With the amazing fresh produce you get with a CSA, take time to learn how to cook seasonally. Get into the practice of using what's fresh and available, and plan your meals accordingly. Doing so can be a little different at first (you may not have a trove of recipes ready that utilize that box of kale, broccoli, and beets you just received), but after you get the hang of it, you may never want to go back.

CSA isn't for everyone. If you're very picky with produce and don't enjoy a wide variety, we suggest sticking to the farmers' market or your grocery store so that you can pick just what you want. Otherwise, you can end up with a box full of veggies you don't enjoy, and it can go to waste.

To find a local CSA, ask some of the vendors at your local farmers' market. Many times, those same vendors offer CSAs from their own farms. You can also search www.localharvest.com, or ask at your local chamber of commerce.

Discovering other hidden food spots

Depending on your community, you may uncover some uncommon places to find foods that work well with a Mediterranean lifestyle. You likely won't do all your shopping at these places, but you may find that fresh seafood is worth the extra trip. Here are some fabulous hot spots we've seen around:

- Seafood sellers
- Butchers
- Bakeries
- Mediterranean markets
- Greek markets
- Italian markets
- Italian or Greek restaurants that also sell groceries

Our local pizza parlor also sells a few Italian groceries. The best way to find out about these special spots is to ask around your community or your chamber of commerce. You can also search on the Internet, but some stores may not have a website, so make sure to include other ways of researching.

Preparing to Shop: Appreciating the Food

Although many Mediterranean areas have become modernized with chain grocery stores, many people still rely on corner bakeries, mini-marts, butchers, and produce stands. No matter where you shop, you can slow down and grasp a new appreciation for the food you're purchasing. With that appreciation, you can start to plan the meals you'll prepare and put together a shopping list to make your shopping trip easier.

The Mediterranean lifestyle we tout here as healthy is really the everyday lifestyle from 50 or so years ago, when running errands like grocery shopping by foot was more prevalent. In most of the United States, taking a walk down the street to buy baked goods, produce, and fish from the local vendors just isn't a reality. So you have to make do in finding the right foods at your local chain or specialty stores.

If you're a person who currently fills your grocery cart with mostly boxed items, this appreciation will happen naturally as you begin to explore more whole-food items such as fresh fruits and vegetables. Why? Because you have to feel and smell for ripeness, which helps you to focus more on what you're buying. If you already purchase fresh foods in abundance, challenge yourself to slow down and focus on seasonal foods to make your meals.

This idea may sound a little strange, but one of the huge differences between those who live in the Mediterranean regions and those who live in fast-paced regions is the former's appreciation and passion for individual foods, recipes, and meals. This section gives you some ideas to create a Mediterranean-style food shopping trip in a fast-paced world.

Meal planning that fits your lifestyle

Before you head to the grocery store, come up with some meals you want to have for the week. Meal planning doesn't have to be a daunting task, and you can make it work for your lifestyle, putting in as much or as little effort as you prefer. The whole goal is to have a plan for your meals during the week so that you can create a complementary grocery list.

Meal planning isn't necessarily something everyone on the Mediterranean coast does, but if you're transitioning to this lifestyle, the planning can certainly make things easier on you as you begin your journey. It's all too easy to run out of time and groceries and end up going back to your old habits. Chapter 4 gives you the nitty-gritty about how to meal plan.

Starting with a list

After you have an idea of what you'll be eating for the week, make yourself a master grocery list. If you're very organized, you can make one column for the staples you use every week and another column for those foods that are specific for recipes you'll be using. That way, you don't have to reinvent the wheel each week.

If you aren't as organized, just jot down a few of the essentials you'll need for the week and use your memory for those items you always have on hand. Either way, some sort of list helps you to get the foods you need and saves you time so that you can enjoy cooking and eating with your family instead of running to the store every night.

Finding the Right Products

Shopping for food the Mediterranean way is probably simpler than your current grocery procedure. As you transition into this lifestyle, your grocery cart should be filled with fresh foods. The boxed, canned, and frozen items you do buy also tend to be simple whole foods such as canned black beans or frozen spinach.

Buying organic is up to you

The term *organic* refers to foods that have been grown with few or no pesticides or other synthetic chemicals and no antibiotics or hormones. Agriculture in the Mediterranean is a mix of both organic and non-organic. In Europe as a whole, about 23 percent of the farmland is organic. To date, the evidence is inconclusive as to whether organic food is better than conventionally grown food, so whether you buy organic is truly a personal choice. Check out the dirty dozen food list from the Environmental Working Group to see which foods have the highest pesticide residue at `www.food news.org/`. This great guide helps you make informed decisions on the different produce you buy.

You certainly still buy some convenience items with the Mediterranean diet, but as you transition to eating a largely plant-based diet with lean meats, nuts, and beans for protein, you find you don't have to rely on counting fat, carbs, and calories as much. As a result, we don't spend much time discussing how to read food labels or count fat and carbs here. In this section, we show you what to look for as you shop for some of your main food items.

Buying produce

As we note earlier in the chapter, choosing produce in the Mediterranean includes three main criteria: freshness, seasonality, and local proximity. Agriculture is big in the Mediterranean, so lots of local farms are available to supply food vendors with fresh produce. The earlier section "Knowing where to Shop" gets you to the right places (even if you don't have the same abundance of local farms), but how do you know what to buy when you're there?

When you go shopping for produce, keep these tips in mind:

- ✔ **Watch out for bruises and wilting.** They can be signs that the produce has been handled improperly or that the food is past its peak.

- ✔ **Consider the ripeness.** If you plan on eating the food later in the week, avoid picking pieces that are too ripe. Similarly, make sure food you plan to eat tonight is ripe enough.

- ✔ **Go for variety.** Try not to get in the rut of eating only the same few fruits and vegetables. More food variety means a better variety of nutrients. Bananas may be high in potassium, but oranges are high in vitamin C. You want to get it all!

Seeking the perfect seafood

Depending on where you live, you can find a good variety of both local fish and shipped-in fish at your local grocery store or fish market. Choose a variety of fish and shellfish each week. ***Remember:*** You don't have to pick seafood unique to the Mediterranean region; rather, you want fish that's fresh, so local is better.

When buying seafood, look for the following to ensure freshness:

- ✔ Flesh should have a vibrant color, with no darkening or dulling of color around the edges.
- ✔ Any skin should look shiny and metallic.
- ✔ Any moisture on the fish should be clear, not milky.
- ✔ Whole fish should have bright eyes and gills that are tight against the body.
- ✔ The flesh should be firm and elastic; don't be afraid to ask whether you can touch the fish!
- ✔ The smell factor should be mild. If the fish has a strong odor, move on.
- ✔ The seafood shouldn't sit in your grocery cart too long.
- ✔ Frozen seafood should be vacuum-packed, or sealed with little to no air.

All seafood is good for you, but fatty fish found in cold waters such as the Pacific Ocean or cold freshwater lakes are higher in healthy omega-3 fatty acids. Leaner fish found in tropical waters may have lower levels of omega-3, but they're still a great source of lean protein.

If you live near a coastal town, take the time to find a local market that sells the freshest catch. Nothing compares to fresh-caught fish for flavor. If you know someone who enjoys fishing, let him or her know that you'd love to share in some of his or her fresh catches! (You may want to propose some bartering, though; catching and cleaning the fish is a lot of work.)

Be aware that fish do contain mercury from pollutants in the water. Check out Chapter 18 to see which fish to limit.

Purchasing beef, pork, and poultry

Finding beef, pork, and poultry in your local grocery store isn't difficult. You can also check out the local butcher shop for great pieces of meat. Follow these tips to make sure you're purchasing the best products you can find:

- ✔ Beef should be a solid color: not too bright red, and with no graying or greenish tinges to it.

- ✔ Poultry should look firm and not have a strong odor. Believe us; you'll know if your chicken meat is old — it has a very bad odor.

- ✔ Pork chops should be firm and may have a little gristle on the ends.

Checking out the dairy case

Dairy is commonly used in the Mediterranean diet and is a good source of calcium. One great characteristic of dairy products is that they contain a great balance of carbohydrates, fat, and protein, making them an easy, satisfying snack. Dairy is also low-glycemic, which makes it a great choice for those watching their weight or blood sugar. (*Low-glycemic* foods release sugar more slowly, helping to keep blood sugar stable.)

The fat in dairy products is saturated fat, which may be linked to heart disease when consumed in large amounts. For items such as yogurt, cottage cheese, and milk, go middle of the road and use 1-percent or 2-percent fat products.

Cheese is common in Mediterranean cooking, and you may be unfamiliar with some of the called-for cheeses (such as feta or goat cheese) or where to find them. Here are a few places to look when you're shopping:

- ✔ You can typically find containers of crumbled goat cheese and/or feta in the back refrigerated section of your local grocery store by the milk and cottage cheese. Check the high, outermost shelves.

- ✔ The grocery's deli cold case is often full of unique cheeses. You can also ask your deli clerk if the cheese you're looking for is behind the counter.

- ✔ You may be fortunate enough to have a store in your town that specializes in cheese. Count yourself lucky; you'll find everything you need there.

- ✔ If you live in a very rural area and can't find these cheeses in your local grocery store, you can always shop online. Pricing varies depending on the stores. Here are a few to get you started: www.amazon.com, www.cheesesupply.com, and www.igourmet.com.

Exploring grains and breads

You notice a lot of pasta and rice in Mediterranean cooking, and you also see many grains you may not be used to cooking with, such as bulgur wheat, pearl barley, and cornmeal.

You should be able to find most grain products in the inner aisles of your grocery store, where you find the rice products. Cornmeal sometimes appears with the baking supplies. The grains that aren't as popular are often on the lower shelves, so be sure to look around. If you don't find the products you're looking for, venture to a gourmet grocer or health food store. You can also find many products at Amazon.com.

Bread is a big staple in Mediterranean cooking, especially in the Italian culture. You can buy the prepackaged breads or head to the bakery for some fresh baked bread.

Look for breads made with whole grains rather than enriched white flour. Whole grains give you more nutrients and fiber and a lower-glycemic product for everyday use. Of course, getting a loaf of crusty white bread once in awhile for a special meal is perfectly fine.

Getting your caffeine fix

Although Italy is the home of coffee (espresso), caffeine isn't all that big in the Mediterranean diet. Traditionally, a cup of espresso in the morning is all the caffeine a person takes in during the day. As with the rest of the diet, this habit is changing in current times and is a far cry from North American lifestyles with coffeehouses on every corner.

Caffeine offers some health benefits and some unhealthy effects (which we cover in Chapter 2), so it's fine to drink in moderation. If you enjoy a cup of tea, coffee, or soda during the day for a little caffeine boost, try keeping your intake to one serving a day.

Stocking Your Kitchen with Must-Have Mediterranean Staples

Figuring out where to buy the foods you need to transition to the Mediterranean diet is most of the battle (see the preceding sections). After that, you just have to buy them. The following sections provide you with a list of food staples to have on hand in your new Mediterranean kitchen so that you can easily prepare convenient meals and healthy snacks any time instead of feeling like you have to run to the grocery store several times a week.

Always keep tabs on when you're running low on staple items. They're called "staples" because you use them all the time, so you want to make sure you don't run out.

Loading up your pantry

The pantry (whether it's an actual pantry or just your cupboards) is the perfect place to start. Open your pantry door and look at what you have on hand. You likely have several of these items already, but you can use the list in this section to beef up your stock based on your tastes. A well-organized and well-stocked food supply gives you the ability to make more food from scratch when you want to slow down or to throw together fast meals when you're short on time.

For example, we always have a large supply of black beans on hand. They're useful to throw into a tortilla with some cheese for a quickie burrito, with leftover rice and some veggies for a fast meal, and as an addition to many recipes. But if you don't like black beans, don't fill your cabinets with them just because they're on this list. Just stock your pantry with the products you enjoy using most often.

Here is a good pantry list to get you started for all your needs:

- ✔ Baking powder, baking soda, and cornstarch
- ✔ Dry yeast
- ✔ Cornmeal
- ✔ Extracts, such as pure vanilla, anise, and almond
- ✔ Flours, including whole wheat, wheat bran, oat, and all-purpose
- ✔ Sugars, including granulated and light or dark brown sugar
- ✔ Unsweetened cocoa
- ✔ Oils, including olive oil, extra-virgin olive oil, canola oil, and nonstick cooking spray
- ✔ Seasonings, including salt, sea salt, black pepper, ground cumin, paprika, garlic powder, chili powder, curry powder, ginger, cinnamon, dill, parsley, tarragon, basil, oregano, thyme, rosemary, and your choice of other dry herbs
- ✔ Canned and/or dried beans, such as black beans, pinto beans, or white beans
- ✔ Lentils
- ✔ Canned soups, such as minestrone, vegetable, or tomato
- ✔ Rice, including wild rice and brown rice
- ✔ Pearl barley, quinoa, or bulgur wheat
- ✔ Pasta
- ✔ Oatmeal
- ✔ Bread

Storing nuts

Nuts are a common staple on the Mediterranean coast, used in salads, side dishes, and desserts. Nuts are a good source of healthy monounsaturated fats, but those fats can go rancid if you don't stow your nuts properly. Use these guidelines for proper nut storage:

✔ Use airtight, plastic or glass containers.

✔ Avoid keeping nuts near high-odor foods such as garlic because nuts absorb the smell from their surroundings.

✔ Keep shelled nuts at room temperature for up to three months or refrigerated for four months. Store unshelled nuts for four months in the refrigerator and up to eight months in the freezer.

✔ Buy nuts from local farmers if available, or at stores that have a high *turnover rate* (sell foods quickly instead of having them sit for long periods), to ensure freshness.

✔ If possible, buy nuts that include a sell-by date to have a better idea of how old they are (buying from bins doesn't necessarily mean they're fresher).

Keeping a few items on hand in your refrigerator

Having a few staples readily available each week in the fridge is important because many convenience snacks and meals need to be kept cold. And of course, you're also incorporating lots of veggies into your diet, and most of them go in the fridge as well. In this section, we provide a few basic fridge foods (including veggies) that you want to always have on hand:

✔ Carton of eggs

✔ Fresh vegetables, such as lettuce for salads; carrots; and celery

✔ Lean deli meats

✔ Cheese

✔ Lowfat Greek yogurt

✔ 1-percent milk or cottage cheese

✔ Nuts (yes, you can store nuts in the refrigerator — see the nearby side-bar for helpful advice on storing nuts)

✔ Natural nut butter like peanut butter or almond butter

✔ Condiments, such as mustard, Worcestershire sauce, salsas, and mayonnaise

Freezing for the future

Stocking your freezer can go a long way as you move from a fast-paced lifestyle to a slower Mediterranean lifestyle. Keeping certain frozen foods on hand for recipes simplifies the cooking process.

The following frozen items come in handy for cooking and for side dishes.

- ✔ Frozen spinach
- ✔ Other frozen vegetables such as cauliflower or broccoli
- ✔ No-sugar-added frozen fruit such as blueberries (great to thaw out in the morning and add to cereals or oatmeal)
- ✔ Boneless, skinless chicken breasts
- ✔ Fish fillets or salmon burgers
- ✔ Frozen shrimp
- ✔ Extra-lean ground beef in one-pound packages
- ✔ Precooked recipes such as soups, stews, and chilis

You can freeze many of the recipes in this book; doing so makes great homemade fast food. If you know you're going to be busy a couple of evenings, prepare a recipe and freeze it. When you come home exhausted later in the week, you can reheat the food and have a quick and easy dinner.

Filling your countertop

If your countertop is empty, it's time to put away the mail and buy a few decorative bowls. One of the primary concepts of Mediterranean cooking is having plenty of fresh fruits and vegetables on hand, and having them literally at hand is even better. Having a big bowl of fresh fruit on your counter is so inviting that it encourages you to eat more fruit.

Many foods, such as tomatoes, lose flavor if you store them in the refrigerator. A good general rule is that if the produce isn't refrigerated at the store, it shouldn't be refrigerated at your home.

Here are some fruits and other items that are good to keep at the ready on the counter:

- ✔ Fruits such as apples, oranges, bananas, and pears. Pick your favorites and stock a beautiful fruit bowl on your counter to pick at during the day.
- ✔ Lemons are always nice to have on hand for recipes, to add to your water, or to enrich the flavor of your salad.

✔ Tomatoes for salads, sandwiches, or other recipes.

✔ Onions and garlic (in a bowl separate from the others; don't mix your fruit and tomatoes with your garlic and onions).

✔ Avocadoes (if you use them often).

Exploring a Few Handy Cooking Tools

Having some commonly used tools and small appliances in your new Mediterranean kitchen makes cooking easier and more efficient — that is, a breeze. The good news: You don't have to go out and spend hundreds of dollars to incorporate these items, nor do you have to have a gourmet kitchen. The following sections list kitchen tools that come in handy as you use the recipes in this book.

Cutting boards

Nearly every recipe in this book (and elsewhere) requires some kind of cutting, so you need a cutting board. We recommend that you have at least two on hand: one for cutting meats and one for cutting produce. (Having two cutting boards helps to eliminate any cross-contamination of dangerous bacteria between raw meats and your other foods.) You can find cutting boards in a variety of materials; the verdict is still out on which kind is the best. See Table 5-1 for the pros and cons of different styles of cutting boards.

Table 5-1	Comparing Types of Cutting Boards	
Type	*Advantages*	*Disadvantages*
Bamboo	Easy on knives	Not dishwasher safe
	Renewable resource	Need to be periodically seasoned with oil
	Attractive and durable	Vary in quality
	Natural bacteria-fighting properties	Will splinter if low in quality
Composite	Dishwasher safe	May give off odor when wet
	Attractive and durable	Harder on knives
	Easy to clean	Not eco-friendly

(continued)

Table 5-1 *(continued)*

Type	Advantages	Disadvantages
Glass	Sanitary	Damage knives
	Easy to clean	Prone to chips and breaks
	Attractive and durable	
Plastic	Easy on knives	Wear out quickly
	Easy to clean	Sustain gouges and scratches that can harbor bacteria
	Inexpensive	Not as attractive as wood or bamboo
	Can be color coded so you can keep track of which board you use for which products (for example, orange for produce, red for meats)	Vary in quality
	Dishwasher safe	Not eco-friendly
Wood	Easy on knives	Prone to nicks and scratches, which can harbor bacteria
	Can be refinished	Need to be periodically seasoned with oil
	Attractive	Not dishwasher safe
		Vary in quality

Electrical appliances

Although you don't have to have the most expensive electrical appliances available, a few are must-haves in order to make several recipes in this book:

- **Blender, stick (immersion) blender, or food processor:** Having at least one of these items in your kitchen is a good idea for nearly any cookbook you buy. Blenders and food processors are often used to blend sauces (such as pesto) or dips. A stick blender is a hand-held device that lets you blend soups in the pot so that you don't have to transfer hot soup to a stand-up blender or food processor.

- **Hand mixer or standing mixer:** A mixer (either kind) is useful for baking. And you often need the speed of a mixer to make whipped creams or meringues.

✔ **Steamer:** Most steamers are called rice steamers or rice cookers, but they work really well for cooking rice and vegetables. Steamers come in many varieties and price ranges, so you want to shop around to see what product will work best for your kitchen. For a quick, nonelectrical solution, you can also purchase a steamer basket that goes into your cooking pots to steam vegetables.

✔ **Griddle:** This tool isn't a must-have, but if you have a big family or entertain a lot, it can save you a ton of time. Instead of cooking two pancakes at once, you can cook six. You can also use it to make grilled or panini sandwiches and other items.

✔ **Slow cooker:** Although you can make do without a slow cooker, these babies can make cooking a lot more convenient. They're great for soups, stews, chilis, and even meat dishes. Basically, you just throw all your ingredients in your slow cooker in the morning, set it to low, and have a meal waiting for you in the evening.

Pots and pans

No kitchen is complete without a few basic pots and pans. We recommend that you purchase the best you can afford because the cheaper cookware doesn't always hold up over time, and you'll end up spending more money because you replace it more often. Buying a few quality pieces will last you a long time. You can prepare just about anything with these kitchen mainstays in your cabinet:

✔ 12-inch skillet with lid

✔ 6- to 8-quart stockpot with lid

✔ 4- to 6-quart cast-iron pot with lid

✔ 4-quart saucepan with lid

✔ 8-inch nonstick skillet

✔ Large roasting pan with lid

The best utility tools

Utility tools are a must-have in your kitchen in order to cook any recipe. After all, you need to measure and stir. You may already have all these items on hand; in that case, you're ready to go.

If you're just starting out, stick with these basics; you can always add to your collection as you spend more time in the kitchen:

- ✔ 8-inch French or chef's knife
- ✔ Paring knife
- ✔ Serrated bread knife
- ✔ 6-inch utility knife
- ✔ Measuring cups and spoons
- ✔ Glass liquid measuring cup
- ✔ Wooden spoon
- ✔ Slotted spoon
- ✔ Soup ladle
- ✔ Silicone spatula and turner
- ✔ Two rubber spatulas (one large, one small)
- ✔ Silicone basting brush
- ✔ Metal whisk

- ✔ Peeler
- ✔ Tongs
- ✔ Kitchen shears
- ✔ Steel or plastic colander
- ✔ Three mixing bowls (small, medium, and large)
- ✔ 9-inch metal baking pan
- ✔ 9-x-13-inch glass baking dish
- ✔ Two baking sheets
- ✔ Garlic press
- ✔ Zester or microplane
- ✔ Can opener
- ✔ Cheese grater

Chapter 6

Mastering Mediterranean Cooking with Helpful Tips and Techniques

....

In This Chapter

▶ Working cooking into your lifestyle

▶ Using and storing oils properly

▶ Discovering the healthy attributes of herbs and spices

▶ Cooking with whole grains and legumes you may not be familiar with

....

*P*reparing foods at home rather than relying on restaurants and convenience foods is certainly a huge part of moving toward a Mediterranean lifestyle. As you take the first steps into this lifestyle choice, a few key things can help make your cooking a breeze. In this chapter, we cover the basics on managing your time in the kitchen; incorporating simple, quick meals; using oils, herbs, and spices; and grasping a few cooking techniques for grains, beans, and lentils.

Setting Yourself Up for Success

Living a Mediterranean lifestyle does incorporate more time picking and preparing your foods than you may have experienced in the past. As a result, you want to strategize with small goals to help you start living this lifestyle. You don't have to cook three meals a day each and every day. You're busy, and no one really cooks every single meal, regardless of the culture. If you look at your own habits, you likely cook part of the time, use quick pull-together meals like cereal or a sandwich other times, and eat out other meals.

You may not see strategizing as an important concept, but failing to plot a course can become a saboteur in the nutrition world. Many people decide that figuring out what they're going to do and how is just too much work and give up all together. We encourage you to find your own path with the Mediterranean lifestyle; making even a few small changes can make a big difference in your health.

As you read this section, take some time to jot down a few notes on how you can make these strategies work in your lifestyle. Change is hard for everyone; humans are creatures of habit. Having a strategy can help ensure that your journey is a successful one. In this section, you can map out how to incorporate time for cooking and save time on busy days by using quick and easy meals and freezer-friendly leftovers.

Scheduling time for cooking

Cooking is a crucial strategy in the Mediterranean lifestyle because it helps you lean more toward eating fresh, plant-based foods and away from depending on prepackaged meals or on restaurants. Cooking may already be a regular part of your world, or it may only happen once a week. Luckily, you don't have to cook every single day to benefit from the Mediterranean diet.

To incorporate cooking into your schedule, choose how often you cook on any given week. Managing your time and figuring out ahead of time how much time you have to cook are key factors. Here are a few ideas:

- ✔ If you only have time a few nights a week, schedule those evenings for cooking and make enough leftovers for the next day. Treat this appointment like an important date you can't break.

- ✔ Short on time every night? Choose recipes that take less than 20 minutes to prepare. For example, a small fillet of fish takes about 8 minutes to cook; pair that with a large salad and some crusty whole-grain bread and you've got a home-cooked dinner in no time.

- ✔ Utilize batch cooking; see the later section "Making good use of batch cooking" for details.

- ✔ Rearrange your schedule to find time to cook dinner several nights a week. Maybe you frequently run errands after work that you can push off to one day a week or the weekend.

Keep the following time-management tips in mind as you figure out how much time you can devote to cooking:

- ✔ **Focus on one cooked dish.** While your dish is cooking, you can rely on gathering fresh ingredients that require no cooking time (only prep time) for the rest of your meal. This strategy can help you avoid feeling overwhelmed in the kitchen. After you get the hang of it, you can slowly add another cooked dish and then another.

  For example, you may cook the Sautéed Shrimp with White Wine and Feta in Chapter 18 and add a big salad, a side of plain canned black beans, and a slice of crusty sourdough bread.

✔ **Look at the prep and cooking times on each recipe.** When you're planning, make sure you allow yourself enough time to follow through as well as time to eat. You may be able to easily cook two to three dishes if they have minimal prep work and short cooking times.

Don't underestimate how long certain tasks take. Cooking takes time. We can't tell you how often we see people abandon the new, healthy changes they were going to make because of time-management problems. Here's what happens: You make a meal plan for the week (see Chapter 4), buy the groceries, and then continue on with your normal schedule. But then you find that recipe you were going to make on Wednesday needs 45 minutes of prep and cooking time, and you only have about 20 minutes to spare. If you find yourself in that situation . . .

✔ **Making changes to your plans is okay.** Life happens to everyone, even the best chefs. If you get home too late one night to prepare your planned dish, postpone your cooking for another night and throw together a quick meal instead.

Finding ways to create quick and easy meals

Living the Mediterranean lifestyle certainly doesn't mean you have to cook every day. Even the folks that live in that region utilize leftovers and quick, easy, pull-together meals.

When you're creating your quickie meals, focus on completing the meal with fresh, simple flavors from produce and/or legumes. For example, perhaps you have a favorite frozen meal like lasagne that you use when time is short. Add a side salad with fresh lettuce, tomatoes, and kidney beans. Or, you can place your heated lasagne on a bed of fresh spinach leaves that will naturally wilt underneath. Chapter 4 gives you several specific ways to plan quick and easy meals.

Making good use of batch cooking

Batch cooking is a great habit to get into, especially if you want to incorporate a Mediterranean-style diet but feel you don't have as much time to cook as you want. With *batch cooking,* you cook up larger amounts of food than you need for one meal and save the leftovers. The end result? A freezer well stocked with homemade items you can pull out for healthy, easy-to-serve meals later when time is short. You can more easily stick to your Mediterranean diet even when you're busy because you don't have to rely on prepackaged foods and eating out to save time.

Depending on your style, you can tackle batch cooking in any of a few ways:

- ✓ **Take a day to cook many items.** Get together three to five recipes, such as soups, stews, chilis, lasagnes, or casseroles. Clear off your calendar for the day and cook, cook, cook. Package your meals in freezer-friendly containers, date them, and place in the freezer for later use. Note that this strategy does take a lot of time and energy during your cooking day.

- ✓ **Spend a day prepping some of your go-to foods.** Instead of cooking several complete recipes at one time, you can get the base ingredients for later meals ready so you don't have to worry about them later. For example, you can precook beans, sauces, or whole grains such as rice or barley. Meri has a friend who makes large pots of brown rice and quinoa every Monday and then uses them up during the week with various meals.

- ✓ **Make extra when cooking freezer-friendly meals.** You can then pack them, date them, and tuck them away in the freezer. For example, if you're grilling chicken, fill up that grill! Make more than you need and let it cool; slice the extras up and put them in individual storage containers. The next time you want to add grilled chicken to salads, burritos, sandwiches, or steamed veggies, you have the hardest part out of the way.

No matter what approach you use, make sure to package your meals in a way that works best for you. If you're single, use single-serving containers so that you don't have to warm up an entire lasagne. (We've all been there.) If you're cooking for a larger family, you can go ahead and freeze the complete meal. Keep a list on the outside of your freezer of the foods/meals you have stashed and dates you stored them. This way, you don't forget about the food you have (even if it gets hidden).

Cooking with Oils

Part of the Mediterranean lifestyle is using healthy, monounsaturated fats, such as olive oil, in place of butter or other fats. Oils are beneficial for cooking because they allow you to cook food at a higher temperature, and they provide flavor and texture to your foods. The following sections give you the lowdown on cooking with oils to assure you get the healthy benefits.

Although the oils typically associated with the Mediterranean diet are healthier than other oils, they can turn your healthy strategy into an unhealthy one quickly if you aren't careful. As with any fat, you don't want to consume large amounts. Additionally, oils that are too old or have been stored at the wrong temperature are no good. Taste your oil immediately when you open it so you can see what it tastes like in its freshest form. Doing so gives you a good comparison when checking oils that may have been sitting on the shelf for awhile.

Understanding smoke points

All oils have what's called a *smoke point,* or the temperature where the fat begins to break down, turning your healthy fat into an unhealthy fat. You want to avoid cooking oils at high temperatures so you don't hit that point of no return.

You know it when your oil has reached the smoke point because you can actually see smoke and smell a burnt oil or burnt pan odor. According to the International Olive Oil Council, olive oil has a high smoke point of about 410 degrees. Canola oil, another monounsaturated fat, has a smoke point around 400 degrees.

Immaculately conceiving olive oil?

When you start to peruse the oil aisle at the grocery store, you see all sorts of language on the labels like virgin, extra-virgin, and like a virgin (okay, that last one is in the music aisle). And then you've got cold-pressed and expeller-pressed to deal with. It's enough terminology to make your head spin. If you're new to reading these labels, the first thing you need to know is about the manufacturing process.

The hand presses that traditionally pressed olive paste into an oil only make a small amount. To increase the output, hot water was added to the presses to get more flow. *Cold-pressed* or *first-pressed* are synonymous labels that indicate that the oil was pressed with little processing. *Expeller-pressing* is similar to cold-pressing (cold-pressing includes a heat-controlled environment) uses heat and friction, but no chemicals or solvents, creating a pure oil with no risk of chemical residues.

Here's a crib sheet of oil terminology so that you can become a master at picking out oils:

- **Extra-virgin olive oil:** All oils produced by the first pressing (the cold pressing) and that contain less than 1 percent acidity, providing rich flavor perfect for drizzling on salads, veggies, or bread.

- **Virgin olive oil:** Not as pure as the extra-virgin simply because it uses riper olives, making the acidity higher at 1½ percent. The flavor is still great, but this oil works best as a cooking oil so that you can save the purer-flavored extra-virgin stuff for drizzling.

- **Refined olive oil:** A lower-grade olive oil where virgin olive oils with a higher acidity are refined using chemical or physical filters, creating a less-tasty oil with a higher acidity of up to 3 percent. Some places deem this unfit for human consumption based on flavor.

- **Olive oil:** Your basic olive oil is a combination of refined olive oil and virgin olive oil, with a higher quality of flavor than the straight refined olive oil and a 1-percent acidity. This oil works well for basic cooking needs.

- **Light olive oil:** The term *light* in this circumstance has nothing to do with calories or fat; rather, it refers to the flavor and color. Light olive oil is made with a fine filtration process and has a very light, almost neutral flavor that won't be so great in your next salad but is a wonderful choice in baking, where you don't want a strong flavor.

- **Olive Oyl:** Goes well with spinach.

Keep in mind that an oil's smoke point will change depending on how many times you've opened your oil (which brings in oxygen) and how long it's been sitting on the shelf. Don't go higher than medium-high heat when using olive or canola oil; if you see smoke coming off your pan, it's time to start over.

Identifying the best oils for different dishes

The world of oils varies greatly in flavor, so you want to have a basic understanding of which oils work best for the different dishes you'll be making in your new Mediterranean lifestyle. You can't go wrong with a basic olive oil or extra-virgin olive oil. (See the nearby sidebar for the lowdown on the differences between olive oils.)

Keep these general tips in mind as you search for oil:

- ✔ When cooking large recipes, stick with a basic olive oil or extra-virgin olive oil.
- ✔ When drizzling olive oil on vegetables or dipping your bread, go with a high-quality extra-virgin olive oil.
- ✔ When you want a little extra punch, try an olive oil flavored with fresh herbs, vinegars, garlic, or lemon juices. Specialty olive oils get pricey, though, so you want to use them lightly.

To find a good olive oil, visit an olive oil store. The tasting room is set up like a wine tasting. Purchase a good all-purpose olive oil for cooking and one or two specialty olive oils for salads and dipping. The store usually provides a pretzel or piece of bread to sample the oils. You can also plan ahead and bring your own veggies to dip into the different oils to figure out what complements their flavors best on your palette. You may love the citrus flavors of lemon-infused olive oil, or a more pungent garlic flavor. Olive oils come in all different types of flavors, so sample and find the ones you like best.

You can also purchase decent olive oil at any major grocery store chain or your local farmers' market. If you're intrigued by the specialty oils but can't find them in your area, one great store is the Temecula Olive Oil Company at www.temeculaoliveoil.com.

Storing oils

To get as much benefit as possible from your oils, make sure you store them appropriately. Keep your oils in a cool, dark cabinet away from sunlight and heat. You can also store your main cooking oils, such as basic olive oil or canola oil, in the refrigerator. To avoid storing your oil for too long, buy only a small- to medium-sized glass bottle so that you use it quickly enough.

 If you have a high-quality extra-virgin olive oil, avoid keeping it in the refrigerator; refrigerating increases the risk of condensation. Put the lid on tightly after each use to avoid oxidation, which can turn olive oil rancid. After you open a bottle of oil, store it for up to 6 months. If you're using it frequently, you won't have to worry about it wasting away on your shelf.

Knowing how much to use

People on the Mediterranean coast use a lot of oil. They drizzle oil on fresh vegetables and breads every day. When adopting this type of lifestyle, knowing how much is too much oil to drizzle is important.

 To gauge your drizzle, measure a teaspoon of oil and drizzle it on a tomato. Get a feel for what the appearance and flavor of that much oil are like. If you feel it's not enough for your taste, add a little vinegar or lemon juice to the mix.

 Oil is a fat with 9 calories per gram, which equates to about 120 calories per tablespoon. Make sure you're careful and don't go overboard on calories and total fat.

Keeping tabs on your oil use is easier with recipes because they give you an exact amount. In this book's recipes, we use a moderate amount of oil. If outside recipes seem to call for a lot of oil, try adding a little less. The change likely won't make a huge difference in flavor.

A Pinch of This and a Pinch of That: Using Herbs and Spices

People in the Mediterranean use an abundant amount of fresh herbs and spices in their cooking, which is another significant component of the lifestyle. Besides providing taste, color, and aroma, herbs and spices also add health benefits to your meals.

Think about your own diet. Do you tend to use a lot of herbs and spices in your cooking, or do you mostly depend on salt and pepper? If you don't use many seasonings, your Mediterranean goal is to cook with more of them, both for the health benefits and to create amazing flavor in your food. This section lets you in on some interesting health benefits simple seasonings provide, how to store the seasonings, and how you can work more of them into your diet.

Looking at the health benefits of herbs and spices

You may have thought that the oregano and basil in your spaghetti sauce just provided a distinct Italian flavor, but those little herbs are plants, which means they have all sorts of health benefits that can make a big impact on your overall health. Simple seasonings such as ginger and oregano contain *phytochemicals,* which are natural health-promoting substances that have been found to protect against conditions such as cancer and heart disease. (Flip to Chapter 2 for more on the powers of phytochemicals.)

You may be surprised to hear that herbs and spices are also loaded with healthy omega-3 fatty acids, which help decrease inflammation in the body. Check out some of the specific health benefits of commonly used herbs and spices:

- ✔ Basil is shown to have anti-inflammatory effects and may be useful for people with chronic inflammation, such as arthritis or inflammatory bowel disease. Basil also protects against bacteria. and is an excellent source of vitamin A, which helps reduce damage to the body from free radicals. (Chapter 2 has more information on vitamin A's benefits.)

- ✔ Cinnamon helps people better control their blood sugars because it slows digestion and therefore the rise of blood sugar. Not to mention that it's a wonderful flavor for baking or in a cup of tea!

- ✔ Oregano is a nutrient-dense spice containing fiber, iron, manganese, calcium, vitamin C, vitamin A, and omega-3 fatty acids. It's shown to have antibacterial and antioxidant properties.

- ✔ Parsley is a rich source of the antioxidants vitamin A and vitamin C, providing protection from heart disease and cancer. And you thought eating your parsley garnish was silly.

- ✔ Turmeric acts as a powerful anti-inflammatory and antioxidant, helping protect against arthritis, heart disease, and certain cancers. Try the Chicken Curry recipe in Chapter 17 to get a healthy dose of turmeric.

Storing fresh and bottled herbs

Herbs are delicate, so you want to make sure you store them properly to retain their best taste and their nutrient value.

Use these tips for storage:

- ✔ **Fresh herbs:** Immediately use them. Just like fruits and vegetables, the longer fresh herbs sit around, the more nutrients they lose. Store them in perforated bags in your refrigerator crisper for up to four days.

- ✔ **Dried herbs and spices:** Use them within a year of purchase. Keep them in airtight containers away from heat and light. You may want to record your date of purchase on the label; forgetting how long that stack of seasonings has been in your cupboard is really easy.

One way to ensure that herbs and seasonings don't sit too long on the shelf is to use them generously in your cooking. If you're running out of herbs every six months or so, you're on the right track! That's a good problem to have.

You may also consider keeping a raised garden for fresh herbs if you will be using them often. Fresh herbs are expensive at the grocery store, and they're relatively easy to grow, even in a city garden on your back porch. Check out *Herb Gardening For Dummies,* 2nd Edition, by Karan Davis Cutler, Kathleen Fisher, and Suzanne DeJohn (John Wiley & Sons) for more on starting up your own herb garden.

Livening up food with herbs and spices

With all the health benefits of herbs and spices we note in the preceding section, figuring out a way to increase the herbs and spices in your diet, whether you currently use a moderate amount or none at all, is a great idea. Doing so adds lots of flavor on top of the health perks, so it really is a win-win situation. Here are some suggestions for getting more herbs and spices in your diet:

- ✔ Add ample amounts of herbs to your stews, soups, and chilis. Don't be shy.

- ✔ Use fresh basil leaves in sandwiches, or spread your bread with basil pesto (see the recipe in Chapter 9) rather than with mayonnaise.

- ✔ Spice up a tuna- or chicken-salad sandwich with some curry, turmeric, and ginger.

- ✔ Let fresh mint, sliced cucumbers, and lemon sit in a pitcher of water for five to ten minutes for a refreshing drink.

- ✔ Mix fresh mint into your next fruit salad.

- ✔ Sprinkle fresh cilantro or basil over black beans and rice for a quick meal.

   ✔ Top off your scrambled eggs with your favorite herb combination.

   ✔ Kick up your lettuce-and-vegetable salads with cilantro and dill.

   ✔ Add fresh dill to fish.

Including Whole Grains

Incorporating whole grains into your daily meal plans provides a great source of complex carbohydrates, fiber, vitamins, and minerals; it also adds flavor and texture to your meals. The trick is to use grains as a smaller side dish to avoid eating too many calories and increasing your blood sugar with too many carbohydrates. Use one-half to one cup of grains with your meals to stay on the healthy side of the fence.

Although people on the Mediterranean coast frequently use pasta, they also consume many other grains, such as bulgur wheat, barley, and cornmeal. When you aren't used to eating these grains, you may not know how to cook them or add them creatively to your meals. Luckily, introducing them isn't difficult or time consuming. This section offers general cooking tips to conquer grain cookery, as well as suggestions for creating flavorful grain side dishes. Chapter 13 gives you some amazing recipes for whole grains to get you started.

Getting a handle on cooking times

Cooking grains is as simple as adding water and simmering. All grains pretty much cook the same way, other than varying cooking times. In fact, you can cook all grains the same way you cook rice.

You can always find the cooking time for a grain on the package, but we also provide cooking times for common whole grains in Table 6-1 to give you a quick reference whenever you need it. The amounts listed are for one cup of dry grain.

Table 6-1	Whole Grain Cooking Chart		
Type of Grain	*Amount of Liquid*	*Simmering Time after Boiling*	*Amount of Grain after Cooking*
Brown rice	2½ cups	45–55 minutes.	3 cups
Bulgur wheat — medium coarseness	2½ cups	None; remove from heat, cover, and let sit for 30 minutes. Drain any excess water.	2½ cups

Type of Grain	Amount of Liquid	Simmering Time after Boiling	Amount of Grain after Cooking
Cornmeal (polenta)	4 cups	25–30 minutes.	2½ cups
Couscous	1 cup	None; remove from heat, cover, and let sit for 5–10 minutes.	2 cups
Pearl barley	3 cups	45–60 minutes.	3½ cups
Quinoa	2 cups	12–15 minutes.	About 3 cups
Wild rice	3 cups	45–55 minutes.	3 cups

Adding flavor to grains

Incorporating grain side dishes in your menu can provide extra flavor to your meals. In fact, your grain side dishes end up tasting just as good as your main dish. In the Mediterranean region, people include a wide variety of grains in their meals; you aren't going to find a whole lot of plates with plain white rice.

Use the following tips to add some flavor and, in some cases, more nutrient value to your grains (with the exception of cornmeal — its sweet flavor doesn't need any doctoring up):

- ✔ Add one to two teaspoons of heart-healthy olive oil or your favorite nut oil to your pot of grains for a light flavor. This idea works well if you have a very flavorful or saucy entree.

- ✔ Instead of cooking your grains in water, cook them in low-sodium chicken or vegetable broth for more flavor.

- ✔ Don't forget your fresh herbs! Try fresh basil, cilantro, or parsley.

- ✔ Throw in some dry spices such as cumin or cayenne pepper for a little kick.

- ✔ Sauté some garlic, onions, and mushrooms and stir them together in your cooked grains. Take it an extra step and add some fresh herbs.

- ✔ Add chopped walnuts or slivered almonds to cooked grains for some crunch.

- ✔ Mix in chopped tomatoes and sliced olives for a savory flavor.

- ✔ Use one to two tablespoons of Parmesan, feta, or crumbled goat cheese in your pot of grains to add flavor and a creamy texture.

After you get the hang of switching up your grain dishes, you'll never be faced with a boring side dish again! Here is an example of how to combine a few of the preceding tips:

> Cook your grain. Sauté a shallot with a teaspoon of olive oil over medium-high heat. Add it to your cooked grain with 1 teaspoon cumin, ½ teaspoon crushed coriander, ¼ teaspoon garlic powder, and salt to taste.

This creation makes a great basic starter dish that you can serve as-is or with veggies, fresh herbs, and/or cheese and nuts mixed in. Don't be afraid to experiment in your kitchen. You may stumble upon something superb!

You can batch cook a few pots of whole grains for the week to save time. Check out the earlier section "Making good use of batch cooking" for more insight.

Discovering Beans and Lentils

Beans and lentils are a big part of Mediterranean eating and provide great health benefits because they're packed with fiber, B vitamins, protein, and phytochemicals. They're also economical and can create amazing flavor and texture in your meals. People in the Mediterranean often eat less meat, so they depend on plant-based protein foods like beans and lentils. Chapter 14 includes recipes dedicated to legumes. This section gives you the skinny on cooking beans (canned and dried) and lentils, including cooking times for different beans.

If you aren't used to eating beans and lentils, gradually add them to your diet and drink lots of water to cut down on the constipation and gas associated with these foods.

Preparing canned and dried beans and lentils

Beans are available dried or canned. Canned beans are easy to use in any dish, saving you time. Dried beans take longer to prepare, but they have better flavor and texture and less sodium than the canned variety. Lentils provide a unique, rich flavor and have the added benefit of quick preparation and cooking compared to dried beans. The following sections give you some tips on getting these Mediterranean staples ready to use.

Canned beans

Canned beans provide a whole lot of convenience and still pack great flavor. You can pretty much open them and serve, but keep these notes in mind:

✔ If you're adding canned beans to a recipe, rinse them in a colander unless the recipe instructs you not to. Doing so removes the saucy liquid and helps decrease about 40 percent of the sodium used as a preservative.

✔ When incorporating canned beans into a hot dish that's cooking on a fairly high heat, add them toward the end of cooking. Otherwise, they can become too soggy and fall apart.

Dried beans

Using dried beans requires a little bit more upfront work than using canned does, but your reward is a richer taste than what canned offers. Here's how it works:

1. **Sort through the beans, discarding any blemished or dirty ones.**

2. **Soak the beans.**

   The second step is, well, a bath. Preparing dried beans for cooking involves soaking them in one of three ways:

   A. Soak them overnight. A leisurely soak is the most common approach. Soak the beans in a large pot of water overnight (at least eight hours). Afterward, simply discard the soaking liquid and cook with fresh water.

   B. Soak them in boiling water. A quicker method is to bring the water to a boil, add the beans, remove the pan from the heat, and let the beans soak in the hot water for three to four hours. Discard the soaking liquid and then cook the beans in fresh water.

   C. Soak them in a pressure cooker. For fast and furious soaking, use a pressure cooker. Add your beans and about four cups of water to the pressure cooker. Lock the lid on and turn the cooker to high pressure. After the cooker is heated to high, reduce the heat to maintain the pressure and cook for two minutes. Release the pressure cooker by running cold water over the lid and then drain the beans; they're now ready to use in your recipe.

Lentils

Lentils require no soaking before cooking. Just sort through them, discarding any that are discolored or have dirt on them. Give them a good rinse in a colander and cook them according to package directions or recipe directions.

Finding cooking times for dried legumes

To cook unsoaked lentils or soaked dried beans, cover about 1 pound of the legumes with 6 cups of fresh water (not the water used for soaking). Simmer the beans or lentils until they're cooked and soft. Table 6-2 shows you some cooking times for various legumes.

Table 6-2	Cooking Times for Legumes	
Type of Legume	*Cooking Time in a Saucepan*	*Cooking Time in a Pressure Cooker*
Black beans	2–3 hours	15–20 minutes
Fava beans	1 hour	10–15 minutes
Chickpeas	2–3 hours	15–20 minutes
Kidney beans	2–3 hours	15–20 minutes
Lima beans	45 minutes	Not recommended
Pinto beans	2–3 hours	15–20 minutes
Lentils	30–45 minutes	Not recommended

Most people enjoy a pretty soft texture to their beans. If you aren't using a pressure cooker, you can try them at the early end of the cooking times to see if they're soft enough for you; if they aren't, continue cooking. You want to use your cooked beans within 5 days; if you can't make that happen, you can freeze them for up to 6 months.

Cooking meats the healthy way

Although the types of meats you eat on a regular basis are important, the way you cook them is equally important. If you deep-fry a lean chicken breast, it's not so lean anymore. So what do you do? Why, look to the Mediterranean, of course. (What did you think we were going to say?) Folks there tend to cook meats by using the following methods, which create a lot of flavor but still keep the meats lean:

✔ **Braise:** Simmering meats over low heat in a liquid (such as water, broth, wine, or fruit juice) in a covered pot for a long period of time. Braising works nicely with chicken, beef, and pork dishes.

✔ **Grill:** Cooking with direct heat over coals or another heat source such gas. Grilling is a delicious option for any kind of meat.

✔ **Poach:** Cooking meats gently in a small amount of liquid (such as broth or water) just below boiling. This method works well with meats that cook quickly, such as fish.

✔ **Roast:** Cooking meats uncovered with dry heat in the oven. Use this method with large pieces of meats, such as a whole chicken, a pot roast, or pork tenderloins.

✔ **Sauté:** Quickly cooking meats in a small amount of fat (such as butter or oil), stirring until the meat is cooked through. Sautéing bite-sized pieces of chicken is easy and tasty.

Part III
Starters and Sides

The 5th Wave   By Rich Tennant

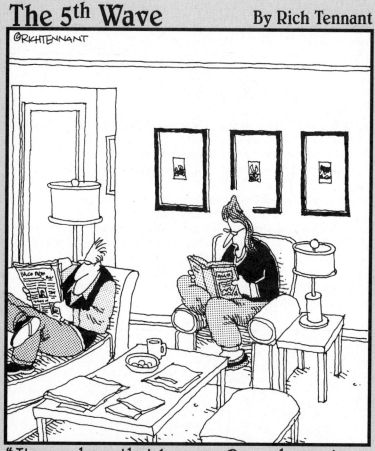

"It says here that because Persephone ate a
pomegranate seed she had to spend all year
in the underworld except for 4 months each
year that she spent with her mother. Some
scholars say it was 6 months. It probably
just _felt_ like 6 months."

In this part . . .

Bland, boring recipes are the one thing you won't find in Mediterranean cooking. The folks who live on the Mediterranean coast are known for big flavor in all their cooking, and the recipes in this part give you a glimpse.

This part includes various breakfast dishes; classic regional dips and appetizers such as hummus and bruschetta; and savory soups, stews, and sauces. If you've wondered how to incorporate more vegetables and whole grains in your diet, this part also offers recipes that demonstrate just how delicious and simple adding these foods can be. Eating more veggies is far easier when they taste amazing!

Chapter 7

Beginning the Day the Right Way

In This Chapter

▶ Exploring quick and easy Mediterranean-style breakfast ideas

▶ Getting started with some amazing egg dishes

▶ Going traditional with unique Mediterranean specialties

*Y*ou may be surprised to hear that a typical Mediterranean breakfast is on the light side. Although people in the Mediterranean region don't skip breakfast outright (doing so may negatively affect your health), they typically rely on quick meals to get them through to the main meal, lunch. Let us repeat that: They don't skip breakfast.

Research shows that beginning your day by eating a healthy breakfast is linked to

✔ Improved energy levels

✔ Weight control

✔ Better endurance for physical activities

✔ Improved concentration at work or in the classroom

Whether you like cereal, eggs, or pancakes, our goal for this chapter is to share some great breakfast recipes so that you can start your day off in a healthy way.

Waking Up to Breakfast, Mediterranean-Style

Beginning your day with breakfast gives your body the energy it needs to get moving. Whether you're in a hurry and need to grab something on the run or have more time to prepare a home-cooked meal, the Mediterranean diet gives you ample options.

A typical workday Mediterranean breakfast is often similar to a snack, usually consisting of two items you can throw together from your pantry. The most traditional Mediterranean breakfast options include the following, typically accompanied by milk, juice, or coffee:

- ✔ Toast with nut butter (like Nutella or peanut butter), fruit preserves, olive oil, or tomatoes
- ✔ Bread with cheese
- ✔ Yogurt
- ✔ Cereal
- ✔ A small pastry

Even though these items are small, they typically include protein and fat (through the nuts and dairy), which help you feel fuller and more satisfied until your next meal or snack. Eating something small is far better than skipping breakfast all together. This tendency is one part of this diet philosophy that works well with the Westernized world, where many people have limited time in the morning or perhaps get a queasy stomach from eating a large breakfast.

Similar to the United States and Canada, the weekends are often a time of cooking more elaborate breakfasts in the Mediterranean. To truly live the Mediterranean experience, choose some simple breakfasts for most of your week and then enjoy a big breakfast a few days a week. Doing so helps you to keep your calorie intake within a good range and allows you to enjoy some amazing foods throughout the week. Remember, people in the Mediterranean love food and eat a large variety during the week. Visit Chapter 4 for sample menus to see how to balance your breakfasts during the week.

Bringing on the Eggs

Eggs are eaten often in the Mediterranean and are a great breakfast choice because they're a wonderful source of protein and offer other healthy vitamins and minerals. Although they're high in cholesterol, eating eggs in moderation hasn't proven to have any adverse affects on heart health. In fact, a review of 224 studies carried out over the last 25 years has determined that eating eggs daily didn't raise cholesterol levels. Don't get too excited, because some information with other studies contradicts this info, and it's still recommended that you limit dietary cholesterol to 300 milligrams per day, for the average healthy person. One large egg has 213 milligrams of cholesterol, all in the yolk making eggs an okay food to eat in moderation.

If you have high cholesterol or heart disease, be sure to follow your physician's specific recommendations in regard to this diet and eggs, because every person's situation is unique.

People of the Mediterranean often use egg scrambles and frittatas as a way to use up leftovers, which is a great idea. Not only does it save you money by not wasting food, but it's also a great way to sneak in some vegetables. This section walks you through the following healthy egg recipes and offers some variations to use what you have on hand.

Choosing the best eggs

Eggs are common in the Mediterranean diet because they're economical and readily available. Eating eggs is a great choice for you because they're a good source of protein and vitamins A, D, and B-12. Although eggs can be part of a healthy diet, you have to handle them carefully because they may be contaminated with *salmonella,* bacteria that can make you very sick. Use the following tips to avoid any problems:

- Open egg cartons before you buy them and avoid any that contain cracked or unclean eggs.

- Avoid purchasing eggs at room temperature, because eggs can spoil quickly when not refrigerated.

- Discard eggs after the expiration date on the package. If you have farm-fresh eggs, you can store them in the refrigerator for four to five weeks.

- Take a good look at your eggs when cooking. The egg white should be thick, and the yolk should sit firm and high rather than flat.

- Don't eat eggs raw. You don't know whether that particular egg contains salmonella, and cooking the eggs is the only way to destroy the bacteria.

Determining when eggs spoil is difficult because they don't change color or have an odor. To check whether your eggs are good, carefully place them in a bowl of cold water. If they sink, they're in good shape. If they float, they're old, and you should toss them out. The more they float, the older they are.

Vegetable Omelet

Prep time: 15 min • **Cook time:** 25 min • **Yield:** 4 servings

Ingredients	*Directions*
1 tablespoon olive oil 2 cups thinly sliced fresh fennel bulb 1 Roma tomato, diced	*1* Preheat the oven to 325 degrees. In a large ovenproof skillet, heat the olive oil over medium-high heat. Add the fennel (see Figure 7-1 for how to slice fennel for this recipe) and sauté for 5 minutes, until soft.
¼ cup pitted green brine-cured olives, chopped	*2* Add in the tomato, olives, and artichoke hearts and sauté for 3 minutes, until softened.
¼ cup artichoke hearts, marinated in water, rinsed, drained, and chopped 6 eggs	*3* Whisk the eggs in a large bowl and season with the salt and pepper. Pour the whisked eggs into the skillet over the vegetables and stir with a heat-proof spoon for 2 minutes.
¼ teaspoon salt ½ teaspoon pepper	*4* Sprinkle the omelet with the cheese and bake for 5 minutes or until the eggs are cooked through and set.
½ cup goat cheese, crumbled 2 tablespoons chopped fresh dill, basil, or parsley	*5* Top with the dill, basil, or parsley. Remove the omelet from the skillet onto a cutting board. Carefully cut the omelet into four wedges, like a pizza, and serve.

Per serving: Calories 152 (From Fat 91); Fat 10g (Saturated 4g); Cholesterol 13mg; Sodium 496mg; Carbohydrate 6g (Dietary Fiber 2g); Protein 11g.

Vary It! You can replace the vegetables in this recipe with whatever you have on hand. Some good fits include mushrooms, broccoli, and spinach. Just make sure you sauté them until they're soft before adding your eggs.

HOW TO SLICE A FENNEL BULB

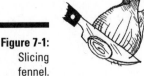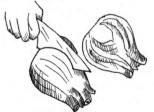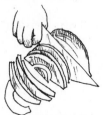

1. CUT A THIN SLICE OFF THE BOTTOM OF THE FENNE BULB TO REMOVE THE ROOT END.

2. CUT THE FENNEL IN HALF FROM TOP TO BOTTOM, LENGTHWISE.

3. FLAT SIDES DOWN, THINLY SLICE THE TWO HALVES, AND LAYER ON THE GREENS.

Figure 7-1: Slicing fennel.

Zucchini and Goat Cheese Frittata

Prep time: 30 min • **Cook time:** 20 min • **Yield:** 4 servings

Ingredients	*Directions*
2 medium zucchinis 8 eggs 2 tablespoons milk ¼ teaspoon salt ⅛ teaspoon pepper 1 tablespoon olive oil 1 clove garlic, crushed 2 ounces goat cheese, crumbled	**1** Preheat the oven to 350 degrees. Slice the zucchinis into ¼-inch-thick round slices. In a large bowl whisk the eggs with the milk, salt, and pepper.
	2 In a heavy, ovenproof skillet (preferably cast iron), heat the olive oil over medium heat. Add the garlic and cook for 30 seconds. Add the zucchini slices and cook for 5 minutes.
	3 Pour the whisked eggs over the zucchini and stir for 1 minute. Top with the cheese and transfer to the oven. Bake for 10 to 12 minutes or until the eggs are set. Remove the pan from the oven and let sit for 3 minutes.
	4 Transfer the frittata to a cutting board, slice into four pie wedges, and serve hot or at room temperature.

Per serving: Calories 134 (From Fat 72); Fat 8g (Saturated 3g); Cholesterol 11mg; Sodium 324mg; Carbohydrate 4g (Dietary Fiber 1g); Protein 12g.

Vary It! You can use yellow squash in place of the zucchini.

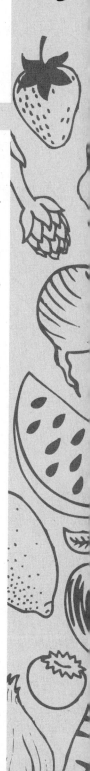

Pancetta and Spinach Frittata

Prep time: 5 min • **Cook time:** 35 min • **Yield:** 4 servings

Ingredients	Directions
Nonstick cooking spray	*1* Preheat the oven to 325 degrees. In a heavy, ovenproof skillet (preferably cast iron), heat 1 tablespoon of the olive oil over medium heat.
1 tablespoon plus 2 teaspoons olive oil	
¼ pound pancetta, diced small	*2* Add in the pancetta and cook for 3 to 5 minutes, until crispy. Add the garlic and cook for 30 seconds. Add the spinach and sauté for 4 minutes or until lightly wilted. Strain the mixture to remove excess liquid.
2 cloves garlic, crushed	
8 cups baby spinach, rinsed and patted dry	
6 eggs, lightly beaten	*3* Heat the remaining olive oil over medium-high heat. Return the vegetable mixture to the skillet and sauté for 1 minute. Spread the vegetables evenly in a layer at the bottom of the pan.
¼ teaspoon salt	
¼ teaspoon pepper	
2 ounces feta, crumbled	*4* Add the eggs and season with the salt and pepper. Gently stir for about a minute. Let the pan set over low heat for a minute or two or until the mixture begins to set, getting firm in the center.
	5 Top with the cheese and transfer to the oven. Bake for 10 to 12 minutes or until the eggs are set. Remove the pan from the oven and let the mixture rest for 3 minutes.
	6 Transfer the frittata to a cutting board, slice into four pie wedges, and serve hot or at room temperature.

Per serving: Calories 256 (From Fat 196); Fat 22g (Saturated 7g); Cholesterol 32mg; Sodium 670mg; Carbohydrate 4g (Dietary Fiber 1g); Protein 12g.

Vary It! In place of pancetta, you can substitute bacon or Canadian bacon; you get a similar taste while using up any meats you have on hand. Simply omit the meat for a vegetarian breakfast.

Dilled Eggs

Prep time: 10 min • **Cook time:** 5 min • **Yield:** 4 servings

Ingredients	Directions
1 tablespoon olive oil	**1** In a large nonstick skillet, heat the olive oil over medium heat. Add in the onions and cook for 3 minutes, until softened. Crack the eggs into a medium bowl and then pour them into the pan.
¼ cup onion, minced	
8 eggs	
2 tablespoons fresh dill	**2** Whisk the eggs in the pan, breaking each yolk. Stir the eggs every 30 seconds until they set and are firm.
2 ounces feta, crumbled	
Salt and pepper to taste	**3** Add in the dill and cheese. Season with salt and pepper to taste and serve.

Per serving: Calories 103 (From Fat 59); Fat 7g (Saturated 3g); Cholesterol 13mg; Sodium 268mg; Carbohydrate 2g (Dietary Fiber 0g); Protein 9g.

Vary It! You can replace the feta with goat cheese. Using goat cheese adds a slightly milder taste but keeps the delicious flavor.

Note: If you prefer a more scrambled egg, simply beat the raw eggs in a small bowl first and then cook them as you would scrambled eggs. Figure 7-2 explains how to mince an onion. You can also see a photo of this recipe in the color insert.

HOW TO MINCE AN ONION

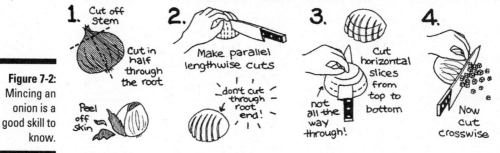

Figure 7-2:
Mincing an onion is a good skill to know.

1. Cut off stem. Cut in half through the root. Peel off skin.

2. Make parallel lengthwise cuts. don't cut through root end!

3. Cut horizontal slices from top to bottom. not all the way through!

4. Now cut crosswise

Mediterranean Egg Scramble

Prep time: 15 min • **Cook time:** 25 min • **Yield:** 4 servings

Ingredients	*Directions*
1 teaspoon olive oil	*1* In a large nonstick skillet, heat the olive oil and butter to medium-high heat. Add the sliced potatoes and sauté for about 15 minutes or until golden. Add the bell pepper and olives and cook for 4 minutes.
1 teaspoon butter	
3 medium-sized new potatoes, thinly sliced	
¼ large red bell pepper, small diced	*2* In a medium bowl, whisk together the parsley, ricotta, and eggs. Pour the egg mixture over the potato mixture, stirring every 30 seconds until firm and set but not dry, about 3 minutes. Salt and pepper the egg scramble to taste.
8 black olives, chopped	
¼ cup fresh parsley, chopped	
¼ cup fresh ricotta cheese	
6 eggs	*3* Serve with crusty bread, lightly toasted and buttered with 1 teaspoon of butter or lightly brushed with 1 teaspoon of extra-virgin olive oil per slice.
Salt and pepper to taste	
4 slices crusty bread	
4 teaspoons butter or extra-virgin olive oil	

Per serving: *Calories 330 (From Fat 113); Fat 13g (Saturated 3g); Cholesterol 9mg; Sodium 364mg; Carbohydrate 43g (Dietary Fiber 4g); Protein 13g.*

Vary It! Replace these vegetables with artichoke hearts and fennel for an Italian scramble.

Egg Panini

Prep time: 18 min • **Cook time:** 6 min • **Yield:** 4 servings

Ingredients	Directions
4 eggs	*1* Place the eggs in a 2-quart saucepan and fill it with cold water. Cook over high heat until the water comes to a boil. Remove the pan from the heat and cover for 15 minutes.
⅛ teaspoon salt	
¼ teaspoon pepper	
8 slices country bread	*2* Meanwhile, wash and slice the tomato into 8 slices (about ⅛-inch thick). Wash and pat dry the basil. Slice the mozzarella ball into 4 slices and halve each slice.
1 tomato	
8 basil leaves	
4 ounces fresh mozzarella	*3* Run cold water over the eggs, shell them, and slice each egg into 4 slices. Assemble the sandwiches: Top 1 slice of bread with 1 egg, 2 tomato slices, 2 basil leaves, 2 mozzarella slices, and another slice of bread.
8 teaspoons olive oil	
	4 Using a pastry brush or your fingers, brush the outer bread slices with one teaspoon of olive oil each. If you have a Panini press, add your sandwich and cook for about 3 minutes until golden brown. If you don't have a Panini press, heat a heavy skillet on medium-high heat and cook the cheese side of one sandwich for 3 minutes or until golden.
	5 Flip the sandwich and place a heavy pan on top (a filled tea pot works well, too) for 2 to 3 minutes or until golden. Repeat until all sandwiches are prepared. Serve.

Per serving: Calories 322 (From Fat 155); Fat 17g (Saturated 5g); Cholesterol 27mg; Sodium 604mg; Carbohydrate 27g (Dietary Fiber 3g); Protein 16g.

Vary It! You can replace the fresh basil with spinach leaves for a more savory flavor.

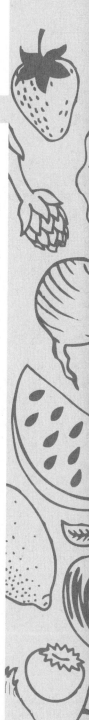

Trying Some Delicious Breakfast Specials

Breakfast in the Mediterranean is usually simple fare, but you can also find many specialties that are unique to the region. Although pancakes and scones are options you may be used to seeing, Greek yogurt bowls, farina, and beans may be a little different. We love opening up the doors to new breakfast foods to take you out of any food ruts so you can kick back and enjoy your first meal of the day.

This section provides you with some amazing recipes that are unique and truly celebrate the Mediterranean region. You just may find some new favorites!

Greek yogurt: The king of yogurts

Although you can find many yogurts lining the shelves of your local grocery store, lowfat plain Greek yogurt reigns over the rest. One reason: All the liquid whey is drained out, leaving a thicker, creamier texture. Face it: Creamier is just better!

Along with the normal health benefits of yogurt (such as calcium, potassium, and vitamins B-6 and B-12), Greek yogurt contains twice the amount of protein of regular yogurt, keeping you feeling fuller longer. Greek yogurt is also lower in sugar and higher in the probiotic

cultures that are helpful for healthy digestion. Choose lowfat plain Greek yogurt to save on fat grams and calories.

If you aren't used to the taste of plain yogurt, mix in some all-fruit spread or fresh berries to add a little sweetness. Try the Greek Yogurt and Fruit Bowls recipe in this chapter for a quick, healthy and delicious breakfast, or the Cucumber Yogurt Sauce in Chapter 9 for a savory addition to pita sandwiches or hot meals. Here's to adding more yogurt into your diet!

Greek Yogurt and Fruit Bowls

Prep time: 10 min • **Yield:** 4 servings

Ingredients	*Directions*
2 cups red or green grapes 4 fresh apricots 2 cups lowfat plain Greek yogurt 4 tablespoons slivered almonds 4 tablespoons raw, old fashioned oats 4 tablespoons honey	*1* Slice the grapes in half and divide into 4 bowls (½ cup per bowl). Slice the apricots and discard the seed; divide equally into the 4 bowls.
	2 Top each fruit bowl with ½ cup lowfat Greek yogurt and sprinkle with the slivered almonds and oats.
	3 Drizzle 1 tablespoon of honey over each bowl and serve.

Per serving: Calories 206 (From Fat 45); Fat 5g (Saturated 0g); Cholesterol 0mg; Sodium 23mg; Carbohydrate 36g (Dietary Fiber 3g); Protein 8g.

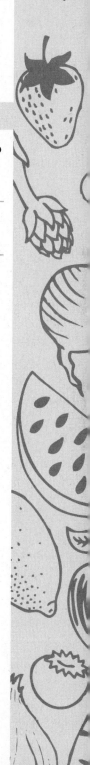

Farina Farina

Prep time: 3 min • **Cook time:** 3 min • **Yield:** 2 servings

Ingredients	*Directions*
2 cups milk	*1* Bring the milk and the salt to a boil in a small saucepan over medium-high heat, stirring constantly to avoid burning the milk.
¼ teaspoon salt	
⅓ cup farina	
2 tablespoons honey	*2* Whisk in the farina; reduce the heat to medium-low and simmer, stirring occasionally, until thickened, 2 to 3 minutes.
2 fresh apricots, diced, or ¼ cup dried	
2 tablespoons walnuts, chopped	*3* Spoon the cooked farina into two bowls and top each with 1 tablespoon of honey, half the apricots, and 1 tablespoon of walnuts.

Per serving: Calories 164 (From Fat 33); Fat 4g (Saturated 1g); Cholesterol 6mg; Sodium 200mg; Carbohydrate 27g (Dietary Fiber 1g); Protein 6g.

Note: Cream of Wheat is a popular brand of farina.

Tip: If you're using dried apricots, soak them in hot water for 5 minutes prior to adding them.

Orange Ricotta Pancakes

Prep time: 10 min • **Cook time:** 15 min • **Yield:** 6 servings

Ingredients	*Directions*
1½ **cups flour**	*1* In a medium bowl, combine the flour, baking powder, and salt until well blended.
1 **teaspoon baking powder**	
½ **teaspoon salt**	*2* In a large bowl, whisk together the egg yolks, milk, ricotta, sugar, vanilla, and orange zest. Add the egg yolk mixture to the dry ingredients, mix well, and set aside.
3 **eggs, separated**	
1¾ **cup milk**	
6 **ounces lowfat ricotta cheese**	
¼ **cup sugar**	*3* Using an electric mixer, beat the egg whites on medium-high speed until frothy and then turn the speed up to high until soft peaks form. Fold the egg white mixture into the batter.
1 **tablespoon vanilla extract**	
2 **tablespoons fresh orange zest**	
Nonstick cooking spray	*4* Spray a griddle or large nonstick skillet with nonstick cooking spray. Heat the pan over medium heat.
½ **cup orange marmalade**	
2 **tablespoons butter**	*5* Pour ¼ cup of the batter onto the pan, evenly spacing as many pancakes as you can fit. When bubbles begin to form, flip and allow the pancakes to finish cooking, about 1 to 2 minutes. Transfer the cooked pancakes to a plate and continue cooking the remaining batter.
	6 Meanwhile, melt the orange marmalade and butter in a small pot over medium-low heat, stirring frequently until they're combined and the sauce is warm. Remove from the heat. Serve the pancakes with about one tablespoon of the orange sauce per serving.

Per serving: Calories 291 (From Fat 64); Fat 7g (Saturated 4g); Cholesterol 23mg; Sodium 412mg; Carbohydrate 47g (Dietary Fiber 1g); Protein 11g.

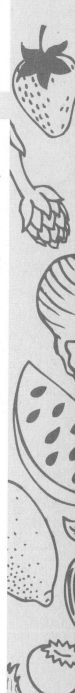

Lemon Scones

Prep time: 15 min • **Cook time:** 15 min • **Yield:** 12 servings

Ingredients	Directions
2 cups plus ¼ cup flour	*1* Heat the oven to 400 degrees. In a medium bowl, combine 2 cups of the flour, the sugar, baking soda, and salt. Using a pastry blender or a food processor, cut in the butter until the mixture resembles fine crumbs.
2 tablespoons sugar	
½ teaspoon baking soda	
½ teaspoon salt	
¼ cup butter	*2* Add the lemon zest and buttermilk, stirring just until mixed. Flour a surface with the remaining flour and turn out the dough; knead gently six times (refer to Figure 7-3). Shape the dough into a ball and then flatten into a ½-inch-thick circle with a rolling pin.
Zest of one lemon	
¾ cup reduced fat buttermilk	
1 cup powdered sugar	*3* Cut the circle into 4 wedges and then cut each wedge into 3 smaller wedges, yielding 12 scones. Place the scones on baking sheet and cook for 12 to 15 minutes or until golden brown.
1 to 2 teaspoons lemon juice	
	4 In a small bowl, mix the powder sugar and just enough lemon juice to make a thin frosting. Drizzle the frosting over the hot scones and serve.

Per serving: *Calories 175 (From Fat 39); Fat 4g (Saturated 3g); Cholesterol 11mg; Sodium 190mg; Carbohydrate 31g (Dietary Fiber 1g); Protein 3g.*

Note: You can use parchment paper to line your cookie sheet prior to serving if you want less browning on the bottom of your scone. Check out the color insert for a photo of this recipe.

KNEADING DOUGH

To knead dough, press down with your palm...

Fold the dough over and rotate ¼ turn

Repeat steps 1 + 2 until dough is soft and elastic.

voila!

Figure 7-3:
How to knead dough.

Savory Fava Beans with Warm Pita Bread

Prep time: 10 min • **Cook time:** 15 min • **Yield:** 4 servings

Ingredients	*Directions*
1½ tablespoons olive oil 1 large onion, chopped 1 large tomato, diced 1 clove garlic, crushed One 15-ounce can fava beans, undrained 1 teaspoon ground cumin	*1* In a large nonstick skillet, heat the olive oil over medium-high heat for 30 seconds. Add the onion, tomato, and garlic and sauté for 3 minutes, until soft. Add the fava beans and their liquid and bring to a boil.
¼ cup chopped fresh parsley ¼ cup lemon juice Salt and pepper to taste	*2* Reduce the heat to medium and add the cumin, parsley, and lemon juice and season with the salt, pepper, and ground red pepper to taste. Cook for 5 minutes on medium heat.
Crushed red pepper flakes, to taste 4 whole-grain pita bread pockets	*3* Meanwhile, heat the pita in a cast-iron skillet over medium-low heat until warm (1 to 2 minutes per side). Serve the warm pita with the fava beans (either on the side or loaded up with the bean mixture).

Per serving: Calories 325 (From Fat 64); Fat 7g (Saturated 1g); Cholesterol 0mg; Sodium 831mg; Carbohydrate 56g (Dietary Fiber 10g); Protein 13g.

Note: You can find canned fava beans in Mediterranean, Indian, or Italian ethnic stores. If you can't find them locally, you can buy them online at www.amazon.com.

Tip: Figure 7-4 shows how you can trim fresh herbs.

CHOPPING PARSLEY & OTHER FRESH HERBS

Figure 7-4: Adding fresh herbs to a dish can add flavor.

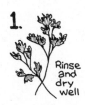

1. Rinse and dry well

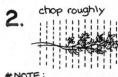

2. chop roughly

*NOTE: For herbs like rosemary and thyme, remove and chop leaves. Discard thick stem.

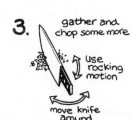

3. gather and chop some more

Use rocking motion

move knife around

Check out chia seeds

Who knew that those same seeds that grow grassy-headed windowsill pets actually have some nutritional value? Chia seeds are an excellent source of omega-3 fatty acids and add a mild, nutty flavor to your meals. You can find chia seeds at most health food stores (don't eat the ones that come with the pet), and you can easily add them to salads, muffins, cereal, granola, smoothies, or yogurt. Unlike flaxseeds, chia seeds don't have to be ground for you to receive their nutritional benefits, even in baking. Chia seeds don't have a strong flavor but rather enhance the flavors you are cooking with.

Chapter 8

Small Appetizers: Starting Off With Tapas, Meze, and Antipasti

In This Chapter

▶ Finding your inner Mediterranean cook with classic appetizers

▶ Serving up some cheesy favorites

▶ Making savory starters for special occasions

Tapas, meze, and *antipasti* are all terms for small dishes, similar to what you think of as appetizers, served in the Mediterranean. Dating back to Roman times, appetizers are traditionally used to whet your appetite or stimulate the gastric juices before a meal. In the Mediterranean, appetizers are seasonal depending on what types of foods are on hand. For example, you see more *dolmas* (stuffed grape leaves) in the summer months while the grape vines are in bloom.

Depending on the exact region, these small appetizers are used in different ways. In some areas, dinner isn't served until 9 p.m. or later, leaving a good amount of time from the end of the work day; small appetizers are often served as a snack between work and dinnertime to compensate. In other regions, people serve several appetizers at once as the dinner meal. However, most homes don't serve this course regularly, and they reserve lavish appetizers for parties and special celebrations.

This chapter shows you simple appetizers you can use as a snack as well as more-elaborate platters, hot dishes, and savory appetizers you can use for your next party or celebration.

The key to adding these small appetizers into your own diet is to make sure doing so makes sense in your day. If you aren't eating dinner late in the evening, you probably don't need to load up on more food right before your meal; you may end up taking in excessive calories and fat, leading to weight gain. However, making something like hummus with pita chips as a snack is a great way to incorporate these recipes into your day. And of course, all the appetizers will go amazingly with your next party!

Creating the Classics

When you think of the Mediterranean, a few classics, such as stuffed grape leaves and hummus, probably come to mind. These kinds of dishes are common throughout parts of the region at family gatherings and in pubs. You can incorporate many of these same classics into your own diet.

If you're having a small gathering, you may want to create a few of the special items, such as the stuffed grape leaves and toasted almonds. We also show you how to put all of this section's recipes together as an entire meze platter for your next blowout. You can't go wrong with this spread!

Cooking up grape leaves

Grape leaves are popular in certain regions of the Mediterranean, particularly Greece and Turkey. Although you may look at grape leaves as a simple wrapper for an appetizer or as something you've never thought about eating before, they actually provide some great health benefits, including the following:

✔ Very low in calories, with only about 14 calories for five leaves or one cup

✔ Loaded with specific nutrients, including iron, calcium, folate, manganese, magnesium, niacin, riboflavin, vitamin A, vitamin B-6, and vitamin C

✔ Good source of dietary fiber, which helps you feel full while eating fewer calories

✔ Rich in flavonoids that benefit heart health

✔ Known to have anti-inflammatory properties, which can be helpful for preventing

and managing many chronic diseases, such as heart disease and diabetes

A common Mediterranean preparation of grape leaves is as *dolmas,* where cooks stuff the leaves with rice, vegetables, herbs, or meat. Whether served hot, warm, or cold, they're delicious! (Check out the dolma recipes in this chapter.) You can pick grape leaves fresh from the vine and preserve them yourself or buy them in bottles. When purchasing bottled grape leaves, make sure to rinse them before using to remove some of the sodium from the brine. If you don't have grapes growing in your backyard and can't find the leaves in your local grocery store, stop by www.amazon.com or www.greekinternetmarket.com to order them online.

Stuffed Grape Leaves (Dolmas)

Prep time: 45 min • **Cook time:** 50 min • **Yield:** 20 servings

Ingredients	Directions
4 Roma tomatoes, small diced	*1* In a large bowl, combine the tomatoes, rice, onion, mint, parsley, fennel seeds, pine nuts, olive oil, and garlic. Rinse the grape leaves under cold water. Cover the bottom of a large (preferably cast-iron) Dutch oven with 5 leaves.
1 cup uncooked basmati rice	
½ medium onion, minced	
½ cup (packed) finely chopped fresh mint	*2* Place 1 grape leaf on your work surface, vein side up, removing the stem if it's still intact. Place a level tablespoon of the rice mixture in center of the leaf near the stem end. (See the recipe, "Meaty Grape Leaves (Meat-Filled Dolmas)" later in this chapter for a drawing on how to wrap grape leaves.)
½ cup (packed) finely chopped fresh parsley	
1½ teaspoons crushed fennel seeds	
½ cup pine nuts, toasted	*3* Fold the sides over the filling and roll up firmly beginning at the stem end, tucking in sides as needed. Place in Dutch oven, seam side down with one end facing the center of pot.
¼ cup extra-virgin olive oil	
2 cloves garlic, minced	
1 16-ounce jar grape leaves	*4* Repeat with the remaining leaves and filling, layering the dolmas along the bottom and starting new layers as necessary. Pour the stock over the dolmas and add the lemon juice. If necessary, add water until the dolmas are just covered with liquid.
3 cups vegetable stock or chicken stock	
Juice of 1 lemon	
	5 Top the dolmas with five more flattened grape leaves and a heatproof plate to hold them down as they cook. Lid the Dutch oven and bring to a boil over high heat. Drop the temperature to low and cook for 50 minutes at a low simmer.
	6 Remove the Dutch oven from the heat, uncover, and cool the dolmas in the pot for 10 minutes. Using tongs, gently remove the dolmas from the Dutch oven onto a serving plate and serve them warm or chilled.

Per serving: Calories 90 (From Fat 47); Fat 5g (Saturated 1g); Cholesterol 0mg; Sodium 201mg; Carbohydrate 10g (Dietary Fiber 0g); Protein 1g.

Tip: Keep the dolmas close together to ensure that they don't unravel while simmering. The more firmly you roll them, the less likely they are to come unraveled during the cooking process.

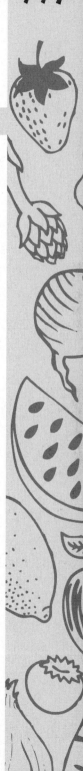

Toasted Almonds

Prep time: 4 min • **Cook time:** 30 min • **Yield:** 16 servings

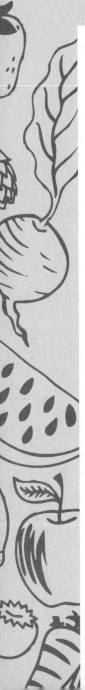

Ingredients	Directions
4 cups whole, raw almonds	*1* Preheat the oven to 300 degrees. Place the almonds in a medium bowl and set aside. In a small bowl, whisk the egg white and water until the egg is broken up. Pour the egg mixture over the almonds and stir. Add the spices and salt and stir until well blended.
1 egg white	
1 tablespoon water	
¼ teaspoon cayenne pepper	
¼ teaspoon ground cumin	*2* Place the almonds on a baking sheet and bake, stirring every 10 minutes, for 30 to 40 minutes or until just toasted and you begin to smell the toasted nuts. Don't let the almonds get too dark, or they'll taste burnt.
½ tablespoon sea salt	
	3 Remove almonds from the oven and immediately transfer them to a heat-proof plate; allow the nuts to cool in a single layer. Serve at room temperature.

Per serving: Calories 205 (From Fat 158); Fat 18g (Saturated 1g); Cholesterol 0mg; Sodium 222mg; Carbohydrate 8g (Dietary Fiber 4g); Protein 8g.

Note: Store in a glass container in the refrigerator and use within 1 to 2 weeks for best quality.

Toasted Pita Chips

Prep time: 5 min • **Cook time:** 12–15 minutes • **Yield:** 4 servings

Ingredients	Directions
4 whole wheat pitas	*1* Preheat the oven to 375 degrees.
4 teaspoons olive oil	*2* Using a pastry brush, brush each pita with 1 teaspoon of olive oil. Sprinkle with sea salt to taste.
Sea salt to taste	*3* Cut each pita into 8 wedges. Arrange the pita wedges on a baking sheet and bake for 12 to 15 minutes. Cool the pita chips to room temperature and serve.

Per serving: Calories 210 (From Fat 55); Fat 6g (Saturated 1g); Cholesterol 0mg; Sodium 341mg; Carbohydrate 35g (Dietary Fiber 5g); Protein 6g.

Note: Serve with any of the tasty dips in this chapter, such as Hummus or Baba Gannoujh. Refer to the color insert in this book for a photo of this recipe.

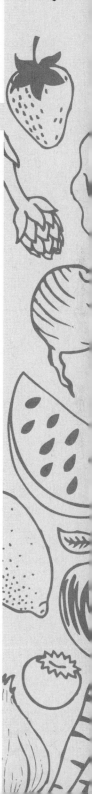

Hummus

Prep time: 10 min • **Yield:** 16 servings

Ingredients	Directions
Two 14.5-ounce cans chickpeas	**1** Drain the chickpeas and reserve ¼ to ½ cup of the liquid. Place the chickpeas in a food processor and puree until smooth.
Juice of 2 lemons	
2 cloves garlic	**2** Add the remaining ingredients and blend until the mixture is creamy. If necessary, add the liquid reserved from the canned chickpeas to create desired creaminess. Transfer the hummus to a bowl and serve.
¼ tablespoon olive oil	
¼ cup tahini paste	
½ teaspoon salt	
Pinch of cayenne pepper	

Per serving: Calories 85 (From Fat 25); Fat 3g (Saturated 0g); Cholesterol 0mg; Sodium 228mg; Carbohydrate 12g (Dietary Fiber 2g); Protein 3g.

Tip: Serve with Toasted Pita Chips or fresh vegetables such as carrots.

Note: Tahini paste is paste made from ground sesame seeds. It is a major component in Hummus and other Middle Eastern dishes. You can find tahini paste at most grocery stores or specialty stores near the cooking oils or possibly in the ethnic sections of the store. If you can't find it in your store, look for it online at www.amazon.com.

Note: Store hummus in a glass container in the refrigerator for up to a week. Cover the surface with a thin layer of olive oil, allowing mixture to be stored in the refrigerator for 1 week. This book's color insert includes a photograph of this recipe.

Roasted Eggplant Dip (Baba Gannoujh)

Prep time: 5 min • **Cook time:** 30 min • **Yield:** 16 servings

Ingredients	Directions
2 large eggplants	**1** Preheat the oven to 450 degrees. Line a baking sheet with foil.
½ cup tahini paste	
2 cloves garlic	**2** Poke the eggplant once with a fork on all sides to allow the steam to escape during cooking. Bake the eggplant on a baking sheet for about 30 minutes or until soft. Remove the eggplant from the oven and cool until you can comfortably touch it.
Juice of 2 lemons	
3 tablespoons water	
1 tablespoon extra-virgin olive oil	
1 teaspoon salt	**3** Cut the eggplant in half. Scoop out the inside of the eggplant with a spoon, discarding the skin.
2 tablespoons fresh parsley, chopped, for serving	
	4 Pulse the cooked eggplant in a food processor for 1 minute. Add the tahini, garlic, lemon juice, water, olive oil, and salt to the eggplant mixture and blend until you achieve a thicker consistency. Transfer to a serving bowl, garnish with the chopped parsley, and serve with pita chips.

Per serving: Calories 68 (From Fat 45); Fat 5g (Saturated 1g); Cholesterol 0mg; Sodium 149mg; Carbohydrate 6g (Dietary Fiber 3g); Protein 2g.

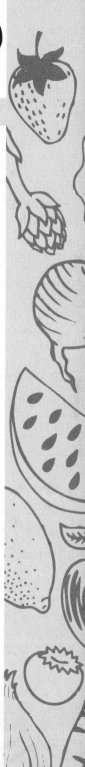

Classic Meze Platter

Prep time: 10 min • **Yield:** 16 servings

Ingredients	*Directions*
Hummus	*1* Arrange the Hummus and Baba Gannoujh in serving dishes on a large platter and position the Toasted Pita Chips around the dips.
Baba Gannoujh	
4 batches Toasted Pita Chips	
Stuffed Grape Leaves	*2* On one side of the platter, layer the Stuffed Grape Leaves. Next to the grape leaves, layer the radishes, cucumbers, and feta.
1 cup radishes, sliced in half	
4 cucumbers, sliced in half and then lengthwise into half-inch spears	
4 ounces feta cheese, cut into 1-inch cubes	*3* Top the feta with chopped parsley and drizzle with the olive oil. Place the olives in a bowl and serve them in the center of the platter.
¼ cup parsley, roughly chopped	
1 tablespoon olive oil	*4* On the other side of the platter, add the Toasted Almonds, grapes, dried apricots, and dates. Serve.
1 cup assorted olives	
Toasted Almonds	
1 bunch grapes	
1 cup dried apricots	
1 cup dates, pitted	

Per serving: Calories 756 (From Fat 361); Fat 40g (Saturated 5g); Cholesterol 6mg; Sodium 1306mg; Carbohydrate 88g (Dietary Fiber 16g); Protein 22g.

Note: You can find the recipes for Hummus, Baba Gannoujh, Toasted Pita Chips, Stuffed Grape Leaves, Toasted Almonds, and Meaty Grape Leaves in this chapter.

Going for the Yum: That's So Cheesy!

Folks in the Mediterranean often serve cheese simply with crackers and bread, but you can also find it with more-detailed appetizer recipes. The United States and Canada don't use as wide a variety of cheeses as people in the Mediterranean do. Although you may be used to aged cheeses like cheddar or American, you find more soft and semi-soft cheeses in Mediterranean cooking, especially with appetizers.

If you haven't ventured very far in your cheese choices, now is the time to explore! This section shows you some simple and wonderful appetizers with an assortment of cheeses. The following recipes are great for snacks or for your nicest party.

Making cheese add to your health, not to your hips

Cheese is a common staple in the Mediterranean diet in all types of dishes. Cheese is a concentrated form of milk (usually cow, sheep, or goat milk). Because it's made from milk, cheese offers a great source of healthy nutrients such as calcium, protein, phosphorus, zinc, vitamin A, riboflavin, and vitamin B-12. However, it also packs a lot of fat and calories. Going overboard with foods like cheese can lead to weight gain and associated health problems such as heart disease or diabetes. The trick is to use the right types of cheese for a particular dish so that you can get a lot of flavor and avoid excessive calories and fat. Use these tips to enjoy cheese in a healthy way:

- When using a large amount of cheese in a recipe like lasagna, choose lower-fat cheeses like lowfat ricotta and part-skim mozzarella.

- Take advantage of part-skim mozzarella when eating cheese with crackers and bread.

- When cooking, use shredded cheese rather than chunks or slices. Most of the time, you end up using less cheese overall.

- With dishes like salads, eggs, or pastas, sprinkle a small amount of strong-flavored cheeses such as goat cheese, Parmesan, or feta. A little goes a long, long way with flavor.

Mini Spanakopita

Prep time: 35 min • **Cook time:** 20 min • **Yield:** 24 servings

Ingredients	*Directions*
Three 10-ounce packages fresh spinach, coarsely chopped	*1* Preheat the oven to 350 degrees. To prepare the filling, microwave the spinach in a microwave-safe bowl for 2 to 3 minutes or until heated. Using a colander, strain and wring out the spinach until it's barely moist; transfer to a large bowl and mix with the feta cheese.
6 ounces (about 1 cup) feta cheese, crumbled	
1 tablespoon plus 2 tablespoons olive oil	*2* In a medium nonstick skillet, heat 1 tablespoon of the olive oil and sauté the chopped onion for 3 minutes. Add the onion, dill, lemon juice, salt, pepper, and eggs to the spinach mixture and stir well.
1 medium onion, minced	
3 tablespoons fresh dill, chopped	
1 tablespoon lemon juice	*3* Combine the remaining olive oil and melted butter in a small bowl. Lightly brush the phyllo sheet with the olive oil and butter and sprinkle with 1 tablespoon of the bread crumbs. Cut 1 phyllo sheet at a time lengthwise into three 4-inch strips.
¼ teaspoon salt	
¼ teaspoon pepper	
2 eggs, lightly beaten	*4* Spoon about 2 to 3 tablespoons of the spinach mixture onto one end of each strip; fold as Figure 8-1 shows.
1 tablespoon butter, melted	
8 sheets frozen phyllo dough, thawed	*5* Place the triangles, seam sides down, on a baking sheet and bake for 20 minutes or until golden. Using tongs, gently place the spanakopitas onto a serving plate. Serve warm.
1½ cups bread crumbs	

Per serving: Calories 78 (From Fat 39); Fat 4g (Saturated 2g); Cholesterol 8mg; Sodium 190mg; Carbohydrate 7g (Dietary Fiber 1g); Protein 3g.

Tip: As you work, cover the unused sheets of phyllo dough with a lightly moistened (not wet) towel to keep them from drying out.

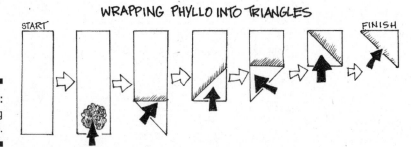

WRAPPING PHYLLO INTO TRIANGLES

START   FINISH

Figure 8-1: Folding Spanakopita.

Goat Cheese with Honey and Fruit

Prep time: 12 min • **Yield:** 8 servings

Ingredients	Directions
32 whole-grain crackers	*1* Arrange the crackers on a serving dish. Spread each cracker with 1 tablespoon of goat cheese and top with an apricot, a fig, or a pear slice.
8 ounces goat cheese	
8 dried apricots	
8 dried figs	*2* In a microwave safe bowl, heat the honey for 30 seconds; drizzle the honey over the fruit and crackers and serve.
1 pear, thinly sliced	
3 tablespoons honey	

Per serving: Calories 249 (From Fat 99); Fat11g (Saturated 6g); Cholesterol 22mg; Carbohydrate 31g (Dietary Fiber 4g); Protein 9g.

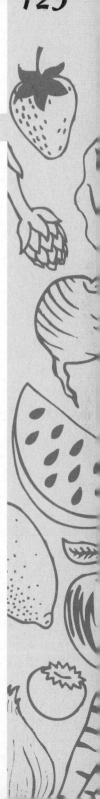

Tomato and Mozzarella Bites

Prep time: 10 min • **Cook time:** 5 min • **Yield:** 16 servings

Ingredients	Directions
¾ **cup balsamic vinegar**	*1* In a small saucepan, cook the vinegar and pomegranate juice over medium heat until it reduces by half, approximately 5 minutes.
¼ **cup pomegranate juice**	
4 vine-ripened tomatoes, sliced ¼-inch thick	
Sea salt to taste	*2* Meanwhile, layer the sliced tomatoes on a serving platter and sprinkle each with sea salt. Layer a basil leaf over each tomato and top with a mozzarella slice. Drizzle the olive oil and the balsamic pomegranate reduction over the tomato and mozzarella bites.
16 fresh basil leaves	
1 pound fresh mozzarella cheese, sliced ¼-inch-thick	
¼ **cup olive oil**	*3* Pierce each mozzarella bite with a toothpick and serve.

Per serving: *Calories133 (From Fat 88); Fat 10g (Saturated 4g); Cholesterol 22mg; Sodium 182mg; Carbohydrate 4g (Dietary Fiber 0g); Protein 7g.*

Note: Flip to the color insert for a photo of this recipe.

Picking your own produce

Although not everyone on the Mediterranean coast has a garden, going to a farm to pick produce is certainly an activity seen more often in those regions. Whether you plant a few fruit trees or a vegetable garden or travel to go apple or berry picking, incorporating this activity several times a year helps you to put more focus on the foods you're choosing to eat. Grabbing some apples at the grocery store isn't nearly as satisfying as picking some off a tree, washing them, and eating them on the spot or baking

some apple pie. The taste of freshly picked apples is better than the store-bought experience, and the whole process is more enjoyable.

Make this a fun tradition in your family to get out to some of your local farms to pick your own produce. Growing up, Meri's family went huckleberry picking in the mountains. Those trips have become some of her best memories, and the resulting huckleberry pancakes are still on her list of top ten favorite foods.

Creating Savory Starters

Cooked, warm appetizers are a perfect fit for parties or intimate gatherings. The following section provides some delicious appetizers that go well with a smaller dinner, such as the entree salads in Chapter 10 or the Lentil Loaf in Chapter 14.

In many Mediterranean regions, the general rule is to serve a hot appetizer before a light meal and a cold appetizer prior to a heavy meal. This strategy is a great health tip; avoiding eating heavy foods on top of heavy foods is one of the ways the people of the Mediterranean naturally balance their calorie and fat intake.

Making meals out of appetizers

Traditional Mediterranean cuisine is quite unique in that many people often don't have a main entrée, but instead they eat a series of small side dishes including a variety of different foods, such as meats, beans, vegetables, grains, and fruits. Lunch is the main meal, so dinner is often something light, such as a meze platter. Making dinner out of appetizers is easy because you have a good variety of foods to choose from. Nowadays, you can find many tapas restaurants sprouting up with this same idea of serving several small appetizers as a meal. Here are a few meal ideas using appetizers from this chapter.

- ✔ Simply Stuffed Grape Leaves with the Pan Grilled Shrimp and some sliced raw tomatoes and radishes

- ✔ Greek meatballs with tomato sauce, Italian Bruschetta, and a small tossed green salad with vinaigrette salad dressing

- ✔ Classic Hummus with Toasted Pita Chips and sliced raw assorted vegetables like carrots and bell peppers and Tuna Stuffed Baby Tomatoes

Italian Bruschetta

Prep time: 12 min • **Cook Time:** 3 min • **Yield:** 16 servings

Ingredients	*Directions*
1 French baguette	***1*** Cut the baguette into ½-inch-thick slices and place 6 inches under the broiler for 2 to 3 minutes until toasted. Watch the baguette so it doesn't burn. Once toasted, take out of the oven and set aside.
¼ cup basil, chopped	
6 Roma tomatoes, chopped	
3 cloves garlic, chopped, plus 1 whole clove for rubbing)	***2*** Combine the basil, tomatoes, chopped garlic, olive oil, and salt.
¼ cup olive oil	
½ teaspoon salt	***3*** Cut the ends off the whole garlic clove. After the bread is done broiling, rub each piece with the garlic. Evenly spread the topping mixture on each slice of bread.
	4 Arrange the slices on a platter or individual plates and serve immediately.

Per serving: Calories 119 (From Fat 36); Fat 4g (Saturated 1g); Cholesterol 0mg; Sodium 265mg; Carbohydrate 17g (Dietary Fiber 1g); Protein 4g.

Tip: If you aren't a garlic fan or want a milder flavor, you can skip the garlic all together or add less chopped garlic to the topping. Check out Figure 8-2 for help in chopping garlic if you do use it.

Note: Refer to the color insert for a photo of this recipe.

MINCING GARLIC

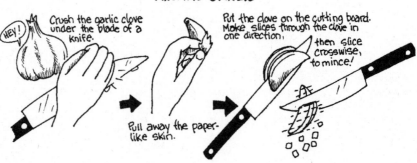

Figure 8-2:
How to chop
garlic.

Pan-Grilled Shrimp

Prep time: 15 min • **Cook time:** 8 min • **Yield:** 6 servings

Ingredients	Directions
24 raw shrimp, peeled and deveined (tail may be intact)	*1* Skewer 4 shrimp ½ inch apart on each of 6 small skewers.
8 cloves garlic, sliced	
¼ cup olive oil	*2* Mix the garlic, olive oil, and cracked pepper in a small skillet. Heat the mixture over medium heat to infuse flavors, about 3 minutes. Remove from the heat and add the lemon zest.
¼ teaspoon cracked red pepper flakes	
1 lemon, zested and cut into 6 wedges	*3* Using a pastry brush, brush both sides of the shrimp skewers with the heated oil mixture.
1 cup parsley, chopped	
Sea salt to taste	*4* Heat a grill pan, cast-iron pan, or griddle over medium high heat. Cook the skewers 1-inch apart for 3 to 4 minutes on each side, or until pink in color. Sprinkle the shrimp evenly with parsley, sea salt, and cracked pepper and serve each with a lemon wedge.
Cracked black pepper to taste	

Per serving: Calories 111 (From Fat 85); Fat 9g (Saturated 1g); Cholesterol 36mg; Sodium 36mg; Carbohydrate 2g (Dietary Fiber 0g); Protein 5g.

Note: If you have to clean and devein your own shrimp, check out Figure 8-3 for guidelines.

CLEANING AND DEVEINING SHRIMP

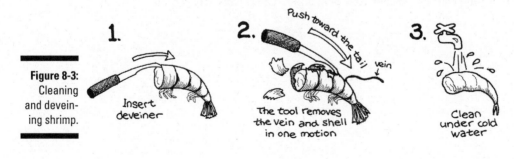

Figure 8-3: Cleaning and deveining shrimp.

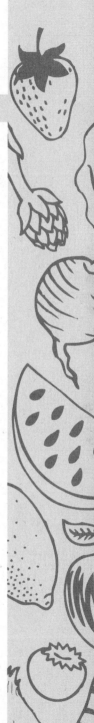

Greek Meatballs in Tomato Sauce

Prep time: 17 min • **Cook time:** 50 min • **Yield:** 10 servings

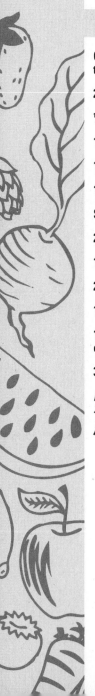

Ingredients	*Directions*
One 28-ounce can diced tomatoes	*1* In a Dutch oven, heat the tomatoes and vegetable stock to a boil over medium-high heat. Reduce the heat to a low simmer and stir in the wine, cumin, coriander, cinnamon, salt, and pepper.
2 cups vegetable stock	
¼ cup dry white wine	
1 teaspoon ground cumin	*2* Meanwhile, combine the ground beef, basmati rice, onions, olive oil, mint, and garlic in a large bowl. Using your hands, knead the mixture and roll into 1-inch balls.
1 teaspoon coriander	
1 teaspoon cinnamon	
Salt and pepper to taste	
2 pounds lean ground beef	*3* Add the meatballs to the sauce and simmer for 40 to 45 minutes or until the meatballs are cooked through, occasionally stirring to coat the meatballs with the sauce. Serve on a warm platter with toothpicks.
1 cup uncooked basmati rice	
2 onions, minced	
1 tablespoon olive oil	
1 teaspoon fresh mint, chopped	
3 cloves garlic, minced	

Per serving: Calories 318 (From Fat 137); Fat 15g (Saturated 6g); Cholesterol 62mg; Sodium 294mg; Carbohydrate 24g (Dietary Fiber 2g); Protein 19g.

Note: If you don't like to cook with alcohol, you can replace it with broth.

Tuna-Stuffed Tomato Bites

Prep time: 20 min • **Yield:** 18 servings

Ingredients	Directions
One 6-ounce can tuna packed in olive oil, drained	**1** Mix the tuna, capers, mayonnaise, vinegar, parsley, and olive oil in a medium bowl. Season the mixture with salt and pepper to taste.
2 tablespoons capers	
1 tablespoon mayonnaise	**2** Cut off the top (stem side) of each tomato and gently remove the insides with a spoon or a grapefruit spoon, being careful not to go through the bottom of the tomato.
1 tablespoon balsamic vinegar	
¼ cup chopped parsley	
Salt and pepper to taste	**3** Fill each tomato with 1 to 2 teaspoons of the tuna mixture; the mixture should be coming out the top. Serve or store in the refrigerator until your guests arrive.
18 large cherry tomatoes (preferably with flat bottoms)	

Per serving: Calories 26 (From Fat 10); Fat 1g (Saturated 0g); Cholesterol 2mg; Sodium 69mg; Carbohydrate 1g (Dietary Fiber 0g); Protein 3g.

Tip: If you can't find flat bottomed tomatoes, you can slice a small sliver off the bottom so that the tomatoes sit flat.

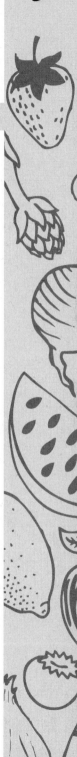

Meaty Grape Leaves (Meat-Filled Dolmas)

Prep time: 20 min • **Cook time:** 55 min • **Yield:** 40 servings

Ingredients	*Directions*
½ **pound lean ground beef**	*1* In a large bowl, mix the beef, rice, onion, mint, parsley, cumin, coriander, olive oil, and garlic.
1 **cup bulgur wheat (small grain) or basmati rice**	
½ **medium onion, minced**	*2* Repeat Steps 2 through 6 of the Stuffed Grape Leaves recipe earlier in this chapter, substituting the meat mixture for the vegetable filling. (See Figure 8-4 for help wrapping grape leaves.)
½ **cup (packed) finely chopped fresh mint**	
½ **cup (packed) finely chopped fresh parsley**	*3* Remove the Dutch oven from the heat, uncover, and cool the dolmas in the pot. Using tongs, gently remove the dolmas from the Dutch oven onto a serving plate and serve them warm or chilled.
1 **teaspoon ground cumin**	
1 **teaspoon coriander**	
¼ **cup extra-virgin olive oil**	
2 **cloves garlic, minced**	
1 **jar grape leaves**	
3 **cups chicken stock**	
Juice of 1 lemon	

Per serving: Calories 46 (From Fat 23); Fat 3g (Saturated 1g); Cholesterol 4mg; Sodium 237mg; Carbohydrate 4g (Dietary Fiber 1g); Protein 3g.

WRAPPING STUFFED GRAPES LEAVES

Figure 8-4:
You can stuff grape leaves with a mixture of your choice.

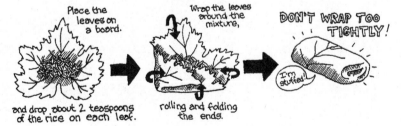

Place the leaves on a board.
and drop about 2 teaspoons of the rice on each leaf.

Wrap the leaves around the mixture,
rolling and folding the ends.

DON'T WRAP TOO TIGHTLY!
I'm stuffed!

Chapter 9

Whipping Up Some Sauces

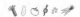
In This Chapter

▶ Making homemade Italian sauces

▶ Crafting classic sauces unique to the Mediterranean coast

You can't have a Mediterranean cookbook without a chapter for sauces to serve with pasta dishes, pizza, and breads. Adding sauces enhances your dish by bringing out amazing flavors and incorporating healthy nutrients from fresh vegetables, herbs, spices, cheese, and yogurt. For example, recipes in this chapter include the following ingredients that create the corresponding health benefits:

✔ **Cooked tomatoes** are high in antioxidants, lycopene, vitamin C, potassium, and folate. These helpful nutrients lower the risk of chronic diseases (such as cardiovascular disease) and certain cancers.

✔ **Basil** (found in pesto) contains vitamin A, an antioxidant that has anti-inflammatory properties and can help reduce your risk of cardiovascular disease, and vitamin K, which can help keep your bones healthy.

✔ **Chickpeas** are a great source of protein, fiber, and folate. Beans of all kinds pack a great nutrient punch to protect you from chronic diseases.

✔ **Yogurt** contains live bacterial cultures, which help keep your gastrointestinal tract in tiptop shape and may also boost your immune system. Plus, yogurt is an excellent source of calcium to help keep your bones strong.

✔ **Almonds** are a great source of protein and healthy fats. They have been shown to help decrease bad cholesterol levels, and their high antioxidant level helps decrease damage to the heart from free radicals. A few studies also show that eating almonds in moderation can help you maintain a trim waistline.

The following chapter shows you some simple homemade sauces. They're so flavorful that a little can go a long way, keeping the flavor strong and the calorie count in check.

We focus on Mediterranean philosophies so the portion sizes of sauce in this section reflect using pasta as a side dish. You can find most of the serving sizes to be around ½ cup to ⅔ cup per serving. If you want to include more sauce, we suggest doubling your sauce recipe accordingly.

Making Classic Italian Sauces

Nothing speaks to the term *sauces* like Italian cooking. Italians use sauces in much of their cooking, from pasta to meat dishes. With Italian cooking, you may hear sauces called by a few different names. *Salsa* refers to meat-less tomato sauces, while *ragu* describes a sauce that has one or two meats added. If you come from an Italian family, you likely also hear the term *gravy* in relation to any sauce. In this section, you get to sample a variety of sauce recipes sure to fill your kitchen with wonderful aromas.

Tomatoes: The best base for sauce

You may be surprised to discover that toma-toes didn't originate in Italy or Europe at all. Tomatoes reached Europe during the 16th century after originating in South America. Although the Spanish were likely the first to use tomatoes for cooking, the Italians are best known for bringing out the tomato's full culinary potential (despite the fact that they originally used the fruit for tabletop decoration). Tomato sauce opened up a world of flavors for pasta and other dishes; the simple addition of differ-ent herbs, meats, and cheeses created a vari-ety of sauces for different occasions and meals.

You can set the stage for meals by tweaking tomato sauce with different ingredients. Try the following variations on the Marinara in this chapter. Just add

- Sautéed mushrooms and kalamata olives
- Blanched broccoli, cauliflower, carrots, and bell peppers
- Cream at the end for a quick cream sauce
- Black olives, capers, and oregano for Sicilian flair
- A little red wine (about ¼ cup)
- Seafood (such as crab meat and shrimp)
- Cooked chicken breast cut into 3-inch pieces
- Prosciutto
- Ground cumin, coriander, and lemon zest for a Greek sauce

You can also add more or less of a spice to get the flavor you desire. Meri's family has always favored a more savory sauce with more oregano and less basil. Experiment in your own kitchen to find your favorites.

Marinara

Prep time: 5 min • **Cook time:** 35 min • **Yield:** 4 servings

Ingredients	*Directions*
12 plum or Roma tomatoes	**1** Bring 4 quarts of water to a boil. Blanch the tomatoes in the water for 1 minute and shock them to halt the cooking process. Remove the skins of the tomatoes and roughly chop.
¼ cup olive oil	
½ small onion, minced	
2 cloves garlic, minced	**2** In a large skillet, heat the olive oil over medium heat. Add the onion, garlic, and celery and sauté for 8 minutes. Add the tomatoes, basil, and parsley and simmer for 20 to 25 minutes. Season with salt and serve.
¼ cup celery, minced	
¼ cup basil leaves, torn	
2 tablespoons parsley, chopped	
Salt to taste	

Per serving: Calories 169 (From Fat 125); Fat 14g (Saturated 2g); Cholesterol 0mg; Sodium 18mg; Carbohydrate 11g (Dietary Fiber 3g); Protein 2g.

Note: To prepare the tomatoes for blanching, cut a T in the bottom of each tomato to just pierce the skin. After blanching, shock the tomatoes by immediately placing them in ice water.

Note: Store sauce in an airtight container in the refrigerator for up to a week or freeze for two to three months.

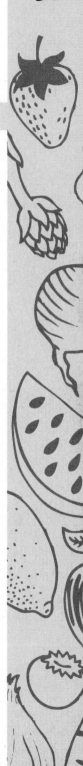

Red Wine Marinara

Prep time: 10 min • **Cook time:** 1 hr • **Yield:** 6 servings

Ingredients	*Directions*
2 tablespoons olive oil	**1** In a large saucepan, heat the olive oil over medium heat. Add the onions and sauté for 5 minutes. Add in the garlic and cook for 5 minutes. Add the tomatoes and black olives and cook for 5 minutes.
1 medium onion, chopped	
6 cloves garlic, chopped	
8 cups plum or Roma tomatoes, chopped	**2** Stir in the wine, tomato paste, parsley, oregano, and red pepper flakes. Bring the mixture to a boil and reduce the heat to a low simmer for 45 minutes or until the sauce has thickened. Season the sauce with salt and pepper before serving.
½ cup black olives, pitted and chopped	
½ cup dry red wine	
2 tablespoons tomato paste	
½ cup parsley, chopped	
2 teaspoons dried oregano	
½ teaspoon red pepper flakes	
Salt and pepper to taste	

Per serving: Calories 107 (From Fat 52); Fat 6g (Saturated 1g); Cholesterol 0mg; Sodium 130mg; Carbohydrate 10g (Dietary Fiber 2g); Protein 2g.

Note: Store sauce in an airtight container in the refrigerator for up to a week or freeze for two to three months.

Garden Sauce

Prep time: 20 min • **Cook time:** 15 min • **Yield:** 4 servings

Ingredients	*Directions*
8 plum or Roma tomatoes **1 carrot, julienned** **(see Figure 9-1)** **2 zucchinis, julienned**	*1* Bring 4 quarts of water to a boil. Blanch the tomatoes in the water for 1 minute and shock them to halt the cooking process. Remove the skins of the tomatoes and roughly chop.
1 yellow squash, seeded and julienned **1 red bell pepper, seeded and julienned** **2 tablespoons olive oil**	*2* Blanch the carrots in the same pot of water for 1 minute; add the zucchini, squash, and bell pepper and blanch for an additional minute. Shock the blanched vegetables to halt cooking.
1 onion, julienned **3 cloves garlic, sliced** **½ cup dry white wine**	*3* In a large skillet, heat the olive oil over medium-high heat for 2 minutes. Add the onion and garlic and sauté for 1 minute. Add the tomatoes, carrots, zucchinis, squash, and bell peppers and sauté for 3 minutes.
¼ cup parsley **Salt and pepper to taste**	*4* Stir in the wine and parsley and bring the mixture to a boil. Reduce the heat to low for 1 minute, add salt and pepper to taste, and serve with pasta.

Per serving: Calories 196 (From Fat 71); Fat 8g (Saturated 1g); Cholesterol 0mg; Sodium 43mg; Carbohydrate 25g (Dietary Fiber 6g); Protein 5g.

Note: To prepare the tomatoes for blanching, cut a T in the bottom of each tomato to just pierce the skin. After blanching, shock the tomatoes by immediately placing them in ice water.

Tip: For a thicker sauce, add 1 to 2 tablespoons of tomato paste when you add the wine. Store sauce in an airtight container in the refrigerator for up to a week or freeze up to two to three months.

JULIENNE A CARROT

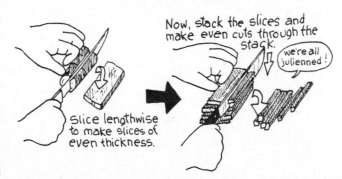

Now, stack the slices and make even cuts through the stack.

we're all julienned!

Figure 9-1: Julienne a carrot by stacking slices and cutting into matchstick-sized pieces.

Slice lengthwise to make slices of even thickness.

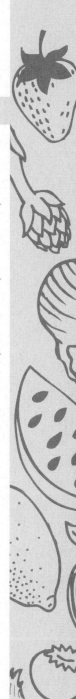

Meat Sauce

Prep time: 10 min • **Cook time:** 46 min • **Yield:** 6 servings

Ingredients

1 tablespoon olive oil

1 pound lean ground beef

½ teaspoon salt

1 large onion, chopped

3 cloves garlic, minced

1 teaspoon dried parsley, or 2 tablespoons fresh

2 teaspoons dried basil, crumbled, or ¼ cup fresh

2 teaspoons dried oregano, crumbled, or ¼ cup fresh

One 28-ounce can Italian diced tomatoes, drained

One 8-ounce can tomato sauce

1 teaspoon sugar

Directions

1 Heat the oil in large, heavy skillet over medium-high heat. Add the ground beef and sprinkle with the salt. Cook the beef until brown about 3 to 5 minutes, breaking it up with fork. Using a slotted spoon, transfer the beef to a plate.

2 Add the onions and garlic to the skillet and sauté until the onion is tender, about 5 minutes. Depending on how lean your beef is, you may need to add a teaspoon of oil to the pan. Stir in the parsley, basil, and oregano and cook 1 minute. Return the beef to the skillet and stir in the tomatoes, tomato sauce, and sugar. Reduce the heat to medium-low and simmer until the sauce is thick, about 45 minutes.

Per serving: Calories 232 (From Fat 125); Fat 14g (Saturated 5g); Cholesterol 51mg; Sodium 545mg; Carbohydrate 12g (Dietary Fiber 2g); Protein 16g.

Tip: Sugar is often added to sauces to decrease the bitterness of the tomatoes. You can eliminate the sugar by adding ½ cup of shredded carrots when you add the onions.

Note: Store sauce in an airtight container in the refrigerator for 3 to 5 days or freeze for up to a month.

Pizza Sauce

Prep time: 5 min • **Cook time:** 40 min • **Yield:** 3–4 pizzas (4 cups, 16 servings)

Ingredients	Directions
3 tablespoons extra-virgin olive oil 1 small onion, minced 3 cloves garlic, minced One 28-ounce can diced tomatoes 2 tablespoons red wine vinegar 1 tablespoon sugar 1 tablespoon fresh thyme ¼ cup fresh parsley, chopped ½ teaspoon red pepper flakes, or to taste Salt and pepper to taste	**1** In a large saucepan, heat the olive oil over medium heat. Add the onions and garlic and sauté for 5 minutes. Strain the diced tomatoes and add to the saucepan, and cook for 5 minutes. **2** Add the vinegar, sugar, thyme, parsley, and red pepper flakes and bring the mixture to a boil. Reduce the heat and simmer for 25 minutes or until the sauce thickens. Season with salt and pepper to taste. **3** Blend the sauce with a blender, stick blender, or food processor until smooth. Cool slightly before adding to pizza dough.

Per serving: Calories 42 (From Fat 24); Fat 3g (Saturated 0g); Cholesterol 0mg; Sodium 73mg; Carbohydrate 5g (Dietary Fiber 1g); Protein 1g.

Tip: You can store this sauce in the refrigerator for 1 week or freeze it for three months to enjoy later. You'll never buy store-bought sauce again.

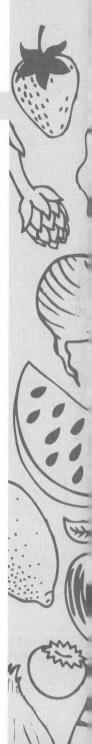

Béchamel

Prep time: 5 min • **Cook time:** 12 min • **Yield:** 8 servings

Ingredients	Directions
¼ cup butter, cut into cubes	**1** Melt the butter in a heavy saucepan. Whisk in the flour and cook over low heat for 3 minutes. Raise the heat to medium and whisk in the milk.
4 tablespoons flour	
2 cups milk	
¼ teaspoon paprika	**2** Continue to whisk the sauce until it thickens, about 6 minutes. Add the paprika and nutmeg. Season with salt and pepper and serve.
⅛ teaspoon nutmeg	
Salt and white pepper to taste	

Per serving: Calories 91 (From Fat 57); Fat 6g (Saturated 4g); Cholesterol 18mg; Sodium 28mg; Carbohydrate 6g (Dietary Fiber 0g); Protein 3g.

Note: Béchamel is a basic white sauce that serves as the base of most cheese sauces. You add your cheese(s) of choice before the salt and pepper; use whatever amounts suit your need and tastes.

Tip: Add more milk to create a thinner sauce.

Note: Store in the refrigerator in an airtight container for 3 to 5 days.

Pesto

Prep time: 10 min • **Yield:** 8 servings

Ingredients	Directions
5 cups basil	**1** In a food processor, pulse the basil, garlic, and red chili pepper flakes ten times. Add the pine nuts and cheese and blend for 1 minute.
3 to 6 cloves garlic, crushed	
¼ teaspoon red pepper flakes	
½ cup pine nuts	**2** Turn the food processor on and slowly drizzle in the olive oil, adding more if needed. Season with salt and serve.
1 cup grated Parmesan cheese	
½ cup olive oil	
Salt to taste	

Per serving: Calories 235 (From Fat 207); Fat 23g (Saturated 4g); Cholesterol 11mg; Sodium 192mg; Carbohydrate 2g (Dietary Fiber 1g); Protein 7g.

Tip: You can keep pesto in the refrigerator for a week; be sure to store with a top layer of olive oil. You can also freeze pesto for three months. Olive oil on the surface is not needed when freezing.

Tip: To preserve the bright green color of the basil in your pesto, drop the leaves in 4 quarts of boiling water for 20 seconds and then quickly strain them and place them into ice water. Drain and pat the leaves dry to remove excess water.

Vary It! Replace half the basil with arugula and the pine nuts with walnuts.

Vary It! Replace the basil with cilantro, the pine nuts with almonds, and the Parmesan with manchego cheese.

Vary It! Replace half the basil with spinach and the pine nuts with walnuts or almonds.

Note: Check out the color insert for a photo of this recipe.

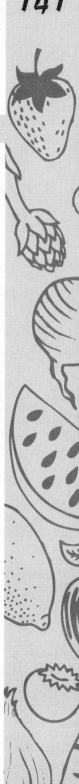

Gremolata

Prep time: 5 min • **Yield:** ½ cup (⅓ cup); 4 servings

Ingredients	*Directions*
1 teaspoon lemon zest (see Figure 9-2)	*1* Combine all the ingredients in a small bowl.
1 tablespoon lemon juice	
¼ cup parsley, chopped	
4 cloves garlic, chopped	
¼ cup olive oil	

Per serving: Calories 127 (From Fat 122); Fat 14g (Saturated 2g); Cholesterol 0mg; Sodium 3mg; Carbohydrate 2g (Dietary Fiber 0g); Protein 0g.

Note: Serve this sauce over pasta with pine nuts or use it with lamb, beef, or fish dishes for a punch of flavor. You can also add it to bean soups or stews.

Note: Store in the refrigerator in an airtight container for up to a week.

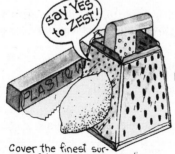
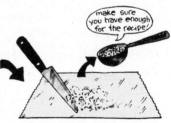

Figure 9-2: You can use a grater to zest lemons and other citrus fruits.

Say YES to ZEST!

Cover the finest surface of the grater with plastic wrap.
Rub the citrus across the plastic-covered surface... (JUST THE COLORED PART! NOT THE BITTER WHITE PITH)!

make sure you have enough for the recipe!

When you think you've grated enough, lift off the plastic and scrape up the zest with a flat edge.
Use a measuring spoon to see if you've grated enough.

Creating the Mediterranean Standbys

You may associate sauces with Italian cooking, but many other regions along the Mediterranean also have some classics of their own. You'd be hard-pressed to find a Greek meal without yogurt sauce nearby. This section shows you some quintessential Greek, Moroccan, and Spanish sauces.

Using your leftover sauce in unexpected ways

One great time-saving tip is to double or triple your sauce recipes and make enough to freeze for later use. While you can continue to use your sauce for pasta dishes, don't limit yourself; be imaginative and use your leftover tomato-based sauces in all sorts of ways. Here are some ideas:

✔ Pour sauce over stuffed peppers or stuffed tomatoes.

✔ Use it in your meatloaf recipe to provide moisture to your meat and amazing flavor.

✔ Stew some chicken pieces in sauce until the chicken are cooked for a full-flavored and tender chicken dish.

✔ Bake mini calzones using pizza crust (see Chapter 16) and your favorite fixings. Use either your leftover pizza sauce or tomato sauce for dipping!

✔ Use overbaked polenta for a flavorful and easy-to-make side dish.

✔ Pour tomato sauce over stuffed Portobello mushrooms.

✔ Use left-over sauce as a base for vegetable soups.

✔ Mix with cooked garbanzo beans for a simple and delicious side dish.

✔ Serve as a dipping sauce for bread sticks.

✔ Layer on a bun with a grilled chicken sandwich for an Italian flavor.

Chickpea Sauce

Prep time: 8 min • **Cook time:** 30 min • **Yield:** 6 servings

Ingredients	*Directions*
One 14.5 ounce can chickpeas, drained and rinsed	*1* Blend the chickpeas in a food processor for 1 minute. Add the water and blend until smooth.
1 cup water	
¼ cup olive oil	*2* In a heavy skillet, heat the olive oil over medium heat. Add the red chili pepper flakes and garlic and cook for 1 minute. Add the onion, parsley, basil, and bay leaf and cook for 8 minutes.
½ teaspoon red chili pepper flakes	
2 cloves garlic	
1 onion, chopped	*3* Add the chickpeas and tomatoes to the skillet and simmer for 20 minutes. Season with salt and pepper. If the sauce is too thick, stir in about ¼ cup hot water to thin it out. Remove the bay leaf and serve.
2 tablespoon parsley, chopped	
½ cup basil leaves, torn	
1 bay leaf	
One 14.5-ounce can diced tomatoes	
Salt and pepper to taste	

Per serving: Calories 192 (From Fat 89); Fat 10g (Saturated 1g); Cholesterol 0mg; Sodium 308mg; Carbohydrate 23g (Dietary Fiber 4g); Protein 4g.

Tip: This rustic sauce is excellent over any pasta. Just dust the dish with manchego or any hard, white cheese.

Note: Store in the refrigerator in an airtight container for up to a week.

Cucumber Yogurt Sauce

Prep time: 5 min • **Yield:** 12 servings

Ingredients	*Directions*
2 cups Greek yogurt	*1* Place yogurt into a bowl. Grate the cucumber into the yogurt and stir. Season the yogurt mixture with the remaining ingredients. Store in the refrigerator until ready to serve.
1 cucumber, peeled and seeded	
Zest and juice of 1 lemon	
¼ cup mint, minced	
2 cloves garlic, minced	

Per serving: Calories 24 (From Fat 0); Fat 0g (Saturated 0g); Cholesterol 0mg; Sodium 18mg; Carbohydrate 2g (Dietary Fiber 0g); Protein 4g.

Tip: If you can't find Greek yogurt, place a container of regular yogurt upside down in a coffee-filter- or cheesecloth-lined strainer and over a bowl. Store the setup in the refrigerator overnight until the yogurt thickens.

Tip: This sauce makes a great addition to any grilled meat or kabobs.

Note: Store in the refrigerator for up to a week.

Focusing on flavor

When many people think of the word "healthy," they immediately think of eating something that tastes like cardboard, but we assure you that that flavor profile isn't the case with the Mediterranean diet. You won't find the people of the Mediterranean coast eating plain baked chicken and white rice. They're known for big flavors that utilize lots of impactful ingredients such as strong cheeses, fresh herbs and spices, vinegars, olives, garlic, and onions.

Even quick, everyday meals are delicious and full of flavor. Cooking up some of the recipes in this book can help take "boring" and "bland" out of your healthy food vocabulary.

Don't wait until your next party to serve something outstanding. You can easily delight your taste buds every night by using the recipes in this book to enjoy healthy food the Mediterranean way!

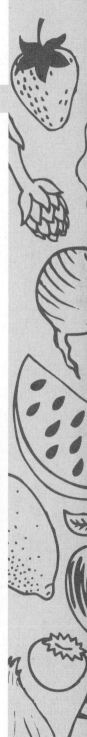

Spanish Almond Sauce

Prep time: 25 min • **Cook time:** 8 min • **Yield:** 10 servings

Ingredients	*Directions*
1 red bell pepper, cut in half and seeded	*1* Preheat the broiler with the rack 5 inches from the heat. Place the bell pepper halves on a baking sheet, cut side down, and broil until the skin is bubbled and slightly blackened.
1 cup almonds, dry-roasted	
½ cup hazelnuts	
2 cloves garlic	*2* Place the roasted peppers in a paper bag or cover with a towel for 5 minutes until they're cool to touch and the skins are easy to remove.
½ teaspoon red pepper flakes	
½ cup olive oil	
2 tablespoons sherry vinegar	*3* Blend the skinned peppers, almonds, hazelnuts, garlic, and red pepper flakes in a food processor for 1 minute. Whisk together the olive oil and vinegar.
¼ cup heavy cream	
Salt to taste	
	4 Turn on the food processor and begin drizzling the vinegar mixture into the nut mixture. Continuing to blend, drizzle in the cream. Season with salt before serving.

Per serving: Calories 247 (From Fat 220); Fat 24g (Saturated 4g); Cholesterol 8mg; Sodium 50mg; Carbohydrate 5g (Dietary Fiber 3g); Protein 4g.

Tip: This sauce is great as a dip for vegetables or grilled shrimp or as a sauce over pasta or fish.

Tip: For a thinner sauce, add more cream or olive oil depending on your tastes.

Note: Freeze this sauce in an airtight container for up to a month. Store in the refrigerator for up to a week.

Chapter 10

Creating Fresh Delicious Salads

*I*n the Mediterranean, farming is big business, which means an abundance of fruits, vegetables, beans, herbs, nuts, and olives are available. Salads are one way folks in the Mediterranean incorporate all this fresh produce into their daily lives. In the Mediterranean, salads are often the starter for a meal, but you can also find some regions that eat the salad after the main course. Bean salads and other vegetable salads make a popular side with a meal, and some salads are big enough to be the entire meal. Healthwise, all these options are great ways to get those extra veggies!

Making salads a regular part of your dining experience is a good habit to get into for several reasons:

✔ They help you feel full even though you're taking in fewer calories (depending on the toppings and amount of dressing).

✔ They increase your intake of vitamins, minerals, and phytochemicals, helping you to prevent diseases.

✔ They add more fiber in your diet, which helps with weight management, colon health, and heart health.

This chapter shows you some amazing salad choices that you can include with your next lunch or dinner.

REMEMBER

Always wash your salad veggies thoroughly in water, especially if you get them fresh from the garden or farmers' market.

Eating Your Veggies Fresh from the Garden

Using salads as a regular part of your diet is a great, easy way to add a variety of healthful, nutrient-rich ingredients. For example, cooking broccoli as a side is a wonderful choice, but that dish only provides the nutrients found in that one food. Salads, on the other hand, offer the nutrients of many different foods, such as greens, tomatoes, cucumbers, and beans, in one dish. And that doesn't even begin to cover the flavors and textures that a variety of foods provides; nothing's better than the sweet taste of a tomato next to the crunchy texture of a cold cucumber.

If you're beginning to get excited at the sound of a fresh, ripe tomato or cucumber adorning your plate, the Mediterranean spirit is beginning to build within you. This section shows you some simple steps to improve your health with amazingly flavorful salads.

Picking the best greens for your next salad

Not too long ago, the main selections of salad greens you'd find in your local grocery store pretty much began and ended with iceberg, romaine, and red leaf lettuces. Now you can find a whole assortment of greens you can purchase separately or prewashed and mixed together in bags. Knowing what flavors to expect can help you pick the right greens for your salads. Use these descriptions to help you navigate the world of salad greens:

✔ **Iceberg lettuce:** Pale, crisp iceberg lettuce has a mild flavor due to its high water content. This salad green is great to add to other salad mixes for a crunchy texture. Although iceberg isn't nutrient-dense, it's low in calories and helps improve your water intake.

✔ **Romaine lettuce:** Romaine is a large leaf with a white stem that provides a crunchier texture to your salad. The flavor is mild and can be a wonderful addition to any salad combination.

✔ **Leaf lettuce:** Green leaf and red leaf lettuce are popular in American cuisine. They have

a light flavor, and their uneven leaves provide lots of great texture for any salad base.

✔ **Arugula:** Arugula originates from the Mediterranean coast and has a bitter, peppery flavor you won't mistake for any other green. If you're looking for strong flavor to add a special kick, arugula's your leaf.

✔ **Butterhead:** *Butterhead,* or *bibb,* lettuce is a head of lettuce with a very soft, delicate texture and a full flavor. This lettuce is a little on the pricey side, so you can also use its sister lettuce, Boston butterhead, which isn't as soft but is similar in texture and taste. You can use these lettuces as a base in any salad; they go very nicely with fruit.

✔ **Dandelion greens:** Dandelion greens have a bitter flavor and delicate texture, adding a big punch of flavor to your next mixed green salad. To balance out the strong flavor, combine these greens with milder flavors such as green leaf or romaine. Dandelion greens also go well with salty flavors such as olives or capers.

Greek Salad

Prep time: 12 min • **Yield:** 4 servings

Ingredients	Directions
8 cups romaine lettuce, torn into bite-sized pieces	*1* Place the torn lettuce leaves into a large salad bowl. Slice the tomatoes into 8 wedges each and place on top of the lettuce. Add the cucumbers, olives, green onions, and parsley.
4 medium tomatoes	
2 medium cucumbers, seeded and diced	
½ cup kalamata olives, pitted and chopped	*2* In a small bowl, whisk together the lemon juice, olive oil, and garlic. Season the dressing with salt and pepper to taste. Pour over the salad and toss. Sprinkle the salad with the feta cheese and serve immediately.
6 green onions, chopped	
¼ cup fresh flat leaf parsley, chopped	
Juice of 1 large lemon	
⅓ cup olive oil	
1 clove garlic, minced	
Salt and pepper to taste	
4 ounces crumbled feta cheese	

Per serving: Calories 264 (From Fat 194); Fat 22g (Saturated 5g); Cholesterol 17mg; Sodium 280mg; Carbohydrate 16g (Dietary Fiber 5g); Protein 6g.

Tip: Use prewashed/pre-torn bagged romaine lettuce from your local grocery store to save a little time. Figure 10-1 demonstrates how to pit an olive.

Note: Flip to the color insert for a photo of this salad.

PITTING OLIVES

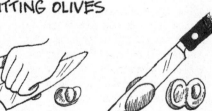

Figure 10-1: How to pit an olive.

SQUEEZE THE OLIVE BETWEEN YOUR THUMB AND FOREFINGER AND SQUEEZE TILL THE PIT COMES OUT.

OR USE A KITCHEN KNIFE TO PRESS DOWN TO SEPARATE THE FLESH FROM THE PIT.

OR USE A SHARP KNIFE TO CUT ALL THE WAY AROUND THE OLIVE AND REMOVE THE PIT WITH YOUR FINGER.

Italian Bread Salad

Prep time: 12 min • **Cook time:** 15 min • **Yield:** 4 servings

Ingredients	*Directions*
½ **pound day-old French bread or other crusty bread**	*1* Cut the bread into one-inch cubes. Heat a cast-iron or heavy skillet over medium-high heat. Place the bread cubes into the skillet and toast until slightly browned.
4 medium tomatoes, large diced	
1 English cucumber, seeded and diced	
½ **small red onion, sliced thin**	*2* In a serving bowl, combine the tomatoes (including the juice), cucumber, and onion. Top with the toasted bread.
½ **cup extra-virgin olive oil**	
¼ **cup red wine vinegar**	
8 basil leaves, sliced into long strips	*3* Mix the oil, vinegar, and basil in a small bowl and season with salt and pepper to taste. Pour over the salad and toss gently before serving.
Salt and pepper to taste	

Per serving: Calories 440 (From Fat 255); Fat 28g (Saturated 4g); Cholesterol 0mg; Sodium 378mg; Carbohydrate 40g (Dietary Fiber 3g); Protein 8g.

Note: Some people prefer to let the salad season for 30 minutes at room temperature prior to adding the toasted bread. Refer to the color insert in this book for a photo of this salad.

(Nearly) 20-minute Mediterranean meals

One of the hardest parts about making diet changes is finding the time to devote to cooking new recipes and trying out a different style of eating. Falling back on your old standby habits, such as prepackaged meals, is easy when you're pressed for time. But in the time you'd take to make that boxed mac and cheese or dump some pre-made sauce on a bunch of spaghetti, you can make a Mediterranean meal that includes a protein, several vegetables, and some grains by using some of the recipes in this book.

The trick to preparing multiple items for one meal in a short period of time is to do all your prep work for all the dishes at once. You can easily work on another dish with all your ingredients on hand. To get you started, here are some sample meals that take around 20 minutes to prepare and utilize recipes in this book:

✔ Smoked Salmon and Arugula Salad (Chapter 10) with a slice of crusty whole-wheat bread dipped in olive oil

✔ Shrimp Pasta with Kalamata Olives and Feta Cheese (Chapter 15) and a mixed green salad with sliced cucumbers and tomatoes and vinaigrette salad dressing

✔ Marsala Scallops (Chapter 18), Black Beans with Tomatoes and Feta (Chapter 14), and a slice of crusty whole-wheat bread dipped in olive oil

✔ Tortellini with Vegetables and Pesto (Chapter 15) with a mixed green side salad topped with walnuts and vinaigrette salad dressing

Pomegranate Salad

Prep time: 8 min • **Cook time:** 7 min • **Yield:** 4 servings

Ingredients	*Directions*
2 tablespoons plus 2 tablespoons olive oil 8 ounces chilled halloumi cheese, cut into ¼-inch-thick slices	*1* In a large, heavy cast-iron or nonstick skillet, heat 2 tablespoons of the oil over medium-high heat. Add the cheese, being careful not to crowd the pan, and lower the temperature to medium-low.
6 cups baby arugula leaves or spinach 1 cup fresh mint leaves, sliced into long, thin strips	*2* Cook the cheese for 2 minutes on each side or until a golden brown crust is achieved. Place the cooked cheese on paper towels to drain; remove the excess oil from the pan and reserve for the salad.
½ cup pistachios ½ cup pomegranate seeds	*3* In a serving bowl, toss together the arugula, mint, pistachios, and pomegranate seeds.
¼ cup bottled pomegranate juice 1 tablespoon lemon juice Salt and pepper to taste	*4* In a small saucepan, heat the pomegranate juice over medium heat until it reduces by half, about 3 minutes. Remove from the heat, add the remaining olive oil and the lemon juice, and season with salt and pepper to taste.
	5 Toss the salad mixture with ¼ cup of the dressing. Arrange the cheese slices on top of the salad, drizzle with the remainder of the dressing, and serve.

Per serving: Calories 419 (From Fat 307); Fat 34g (Saturated 10g); Cholesterol 45mg; Sodium 418mg; Carbohydrate 14g (Dietary Fiber 4g); Protein 18g.

Note: Halloumi cheese is a popular cheese used in Greece and found in specialty stores. You can also buy it online. If you can't find it, buy slices of mozzarella cheese; brush them with egg whites and dust with bread crumbs prior to cooking so they don't melt.

Tip: Take a look at Figure 10-2 for help seeding a pomegranate.

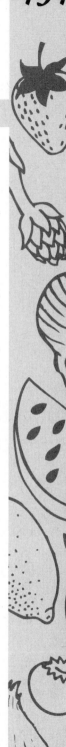

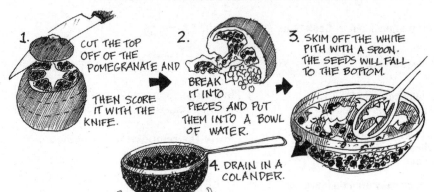

REMOVING SEEDS FROM A POMEGRANATE

1. CUT THE TOP OFF OF THE POMEGRANATE AND THEN SCORE IT WITH THE KNIFE.

2. BREAK IT INTO PIECES AND PUT THEM INTO A BOWL OF WATER.

3. SKIM OFF THE WHITE PITH WITH A SPOON. THE SEEDS WILL FALL TO THE BOTTOM.

4. DRAIN IN A COLANDER.

Figure 10-2:
Seeding a
pomegranate.

Making room for pomegranates

Pomegranates are common in Mediterranean cooking for both their seeds and their juice. Pomegranates are actually an ancient fruit mentioned in early Greek literature; their long history makes the lack of pomegranates in the average American's diet somewhat surprising. For many, using pomegranates may seem a little intimidating. After all, how often do you cut open a fruit to have gobs of juicy, bright red seeds seeds spill out?

Pomegranate juice and seeds are both good sources of vitamin C, potassium, and phytochemicals. Eating the seeds gives you an extra benefit in the form of fiber that you can't get from the juice alone. Limited research has been done in respect to pomegranates, but a few studies indicate that they can increase antioxidant activity in the body and decrease blood pressure.

Here are some delicious ways to enjoy pomegranates more often in your day-to-day routine:

- Eat the seeds as a snack; just keep some napkins handy because they can get messy!

- Add the seeds to your yogurt for a sweet crunch.

- Toss the seeds with a green salad to add sweetness, texture, and beautiful color

- Mix the juice with carbonated water for a delightful drink.

- Combine the juice with oil and seasonings for a fresh salad dressing. Check out the Pomegranate Salad recipe in this chapter to see how it's done!

Tomato, Cucumber, and Basil Salad

Prep time: 12 min • **Yield:** 8 servings

Ingredients	*Directions*
8 Roma tomatoes	**1** Slice each tomato into 6 wedges. Cut off both ends of the cucumber and slice it lengthwise down the middle. With a spoon, scrape out the seeds. Slice the cucumber into half moons about ¼-inch thick.
1 large cucumber	
¼ cup red onion, cut into ⅛-inch slices and then halved	
¼ cup fresh basil leaves, cut into thin strips	**2** In a large serving bowl, toss together everything but the salt and pepper. Season with salt and pepper and serve.
2 tablespoons olive oil	
3 tablespoons balsamic vinegar	
¼ cup feta cheese	
Salt and pepper to taste	

Per serving: Calories 65 (From Fat 41); Fat 5g (Saturated 1g); Cholesterol 4mg; Sodium 58mg; Carbohydrate 5g (Dietary Fiber 1g); Protein 2g.

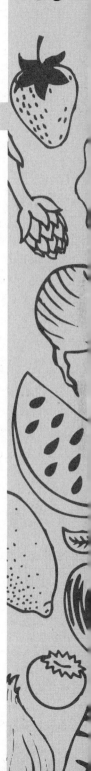

Eggplant and Tomato Stacks with Pesto

Prep time: 30 min • **Cook time:** 8 min • **Yield:** 4 servings

Ingredients	Directions
1½ teaspoons sea salt	**1** To extract the bitterness from the eggplant, layer several paper towels on a plate. Place about 1 teaspoon of the sea salt on the towels and stack the eggplant rounds in a single layer. Sprinkle the remaining ½ teaspoon of sea salt on top of the eggplant slices.
1 eggplant, sliced into ½-inch rounds	
1 cup basil leaves, plus 12 to 15 more leaves for stacking	
2 tablespoons pine nuts	**2** Top the eggplant with another layer of paper towels and then stack a plate on top of that. Weigh the plate down and allow to sit for 20 to 30 minutes.
1 clove garlic	
2 tablespoons olive oil	
Juice and zest of 1 lemon	**3** Meanwhile, to create the pesto, blend 1 cup of the basil leaves, pine nuts, garlic, olive oil, lemon juice and zest, and salt and pepper to taste in a food processor or blender for 2 to 3 minutes or until smooth. Set aside.
Salt and pepper to taste	
Nonstick cooking spray	
2 to 3 beefsteak or Roma tomatoes, sliced into ½-inch rounds	**4** Rinse the eggplant well and pat dry. Spray the eggplant (lightly) and the grill with nonstick cooking spray and heat the grill to medium-high heat. Grill each eggplant round about 3 to 5 minutes on each side or until you achieve the desired texture.
⅓ cup freshly grated Parmesan cheese	
	5 On a serving plate, stack a grilled eggplant round, 1 teaspoon of the pesto, 1 tomato slice, and 1 teaspoon pesto. Top with a basil leaf. Repeat until you use all the eggplant. Top with the freshly grated Parmesan cheese and serve.

Per serving: Calories 174 (From Fat 111); Fat 12g (Saturated 3g); Cholesterol 7mg; Sodium 996mg; Carbohydrate 13g (Dietary Fiber 6g); Protein 6g.

Note: You can use one eggplant round per stack, or add visual height to your plate by making double-decker stacks (although doing so will reduce the number of stacks).

Chickpea Salad

Prep time: 20 min • **Cook time:** 5 min • **Yield:** 6 servings

Ingredients	*Directions*
1 cup chicken or vegetable broth	*1* In a small saucepan, bring the broth to a boil over high heat. Add the barley, cover, and remove the pot from the heat to rest for 15 minutes.
½ cup pearl barley	
One 15-ounce can chickpeas, rinsed and drained	*2* Meanwhile, combine the chickpeas, apricots, onion, parsley, lemon zest and juice, olive oil, and spices in a bowl.
1 cup diced dried apricots	
1 small red onion, thinly sliced	*3* Add the cooked barley and stir to mix well. Add the hot sauce and sea salt to taste. Place the baby spinach leaves on a serving platter and spoon the warmed chickpea/barley mixture over the top. Top the salad with the pistachios and serve.
1 cup parsley, chopped and stems discarded	
Zest and juice of 2 lemons	
¼ cup olive oil	
¼ teaspoon pepper	
¼ teaspoon cardamom	
⅛ teaspoon ginger	
⅛ teaspoon cinnamon	
¼ teaspoon turmeric	
Dash of hot sauce	
Sea salt to taste	
8 cups baby spinach leaves	
1 cup shelled pistachios	

Per serving: Calories 368 (From Fat 184); Fat 20g (Saturated 3g); Cholesterol 0mg; Sodium 580mg; Carbohydrate 39g (Dietary Fiber 8g); Protein 12g.

Getting to the Fruit of Things

Fruit grows in abundance in the Mediterranean, and people who live along the Mediterranean coast eat more fruits in general than Americans do, which contributes to the Mediterranean's higher levels of disease prevention. Fruits are often a breakfast component, a midmorning snack, or even a dessert. In the Mediterranean, you actually see vendors selling fruits on street corners, which makes snacking on fruit while moving through your day easy. The following section demonstrates a few ways to create healthy side-dish fruit salads for your next meal or party.

Fresh from the branch: Fruits of the Mediterranean

Fruits grow plentifully in the Mediterranean climate, but some are more popular than others. Although you may readily find some of these fruits in your local grocery store, many of them are only available during certain seasons, and some may be hard to find in your area. Here are the most commonly planted fruit trees of the Mediterranean and some tips on where you can find these fruits without hopping across the pond:

✔ *Mandarin oranges* are known as *easy-peel* oranges because their skin is loose and easy to peel into segments. They have a sweet flavor and a fresh citrus aroma. Harvest begins in mid-September, and the season lasts until April or May. In the United States, you can find Clementine and Satsuma varieties in most chain grocery stores during the winter months, often beginning in December and going through March.

✔ *Figs* are a small fruit with a mild, sweet flavor. Most people think of figs as the sticky sweet spread in certain cookies or as dried figs, but if you've never eaten a fresh fig, you may be pleasantly surprised by its milder, less-sweet taste. Figs are ready to pick during the summer months in warm climates such as California. Fresh figs may not be easy to find in your local grocery store or farmers' market, but don't worry; you can order fresh figs and have them sent to your door from www.figlady.com/.

✔ *Persimmons* are native to East Asia and have been grown in the Mediterranean for a century. These yellow, orange, or red fruits look like a cross between an orange and a tomato, and if you've ever seen one in the store, you've probably wondered which of the two it was. They're sweet when fully ripened but can be a bit bitter if you eat them too early. The persimmon harvest is from late September to early December. Persimmons are tasty when mixed with other fall fruits, such as raisins or sliced apples. If you can't find them in your local grocery store, you can order them online at www.agbase.com under "Fruit."

Apple and Walnut Salad

Prep time: 15 min • **Yield:** 6 servings

Ingredients	Directions
Juice and zest of ½ an orange	**1** In a serving bowl, whisk together the orange juice and zest, honey, and olive oil. Add the apples and apricots and toss to coat. Add the walnuts, toss again, and serve.
2 tablespoons honey	
1 tablespoon olive oil	
4 medium Rome or Gala apples, diced into ½-inch cubes	
8 dried apricots, chopped	
¼ cup walnuts, toasted and chopped	

Per serving: Calories 163 (From Fat 52); Fat 6g (Saturated 1g); Cholesterol 0mg; Sodium 3mg; Carbohydrate 30g (Dietary Fiber 4g); Protein 1g.

Note: The color insert has a photo of this recipe.

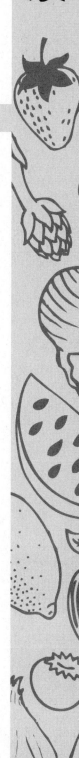

Mediterranean-Style Fruit Salad

Prep time: 7 min • **Yield:** 6 serving

Ingredients	*Directions*
4 Fuyu persimmons, sliced into 10 wedges each (see Figure 10-3)	*1* Combine all ingredients in a serving bowl; toss and serve.
1½ cups grapes, halved	
8 mint leaves, rolled and thinly sliced	
1 tablespoon lemon juice	
1 tablespoon honey	
½ cup almonds, chopped and toasted	

Per serving: Calories 159 (From Fat 37); Fat 4g (Saturated 0g); Cholesterol 0mg; Sodium 2mg; Carbohydrate 32g (Dietary Fiber 5g); Protein 3g.

Tip: You can use all green or all red grapes, but we prefer to use a blend of the two.

SLICING PERSIMMONS

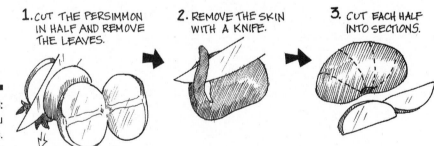

1. CUT THE PERSIMMON IN HALF AND REMOVE THE LEAVES.
2. REMOVE THE SKIN WITH A KNIFE.
3. CUT EACH HALF INTO SECTIONS.

Figure 10-3: Slicing Fuyu persimmons.

Moroccan Fruit Salad with Orange Blossom Water

Prep time: 10 min, plus resting time • **Yield:** 8 servings

Ingredients	*Directions*
4 oranges, peeled and cut into bite-sized pieces	**1** In a serving bowl, toss the oranges, figs, dates, and pomegranate seeds. Drizzle the mixture with the honey and the orange blossom water and gently stir.
8 dried or fresh figs, quartered	
2 Medjool dates, pitted and small diced (see Figure 10-4 for how to pit dates)	**2** Allow the fruit to rest for 2 to 8 hours in the refrigerator. Prior to serving, add in the bananas and toss to coat. Garnish with the toasted pistachios and serve.
½ cup pomegranate seeds	
2 tablespoons honey	
2 tablespoons orange blossom water	
2 bananas, peeled and cut into ½-inch rounds	
¼ cup shelled pistachios, chopped and toasted	

Per serving: Calories 185 (From Fat 22); Fat 2g (Saturated 0g); Cholesterol 0mg; Sodium 14mg; Carbohydrate 43g (Dietary Fiber 6g); Protein 3g.

Tip: You can find orange blossom water at a Mediterranean or specialty market. You can also substitute with 1 tablespoon orange zest, ¼ teaspoon sugar, and 1 teaspoon water.

PITTING AND SLICING A DATE

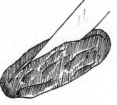

SLICE DOWN THE CENTER OF THE DATE LENGTHWISE UNTIL YOU GET TO THE PIT.

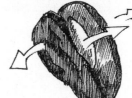

PUSH OPEN AND REMOVE THE PIT.

Figure 10-4: How to pit and slice dates.

Pushing Side Salads Aside: Delicious Entree Salads

Sometimes, you want to make a salad a meal, but you also want it to be satisfying. Enter entree salads. Although the entree salad is more popular in the United States and Canada, you can still create a Mediterranean–inspired meal by combining fresh produce with protein sources like salmon or chicken. Entree salads are also a great summer meal for celebrating the foods that are in season. Grilling is one of the ways Americans enjoy their food to the fullest, and giving your next cookout a Mediterranean look and feel is simple and fun. Cooking up some grilled salmon and laying it over fresh greens and veggies is easy, healthy, and delicious.

This section combines a few fun summer grilling recipes along with some amazing seared and smoked seafood salad options.

Mixing up salad dressings the Mediterranean way

One thing you won't find in the traditional Mediterranean refrigerator is several bottles of salad dressings such as ranch, Thousand Island, or even Italian. Instead, people in that region make their own dressings out of basic ingredients each time they prepare a salad. Although this practice may seem like too much work to you, we promise you it's really simple. Most Mediterranean salad dressings include the following:

✔ A high quality extra-virgin olive oil

✔ Vinegar (red wine, balsamic, or other infused or flavored vinegars)

✔ Salt

That about sums it up. The flavors and acidity level of your vinegar will dictate how much you use, but start with your olive oil, add a little vinegar and a pinch of salt, whisk it together in a small bowl or shake in a bottle, and see how it tastes by dipping a leaf of lettuce. Although you can find some specific recipes on the Internet, you'll probably do best by playing around with this basic recipe, in true Mediterranean fashion, until you perfect it to your specific taste. If you're feeling really crazy, you can try adding lemon juice, garlic, or a dash of mustard. Before you know it, you'll have your own perfected signature salad dressing. ***Remember:*** Add fresh herbs and strong flavors such as sliced onions directly to your salads instead of adding these elements to your dressing.

Grilled Salmon with Caramelized Onions over Mixed Greens

Prep time: 15 min, plus marinating time • **Cook time:** 40 min • **Yield:** 4 servings

Ingredients	*Directions*
1 tablespoon plus ¼ cup olive oil	**1** In a heavy skillet, heat 1 tablespoon of the olive oil and 1 tablespoon of butter over medium-high heat. Add the onions and sauté over medium-high heat until slightly soft and caramelized, being careful not to fully brown, for 3 minutes, tossing with tongs to separate pieces and evenly coat with oil mixture.
1 tablespoon butter	
2 large sweet or yellow onions, sliced thinly	
2 tablespoons fresh dill, chopped	**2** Reduce the heat to medium-low and continue sauté-ing uncovered for 20 to 25 minutes or until golden.
3 cloves garlic, minced	
Zest and juice of 1 lemon	**3** Mix the dill, garlic, lemon zest and juice, remaining olive oil, and melted butter and season with the sea salt to taste. Place all but ¼ cup of the dressing into another bowl and use the ¼ cup to brush both sides of the salmon; marinate for 10 minutes. Discard this portion of the dressing.
1 tablespoon butter, melted	
¼ teaspoon sea salt, or to taste	
1 pound salmon filet	
4 cups romaine lettuce	**4** Heat a grill or grill pan to medium-high heat. Grill the salmon on each side for 4 minutes or until it achieves the desired doneness.
4 cups red leaf lettuce	
¼ cup walnuts or almonds, chopped	**5** In a large mixing bowl, lightly toss the greens with the reserved dressing and plate on four dinner plates.
	6 Divide the caramelized onions evenly among the four plates. Cut the salmon into four equal pieces and plate them over the onions; sprinkle with the chopped walnuts and serve hot.

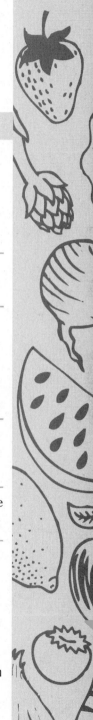

Per serving: Calories 322 (From Fat 161); Fat 18g (Saturated 5g); Cholesterol 74mg; Sodium 290mg; Carbohydrate 15g (Dietary Fiber 3g); Protein 27g.

Tip: You can use 8 cups of salad green mix in place of the romaine and red leaf lettuces. You can also use smaller pieces of salmon rather than one large filet, although doing so will affect their cooking time.

Char-Grilled Chicken with Feta over Mixed Greens

Prep time: 40 min, plus marinating time • **Cook time:** 20 min • **Yield:** 4 servings

Ingredients	Directions
Four 4- to 6-ounce boneless, skinless chicken breasts	**1** Place the chicken breasts in a 9-x-11-inch glass baking dish.
½ cup red wine vinegar	
1 cup olive oil	**2** In a small bowl, whisk together the vinegar, olive oil, garlic, mustard, oregano, fennel seed, coriander, and honey. Pour 1 cup of the dressing over the chicken and coat each breast. Marinate the chicken in the refrigerator for 30 minutes to 4 hours. Discard this portion of the dressing.
2 cloves garlic, chopped	
2 teaspoons yellow mustard	
1 teaspoon dried oregano	
¼ teaspoon fennel seed	**3** Divide the mixed greens among four plates. Halve each tomato and cut it into ½-inch wedges. Divide the tomatoes, olives, and feta evenly among the plates.
¼ teaspoon coriander	
2 teaspoons honey	
8 cups mixed salad greens	**4** Remove the chicken from the refrigerator and discard the marinade. Heat a grill or grill pan to medium-high heat. Grill the chicken for 10 minutes on each side or until the internal temperature reaches 165 degrees.
2 Roma tomatoes	
16 black olives	
4 ounces feta, crumbled	
	5 Allow the chicken to rest on a cutting board for 5 minutes prior to slicing. Slice each chicken breast on an angle in ½-inch-thick slices. Fan one breast over each salad.
	6 Drizzle 1 to 2 tablespoons of the remaining dressing over each salad and serve.

Per serving: Calories 290 (From Fat 92); Fat 10g (Saturated 4g); Cholesterol 126mg; Sodium 576mg; Carbohydrate 7g (Dietary Fiber 1g); Protein 41g.

Seared Tuna with Lemon Dill Sauce over Mixed Greens

Prep time: 25 min, plus marinating time • **Cook time:** 25 min • **Yield:** 4 servings

Ingredients	*Directions*
8 small new potatoes	*1* In a medium saucepan, cover the potatoes with cold water. Bring to a boil over high heat and cover; reduce the heat to low and simmer for 15 minutes or until the potatoes are fork tender. Strain the potatoes in a colander and run under cold water to halt the cooking. Set aside.
½ pound green beans, cleaned, with stems and ends removed	
Zest and juice of 2 lemons	
¼ cup parsley, chopped	*2* In the same saucepan, boil 3 cups of water and add the green beans; boil for 3 minutes. Strain the beans in a colander and run under cold water for 1 minute. Set aside.
1 clove garlic, minced	
1 tablespoon plus 2 tablespoons dill, chopped	*3* In a shallow dish, combine the lemon zest, 2 tablespoons of the lemon juice, the parsley, garlic, 1 tablespoon of the dill, and 2 tablespoons of the onion. Season with salt and pepper to taste.
¼ cup onion, minced, divided	
Salt and pepper to taste	
1 pound 1-inch-thick tuna steaks	*4* Add the tuna to the marinade from Step 3 and coat on both sides. Allow the tuna to marinate for at least 10 minutes while you assemble your salad.
6 cups green leaf or red leaf lettuce, washed and torn	*5* Place the lettuce in a large salad bowl and layer with the green beans, whole potatoes, and carrots.
¼ cup olive oil, divided	
1 carrot, grated	*6* Spray a cast-iron grill pan with nonstick cooking spray (if desired) and heat it over medium-high heat. Sear the tuna for 4 minutes on each side or until it reaches the desired doneness.
Nonstick cooking spray (optional)	
2 tablespoons capers	*7* Place the tuna on a cutting board. In a shallow bowl, whisk the remaining lemon juice, olive oil, dill, and onion and the capers. Whisk and pour the dressing over the salad. Slice the tuna steaks into ½-inch slices and serve over the salad mixture.

Per serving: Calories 397 (From Fat 136); Fat 15g (Saturated 2g); Cholesterol 51mg; Sodium 213mg; Carbohydrate 34g (Dietary Fiber 5g); Protein 32g.

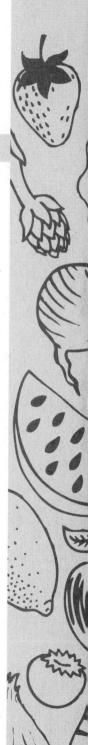

Smoked Salmon and Arugula Salad

Prep time: 15 min • **Yield:** 4 servings

Ingredients	*Directions*
Juice of 1 lemon	*1* In a small glass bowl, whisk the lemon juice, vinegar, olive oil, capers, garlic, and egg yolks. Set aside.
1 tablespoon red wine vinegar	
¼ cup olive oil	*2* Arrange the arugula on a serving plate and top with the smoked salmon, fennel, egg whites, and parsley.
2 tablespoons capers, chopped	
1 clove garlic, minced	*3* Drizzle with the dressing, season with salt and pepper to taste, and serve.
2 hard-boiled eggs, yolks separated from whites and whites chopped	
6 cups arugula	
8 ounces smoked salmon, thinly sliced (⅛ inch)	
½ a fennel bulb, sliced paper thin	
2 tablespoons fresh parsley, chopped	
Salt and pepper to taste	

Per serving: Calories 211 (From Fat 146); Fat 16g (Saturated 2g); Cholesterol 13mg; Sodium 623mg; Carbohydrate 4g (Dietary Fiber 2g); Protein 13g.

Chapter 11

Savoring Soups and Stews

In This Chapter

▶ Adding variety to your diet with classic Mediterranean-inspired soups

▶ Warming up those chilly days with hearty stews

> **Recipes in This Chapter**
>
> ↻ Tomato Basil Soup
> ▶ Italian Leek and Potato Soup
> ▶ Minestrone
> ▶ Cabbage and Bean Soup
> ▶ Lentil Soup with Tomatoes and Spinach
> ▶ Pasta Fagioli
> ▶ Lemony Soup
> ▶ Chicken Stew with Chickpeas and Plum Tomatoes
> ▶ Seafood Stew with Shrimp, Cod, and Tomatoes
> ▶ Tagine Stew
> ▶ Beef Stew with Red Wine
>
>

Although many dinners are ho-hum and don't invoke much excitement, a great cup of soup or stew on a cold winter's day can add some special ka-pow to the doldrums. It truly warms the soul! If you're tired of your old standby soup recipes or the canned varieties in your pantry, check out the classic, flavorful Mediterranean soup and stew recipes in this chapter. No one does soup better than the people who live on the coast of the Mediterranean. The flavors in these recipes are so unique to this region and celebrate all its main crops, from vegetables and herbs to legumes.

Not only do soups and stews speak to the flavor of the Mediterranean, but they also have many health benefits, including the following:

✔ Soups and stews that include vegetables, beans, and/or lentils are full of fiber, which helps with weight management (because it helps you feel full on fewer calories), lowers bad cholesterol, and manages blood sugar levels.

✔ Hot soups cause you to eat more slowly, which gives your brain time to feel more satisfied with fewer calories.

✔ The variety of vegetables, herbs, lentils, and beans in many soups gives you a big dose of vitamins, minerals, and phytonutrients for disease prevention and general wellness.

In addition to the health benefits, soups and stews are economical. The ingredients are usually inexpensive, and each recipe yields a plentiful amount of food. They also freeze well, so you can create your own healthy frozen dinners for those busy days.

Use these recipes as they are or feel free to celebrate the way the people of the Mediterranean live by substituting vegetables and herbs according to your taste and what you have on hand.

Warming Up with a Great Cup of Soup

Peasants originally created soups as a way to put together a meal from the scraps of food they had on hand. Finding eggs or cheese was a great way to enrich soups to add more protein, but the cooks often depended on vegetables, beans, and lentils to add more bulk to the pot. Herbs were easy to find, so soup-makers used plenty of them as seasoning.

Today, soups are used as a starter or as the entire meal in itself and are a great way to add a variety of nutrients to your diet. In this section, you can find soups that include the bountiful crops and unique flavors of the Mediterranean. The soups in this section fall into two basic categories:

✔ **Vegetable soups:** Vegetable soups are a great way to get a variety of vegetables into your diet each day. Remember, the more vegetables you eat, the more disease-fighting nutrients you're consuming on a daily basis. These soups are a perfect accompaniment to your meal, either as a starter or as your main vegetable. (*Remember:* "Vegetable soup" doesn't necessarily mean "vegetarian soup.")

✔ **Soups with beans, lentils, and meats:** Adding beans, lentils, and meats to your soups creates a heartier soup that can often serve as a complete meal. Serve these soups in a bowl with some crusty whole-wheat bread to make a one-pot meal on a cold day.

A soup-er weight-loss tip

Enjoying a cup of soup before your meal may just help you lose weight, according to researchers at Pennsylvania State University. They found that participants who ate a low-calorie vegetable/broth based soup prior to a meal ate one-fifth fewer calories for the total meal than those who ate the entree alone.

This finding makes sense because as you begin to eat, hormones begin releasing that tell your brain you are full. Of course, this strategy only works if you eat a low-calorie soup; otherwise, the calories add up, and you don't really reduce the calorie count of your meal.

Tomato Basil Soup

Prep time: 18 min • **Cook time:** 50 min • **Yield:** 8 servings

Ingredients	*Directions*
4 pounds tomatoes, halved across the hemisphere	*1* Heat the grill or grill pan over high heat to 400 degrees. Remove the tomato seeds; brush the tomato halves with 2 tablespoons of the olive oil and sprinkle them with salt Grill skin side down for 15 to 20 minutes or until slightly blackened.
2 tablespoons plus 2 teaspoons olive oil	
1½ teaspoons sea salt	
1 large onion, chopped	*2* Meanwhile, heat the remaining 2 teaspoons olive oil in a large stock pot over medium heat. Add the onions and garlic and sauté for 4 minutes. Pour in the stock, red pepper flakes, and roasted tomatoes.
6 cloves garlic, sliced	
4 cups low-sodium vegetable or chicken stock	
½ teaspoon red pepper flakes	*3* Bring the stock to a boil and reduce the heat to a simmer for 30 minutes. Add the butter and stir until melted. Blend the soup in a blender or in the pot with a stick blender until it's the desired texture.
1 tablespoon butter	
Salt and pepper, to taste	
½ cup basil, sliced thinly	*4* In the pot, season the blended soup with salt and pepper to taste. Divide the soup into eight bowls, top each serving with 1 tablespoon of sliced basil and 1 tablespoon of Parmesan, and serve.
½ cup freshly grated Parmesan cheese	

Per serving: *Calories 233 (From Fat 126); Fat 14g (Saturated 4g); Cholesterol 12mg; Sodium 967mg; Carbohydrate 22g (Dietary Fiber 6g); Protein 7g.*

Tip: If you're using a traditional blender, blend the soup in small (1-to-2-cup) batches to avoid splattering soup everywhere.

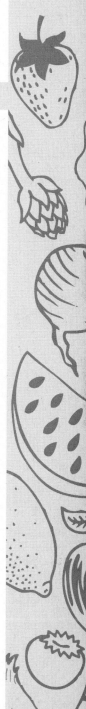

Italian Leek and Potato Soup

Prep time: 8 min • **Cook time:** 30 min • **Yield:** 6 servings

Ingredients	Directions
3 large leeks (about 1½ pounds) **2 tablespoons extra-virgin olive oil** **1 tablespoon butter** **1 medium sweet or yellow onion, chopped** **1 cup dry white wine** **3 pounds Yukon gold or russet potatoes, peeled and diced large** **5 to 6 cups chicken stock** **½ cup whipping cream** **Salt and white pepper to taste**	*1* Thinly slice the leeks (the white portion and the tender part of the green). Soak the leeks in the water and drain twice to ensure all the sand is off the leek; drain and pat the leeks dry. *2* In a large stock pot, heat the olive oil and butter over medium heat until foamy. Add the leeks and onions and sauté for 10 minutes. Add the wine and continue to cook for 5 minutes. *3* Add the potatoes and enough stock to cover the potatoes. Simmer for 20 to 25 minutes until the potatoes are fork tender. *4* Using a blender or stick blender, puree the mixture until creamy. Pour the blended mixture back into the stock pot. Add the cream and simmer for 2 to 3 minutes. Season with the salt and white pepper and serve.

Per serving: Calories 453 (From Fat 149); Fat 17g (Saturated 7g); Cholesterol 38mg; Sodium 334mg; Carbohydrate 60g (Dietary Fiber 4g); Protein 11g.

Tip: If you're using a traditional blender, blend the soup in small (1-to-2-cup) batches to avoid splattering soup everywhere.

Minestrone

Prep time: 15 min • **Cook time:** 6–8 hr • **Yield:** 8 servings

Ingredients	*Directions*
1 onion, diced	*1* Stir the onions, carrots, celery, beans, tomatoes, stock, sausage, thyme, bay leaves, and sage together in a 4- to 5-quart slow cooker.
3 carrots, washed, quartered and sliced into ½-inch slices	
3 celery stalks, quartered and sliced into ½-inch slices	*2* Cook on low for 6 to 8 hours. During the last 30 minutes of cooking, add the orzo and zucchini and cook for 30 minutes on high or until you're ready to serve. Add salt to taste (if desired).
Two 14.5-ounce cans navy beans, drained and rinsed	
One 28-ounce can diced tomatoes	*3* Divide the soup among eight bowls, removing the bay leaves. Top each bowl with 1 tablespoon of the grated Parmesan and serve.
4 cups low-sodium chicken stock	
4 Italian chicken sausage links, quartered and sliced into ½-inch slices	
2 sprigs thyme, or ½ teaspoon dried thyme	
2 bay leaves	
½ teaspoon dried sage	
1 cup orzo or other small pasta	
3 zucchinis, quartered and sliced into ½-inch slices	
½ cup freshly grated Parmesan for serving	
Salt to taste (optional)	

Per serving: Calories 382 (From Fat 98); Fat 11g (Saturated 4g); Cholesterol 25mg; Sodium 1178mg; Carbohydrate 50g (Dietary Fiber 10g); Protein 23g.

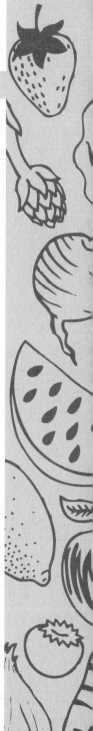

Cabbage and Bean Soup

Prep time: 10 min • **Cook time:** 50 min • **Yield:** 6 servings

Ingredients	*Directions*
¼ cup olive oil 1 medium onion, chopped 2 carrots, chopped 2 celery stalks, chopped 6 sprigs parsley 1 bay leaf ¼ teaspoon dried sage	*1* Heat the olive oil in a large stock pot over medium heat for 1 minute. Add the onions, carrots, and celery and cook until the onions are translucent, about 6 to 7 minutes.
One 14.5-ounce can diced tomatoes 8 cups water	*2* Add the tomatoes (with juice), parsley, bay leaf, and sage; lower the heat to low and simmer for 10 minutes.
½ pound Yukon gold potatoes, cut into bite-sized pieces 1 pound green cabbage, chopped (about 6 cups) ½ pound baked ham, cut into 1-inch cubes	*3* Raise the heat to medium-high, add the water, and bring the mixture to a boil. Add the potatoes, cabbage, ham, and beans. Cover and drop the heat to simmer for 20 minutes or until the potatoes are tender.
One 14.5-ounce can cannellini beans, drained ¼ cup instant polenta Salt and pepper to taste	*4* Whisk in the polenta and continue whisking for 4 to 5 minutes. Season with salt and pepper. Serve.

Per serving: Calories 345 (From Fat 110); Fat 12g (Saturated 2g); Cholesterol 21mg; Sodium 754mg; Carbohydrate 44g (Dietary Fiber 8g); Protein 17g.

Tip: Figure 11-1 shows you how to prepare the cabbage.

CHOPPING CABBAGE

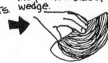
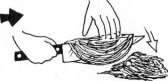

1. Cut the cabbage into halves and then into quarters. Start with one quarter.

2. Put the round side down on the cutting board and hold it by the pointed side of the wedge.

3. Use a big, sharp knife and cut thin slices along the angle of the wedge.

Figure 11-1: Chopping cabbage.

Lentil Soup with Tomatoes and Spinach

Prep time: 8 min • **Cook time:** 45 min • **Yield:** 8 servings

Ingredients	Directions
1 tablespoon olive oil	*1* Heat the olive oil into a large stock pot over medium heat. After 1 minute, add the onions, carrot, and celery and cook until the onions are translucent, about 6 to 7 minutes.
1 cup chopped onion	
½ cup carrot, diced small	
½ cup celery, diced small	*2* Add the salt, lentils, tomatoes, broth, coriander, cumin, and bay leaf and stir to combine. Increase the heat to high and bring just to a boil.
1½ teaspoon salt	
1 pound orange or brown lentils	
One 14.5-ounce can unsalted chopped tomatoes	*3* Reduce the heat to low, cover, and cook at a low simmer until the lentils are tender, about 35 to 40 minutes. Add the spinach in the last 15 minutes or simply add to each bowl for serving. Season with salt and pepper to taste and serve immediately.
8 cups chicken or vegetable broth	
½ teaspoon ground coriander	
½ teaspoon ground cumin	
1 bay leaf	
5 ounces baby spinach leaves	
Salt and pepper to taste	

Per serving: *Calories 285 (From Fat 35); Fat 4g (Saturated 1g); Cholesterol 0mg; Sodium 959mg; Carbohydrate 42g (Dietary Fiber 19g); Protein 21g.*

Tip: If you want to use a slow cooker, combine all the ingredients except the spinach in the slow cooker and cook for 6 hours on low. Add the spinach during the last 15 minutes of cooking or to each bowl for serving.

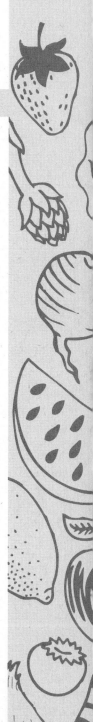

Pasta Fagioli

Prep time: 10 min • **Cook time:** 30 min • **Yield:** 8 servings

Ingredients	Directions
1 tablespoon olive oil	*1* In a large stock pot, heat the olive oil over medium heat for 2 minutes. Add the pancetta and sauté for 3 to 5 minutes. Add the rosemary, thyme, bay leaf, red pepper flakes, onions, carrots, celery, and garlic.
2 ounces pancetta, diced small	
1 teaspoon dried rosemary, minced	
½ teaspoon dried thyme, or 2 sprigs fresh thyme	*2* Continue to sauté for 7 minutes or until the onions are translucent. Add the beans, tomatoes (juice included), and stock. Bring soup to a boil and lower the heat to simmer.
1 bay leaf	
¼ teaspoon red pepper flakes	
1 medium onion, chopped small	*3* Add the Parmesan rind (if desired) and pasta and continue to cook for 20 minutes or until the pasta and vegetables are tender. Remove the rind and discard.
2 medium carrots, diced small	
2 celery stalks, diced small	*4* Season the soup with salt and pepper. Serve each bowl with 1 tablespoon of freshly grated Parmesan cheese.
6 cloves garlic, sliced	
Two 14.5-ounce cans cannellini or navy beans, drained and rinsed	
One 14.5-ounce can diced tomatoes, undrained	
8 cups low-sodium chicken or vegetable stock	
2 inches Parmesan rind (optional)	
1 cup ditalini or other small pasta	
Salt and pepper to taste	
½ cup freshly grated Parmesan cheese	

Per serving: Calories 290 (From Fat 60); Fat 7g (Saturated 2g); Cholesterol 8mg; Sodium 796mg; Carbohydrate 42g (Dietary Fiber 7g); Protein 18g.

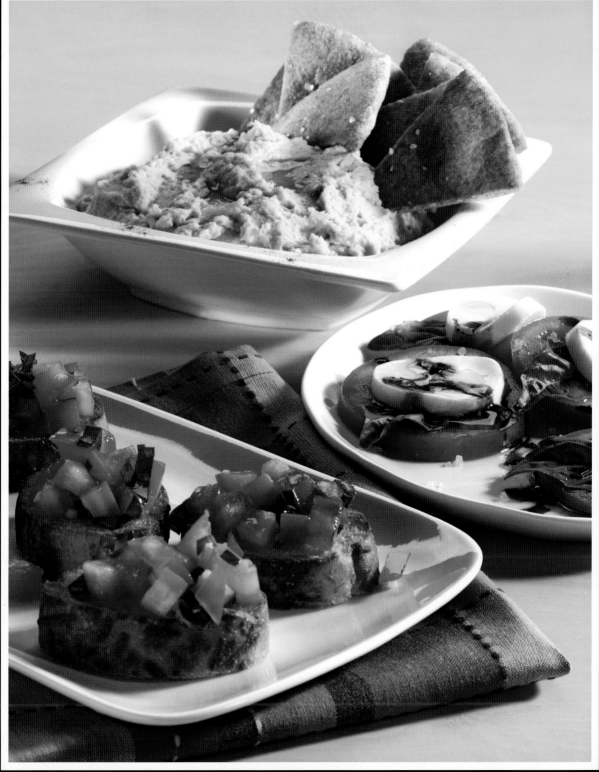

You can make an entire meal or put together a spread for the big game from an assortment of appetizers and starters with the Mediterranean diet. Chapter 8 has numerous recipes including the Hummus, Toasted Pita Chips, Tomato and Mozzarella Bites, and Italian Bruschetta.

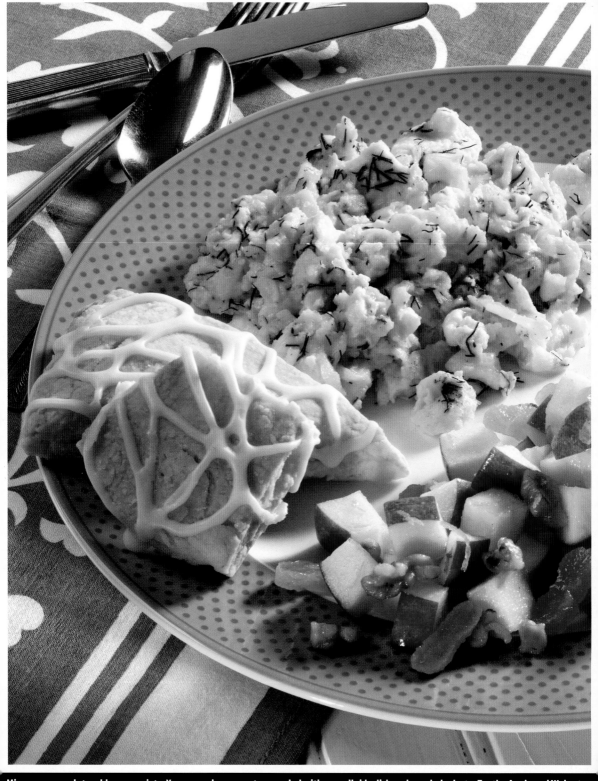

Mix up your meals to add some variety. You can make your entree a salad with a small side dish and a carbohydrate. Try the Apple and Walnut Salad (Chapter 10) with a side of the Dilled Eggs (Chapter 7). You can add one or two Lemon Scones (Chapter 7) for a touch of sweetness.

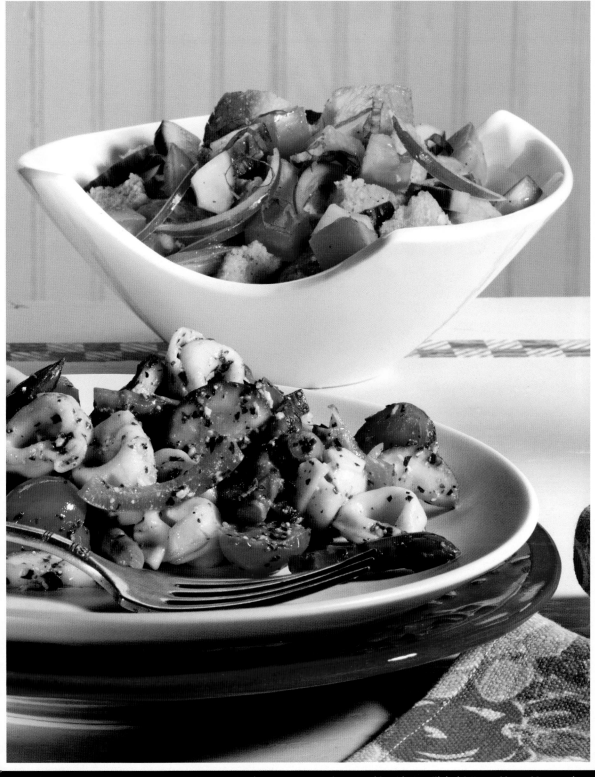

The Mediterranean diet includes pasta and other favorites in reasonable portions. Consider this Tortellini with Vegetables and Pesto recipe from Chapter 15 (with the separate Pesto recipe in Chapter 9). Add Italian Bread Salad from Chapter 10 to transport you to Italia.

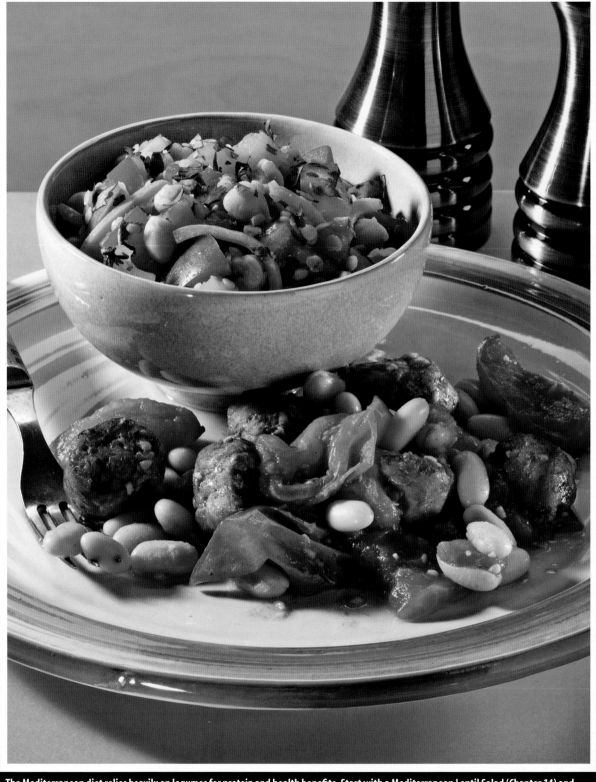

The Mediterranean diet relies heavily on legumes for protein and health benefits. Start with a Mediterranean Lentil Salad (Chapter 14) and make your main course the Pork Sausage with White Beans and Tomatoes (Chapter 19).

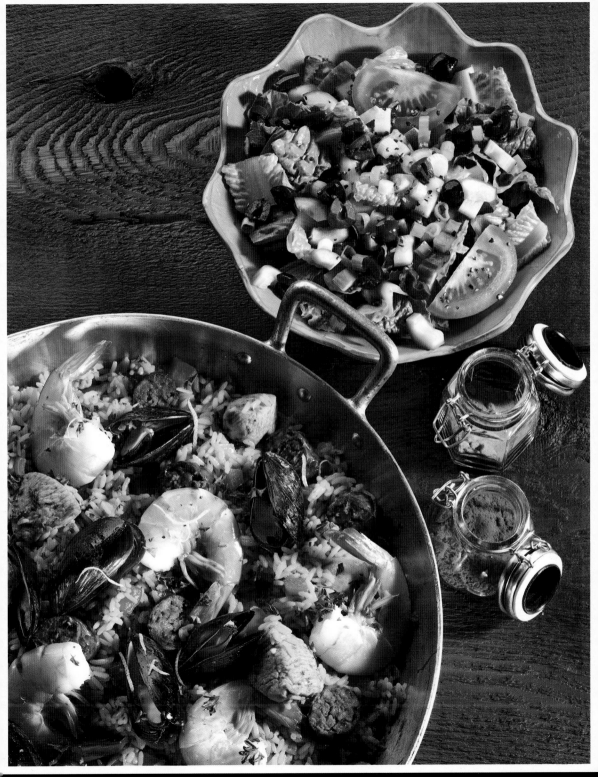

With the Mediterranean diet, you can fuse different countries from the region together to make your own unique, delicious meals. Start with a Greek Salad from Chapter 19 and include the Paella from Chapter 18. You get your ono and your olé all in one meal.

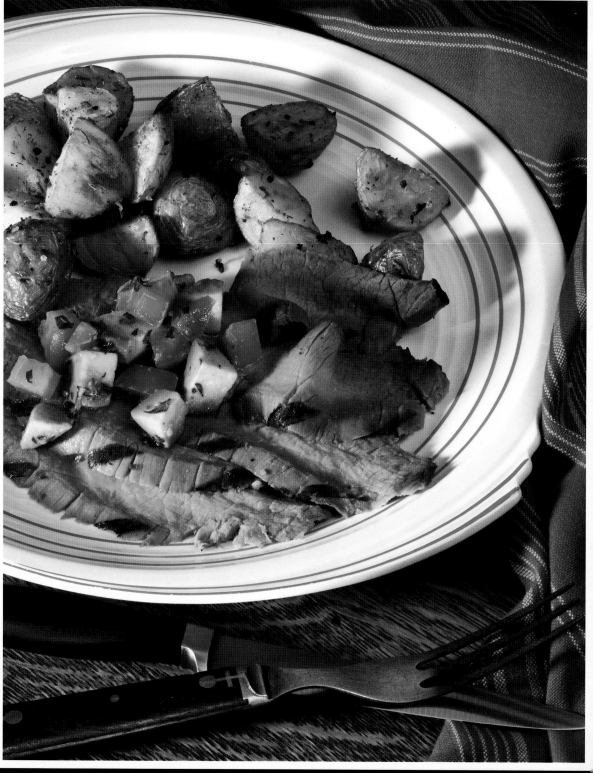

If your family is more into meat and potatoes, you can still embrace the Mediterranean diet. Whip up the Zesty Mediterranean Flank Steak recipe (Chapter 19) with a side of the Garlic and Lemon Roasted Potatoes (Chapter 12) for those hearty souls.

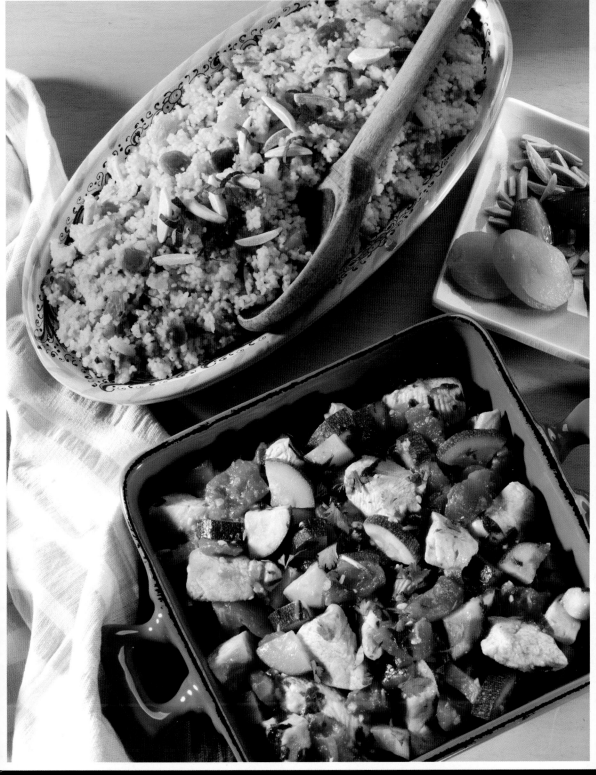

Introduce your family and friends to a North African dinner with the Moroccan Chicken with Tomato and Zucchini recipe in Chapter 17 over a

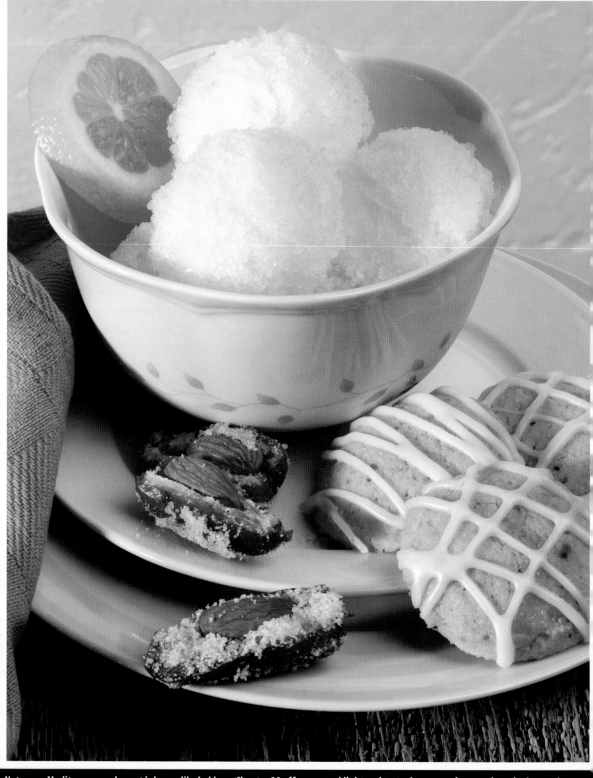

Not every Mediterranean dessert is heavy like baklava. Chapter 20 offers several light and tasty dessert options, such as the Lemon Ices,

Lemony Soup

Prep time: 5 min • **Cook time:** 23 min • **Yield:** 8 servings

Ingredients	*Directions*
8 cups low-sodium chicken stock or vegetable stock	*1* In a large stock pot, heat the chicken stock to a boil over medium-high heat. Drop the heat to a low simmer.
¼ teaspoon ground white pepper	
2 tablespoons olive oil	*2* Combine the olive oil, butter, and flour. Add 2 cups of hot stock to the flour mixture and whisk until blended. Gradually add the flour mixture to the soup and simmer for 10 minutes. Add the orzo and continue simmering for 5 minutes.
2 tablespoons butter	
¼ cup flour	
1 cup orzo	
4 eggs	*3* Meanwhile, whisk the eggs and lemon juice until foamy and blended. Slowly drizzle 1 cup of the hot soup into the egg mixture, stirring constantly.
¾ cup lemon juice	
8 lemon slices	
Salt to taste	*4* Slowly return the egg mixture to the soup pot and continue to simmer for 10 minutes. Add salt to taste. Ladle hot soup into bowls, garnish with lemon slices, and serve.

Per serving: Calories 191 (From Fat 74); Fat 8g (Saturated 3g); Cholesterol 8mg; Sodium 223mg; Carbohydrate 22g (Dietary Fiber 1g); Protein 10g.

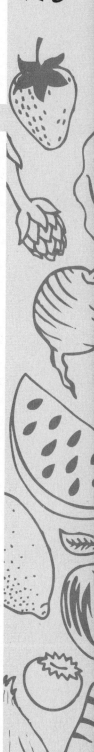

Creating Hearty Stews to Warm Your Heart

Stews are a great one-pot meal. Even though they often take awhile to cook, they're usually very simple to prepare. They're the perfect meal to quickly throw together on a Sunday afternoon and then enjoy the wonderful aroma as the pot simmers all afternoon. And like soups (see the preceding section), they can add a great variety of vegetables, grains, herbs, beans, and lentils to your diet and make for a tasty warm dish when the temperature is chilly.

The following stews have one thing in common: Flavor. From Morocco to Italy, you can find some amazing new stews to bring to the family table.

Taking a look at the Moroccan tagine

Morocco is known for robust flavors, and much of that flavor often comes from using a *tagine*, a slow-cooking clay pot unique to the area. The bottom part of the tagine contains a large, circular dish where you place the food for cooking and serving, while the top part is a rounded cone.

Tagines are typically used to slow cook stews (also known as *tagine stews*) that contain poultry, fish, or beef and often vegetables and fruit.

The cone-shaped top traps steam and recirculates the moisture during cooking so that little liquid is needed. Traditionally, the tagine goes over heated coals for cooking, although you can also use them in the oven or on the stove top. If you want to give tagine cooking a try, you can purchase a tagine at www.tagines.com. Don't worry; you don't have to purchase a tagine to make an amazing tagine stew. Just follow the recipe in this chapter.

Chicken Stew with Chickpeas and Plum Tomatoes

Prep time: 12 min • **Cook time:** 1 hr, 15 min • **Yield:** 6 servings

Ingredients	Directions
2 tablespoons olive oil	*1* In a large stock pot, heat the olive oil over medium high heat. Add the chicken thighs and cook for 3 minutes on each side. Add the onion, celery, spices, and chickpeas and cook for 3 minutes to heat the spices.
4 skinless chicken thighs	
1 small onion, chopped	
1 celery stalk, chopped	
½ teaspoon cinnamon	*2* Pour in the tomatoes (with their juice), stock, lentils, and rice. Bring the mixture to a boil over medium-high heat, cover, reduce the heat to low, and simmer for 1 hour and 15 minutes.
¼ teaspoon ginger	
1 teaspoon turmeric	
1 teaspoon pepper	
½ teaspoon salt	*3* Stir in the lemon juice and divide the stew into six bowls. Garnish each bowl with 2 tablespoons of chopped cilantro and serve.
One 14.5-ounce can chickpeas, drained	
One 28-ounce can whole plum tomatoes, with juice	
6 cups low-sodium chicken stock	
¼ cup red lentils	
½ cup long-grain rice	
¼ cup lemon juice	
½ cup cilantro, chopped	

Per serving: Calories 346 (From Fat 82); Fat 9g (Saturated 2g); Cholesterol 38mg; Sodium 721mg; Carbohydrate 47g (Dietary Fiber 6g); Protein 22g.

Seafood Stew with Shrimp, Cod, and Tomatoes

Prep time: 10 min • **Cook time:** 50 min • **Yield:** 6 servings

Ingredients	Directions
1 tablespoon extra-virgin olive oil	*1* In a large stock pot, heat the olive oil over medium heat. Add the onions, sliced garlic, and red pepper flakes and cook for 8 minutes, stirring every minute.
1 medium onion, chopped	
3 cloves garlic, sliced, plus 1 whole clove	
½ teaspoon crushed red pepper flakes	*2* Stir in the tomato paste and cook for 1 minute. Add the tomatoes, wine, clam juice, bay leaf, thyme, zest, and fennel seeds. Bring the mixture to a boil, cover, and simmer for 30 minutes.
2 tablespoons tomato paste	
One 28-ounce can diced tomatoes	
1½ cups dry white wine	*3* Add the fish and shrimp and cook for 10 minutes. Meanwhile, broil the bread until lightly toasted on both sides, 4 to 6 minutes. Rub the raw garlic clove over each piece.
One 8-ounce bottle clam juice	
1 bay leaf	
1 tablespoon chopped fresh thyme	*4* Season the soup with salt, stir in the parsley, and serve along with the bread.
Zest of 1 small orange	
1 teaspoon fennel seeds, crushed	
2 pounds cod fillets, cut into 2-inch pieces	
1 pound uncooked large shrimp, peeled and deveined	
6 slices French bread or crusty whole-grain bread	
Salt to taste	
1 cup parsley, chopped	

Per serving: Calories 417 (From Fat 49); Fat 5g (Saturated 1g); Cholesterol 180mg; Sodium 790mg; Carbohydrate 32g (Dietary Fiber 3g); Protein 49g.

Tagine Stew

Prep time: 12 min, plus refrigeration time • **Cook time:** 1 hr, 20 min • **Yield:** 6 servings

Ingredients	Directions
1 teaspoon ground cumin	*1* Combine the first eight ingredients and rub the mixture on the chicken. Allow the chicken to sit in the refrigerator for at least 2 hours; afterward, sprinkle the chicken lightly with flour.
½ teaspoon coriander	
1 teaspoon paprika	
½ teaspoon ginger	
1 teaspoon pepper	
½ teaspoon red pepper flakes	*2* Heat the olive oil in a large cast-iron Dutch oven over medium-high heat. Add half the chicken and cook for 3 minutes on each side or until lightly browned. Remove from the pan and repeat with the remaining chicken. Drain the chicken on paper towels.
1 teaspoon garlic powder	
¼ teaspoon turmeric	
8 boneless, skinless chicken thighs	
¼ cup flour	
1 tablespoon olive oil	*3* Add the onion, ginger, and garlic to the hot pan and sauté for 5 minutes or until tender. Add the lemon peel strips to the pan and then return the chicken to the pan.
1 large onion, chopped	
One ½-inch piece ginger, grated or minced	
2 cloves garlic, sliced	
Peel of 1 preserved lemon, or 1 tablespoon preserved lemon peel, chopped	*4* Add the stock, olives, bay leaf, and cinnamon stick and bring to a boil. Cover, reduce the heat, and simmer for 1 hour or until the chicken is tender. Remove the cinnamon stick and bay leaf and stir in the cilantro; add salt and pepper to taste and serve.
4 cups low-sodium chicken stock	
1 cup pitted green olives, halved	
1 bay leaf	
One 2-inch cinnamon stick	
¼ cup fresh cilantro, chopped	
Salt and pepper to taste	

Per serving: Calories 228 (From Fat 93); Fat 10g (Saturated 2g); Cholesterol 76mg; Sodium 499mg; Carbohydrate 11g (Dietary Fiber 1g); Protein 23g.

Note: Preserved lemons are lemons that have been pickled in salt and their own juices; they're common in Middle Eastern and Moroccan cooking. You can also buy just the preserved lemon peel so that you don't have to deal with the rest of the lemon. Look for these products in ethnic grocery stores or online at www.amazon.com.

Tip: You can use 1 tablespoon of lemon zest to replace the preserved lemon peel.

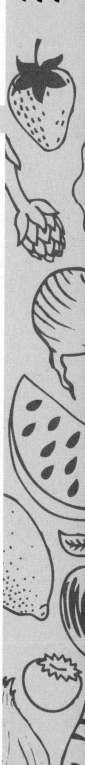

Beef Stew with Red Wine

Prep time: 10 min • **Cook time:** 2 hr, 45 min • **Yield:** 6 servings

Ingredients	*Directions*
1 tablespoon olive oil	*1* Heat the olive oil in a large Dutch oven over medium-high heat until hot. Brown the onions in the oil for 5 minutes and remove them from the pan with tongs.
1 medium onion, cut into 8 wedges	
½ cup flour	*2* Meanwhile, combine the flour, salt, and pepper; dredge the beef in the flour mixture, shaking off the excess. Add the meat to the pan and brown on all sides, about 10 minutes total.
½ teaspoon salt	
1 teaspoon pepper	
2 pounds beef chuck shoulder, cut into 2-inch pieces	
2 carrots, sliced into ½-inch rounds	*3* Return the onions to the pot and stir in the carrots, celery, mushrooms, garlic, bay leaf, thyme, and oregano. Add the wine, tomatoes, stock, and sugar, stirring to blend.
2 celery stalks, sliced into ½-inch pieces	
2 cups crimini mushrooms, quartered	*4* Bring the mixture to a boil and cover; drop the temperature to low and continue to cook for 2½ to 3 hours or until the meat is tender. Stir in the parsley and serve.
2 cloves garlic	
1 bay leaf	
2 sprigs thyme, or ½ teaspoon dried thyme	
½ teaspoon dried oregano	
2 cups red wine	
One 14.5-ounce can diced or petite diced tomatoes	
2 cups low-sodium beef stock	
1 teaspoon granulated sugar	
1 cup parsley	

Per serving: Calories 291 (From Fat 73); Fat 8g (Saturated 2g); Cholesterol 47mg; Sodium 418mg; Carbohydrate 20g (Dietary Fiber 3g); Protein 21g.

Tip: Serve over polenta, mashed potatoes, or orzo for a wonderful meal.

Chapter 12

Bringing New Flavor to Vegetable Sides

In This Chapter

▶ Setting the table with fresh fall harvest vegetables

▶ Finding new ways to cook winter vegetables

▶ Discovering spectacular springtime recipes

▶ Lightening up with summer vegetable recipes

*F*resh vegetables are one of the main reasons that the Mediterranean diet is so healthy. You've probably heard the message that vegetables are good for you numerous times, yet many Americans still aren't eating the recommended two to three cups of vegetables a day. People in the Mediterranean enjoy five to nine servings of vegetables a day on average, which is a good goal to strive for. Consuming more of this one food group has many health benefits, which we discuss in Chapter 2.

Although you can find all types of vegetables in the United States and Canada all year round, you see more seasonal eating in the Mediterranean because inhabitants utilize their crops right after harvest, a few miles from home, instead of shipping in foods from other countries all year round. This practice has the added benefit of being a cheaper way to eat veggies.

But eating seasonally can be tough, especially when you don't like or know how to cook what's in season. This chapter's recipes give you some new ideas to spruce up tried-and-true vegetables and offer new dishes you may have never tried. We divide this chapter into four sections, one for each season, so that you have a plan to buy the freshest produce at the right time of year. Now you have no excuse not to serve several vegetables with each meal rather than just one (or none)!

Introducing Fall Favorites into Your Mediterranean Diet

Although the fall isn't as big a veggie season as summer, you can find several choices, including broccoli, cauliflower, and late summer eggplants and squash. This section highlights some of the vegetables you can find from September to November, adding a punch of flavor with fresh herbs, spices, olive oil, and cheeses.

You are what (vegetables) you eat

You've probably heard the saying "You are what you eat," meaning that if your food is full of sugars and unhealthy fats, that's what you have coursing through your body. Vivid description, but true! Luckily, the same is true for eating vegetables; you may be surprised how healthy a simple serving of vegetables really is for your body. Here are the health benefits of some popular Mediterranean veggie crops so that you can feel great about loading them up on your plate:

✔ **Broccoli:** Broccoli is truly loaded in vitamins and minerals. In fact, it has too many to list here (just take our word for it). Broccoli is chock-full of vitamins C, K, and A as well as folate. Broccoli is known for its anti-inflammatory, antioxidant capabilities and helps enhance the body's detoxification system. This little green tree can help you fight off chronic diseases such as heart disease and even some forms of cancers.

✔ **Eggplant:** Eggplant is very popular in the Mediterranean; it provides a unique flavor and a beautiful, rich purple color. Eggplant is a good source of phenolic compounds that protect the plant from weather and bugs and help you prevent heart disease and cancers.

✔ **Cucumbers:** Cucumbers are on just about every menu in Crete and southern Italy, and they're better for you than you may expect. The skin of cucumbers contains both vitamin C and caffeic acid, which help reduce water retention and skin swelling (hence their popularity as an eye mask). They're also a good source of potassium and magnesium, which help maintain healthy blood pressure. Plus, cucumbers provide high water and fiber contents and few calories, making them a great food to help you feel satisfied and refreshed.

Roasted Broccoli and Tomatoes

Prep time: 8 min • **Cook time:** 15 min • **Yield:** 4 servings

Ingredients	*Directions*
1 pound broccoli	*1* Preheat the oven to 450 degrees. Cut off the broccoli florets with a 1-inch stem on each crown. Peel the remaining stalk with a vegetable peeler and cut into 1-inch-long pieces.
2 cups Roma or cherry tomatoes	
1 tablespoon olive oil	
2 tablespoons balsamic vinegar	*2* Place the broccoli and ¼ cup of water into a microwave-safe bowl; microwave the broccoli for 3 minutes to soften. Drain and pat dry.
¼ teaspoon sugar or honey	
1 teaspoon dried oregano	*3* Quarter the tomatoes and toss with the broccoli. Drizzle the veggies with olive oil, toss, and spread onto a baking sheet. Roast for 12 to 15 minutes or until the broccoli begins to lightly brown.
1 clove garlic, minced	
Salt to taste	
	4 Meanwhile, combine the balsamic vinegar, sugar, oregano, and garlic. As soon as the vegetables come out of the oven, place them in a serving bowl and drizzle with the balsamic dressing. Toss and serve.

Per serving: Calories 90 (From Fat 35); Fat 4g (Saturated 1g); Cholesterol 0mg; Sodium 43mg; Carbohydrate 12g (Dietary Fiber 4g); Protein 4g.

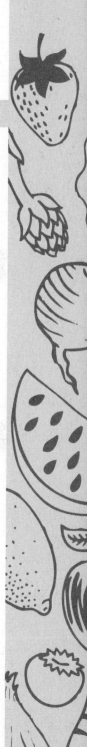

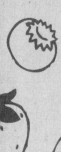

Roasted Vegetables with Béchamel Sauce

Prep time: 13 min • **Cook time:** 30 min • **Yield:** 8 servings

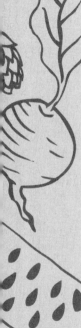

Ingredients	Directions
1 head cauliflower	**1** Heat the oven to 350 degrees. Cut the cauliflower into 1-inch pieces, including the stem and leaves. Cut the zucchini into 2-inch rounds and then quarter lengthwise.
4 small zucchinis	
Nonstick cooking spray	
1 teaspoon chicken base	**2** Spray a 9-x-11-inch baking sheet with the nonstick cooking spray. In a 6-quart stock pot, bring the chicken base and 8 cups of water to a boil. Parboil the cauliflower for 5 minutes and then place on a baking sheet.
3 cups Béchamel	
½ teaspoon pepper	
¼ cup grated Parmesan	
Pepper to taste	**3** Parboil the zucchini for 1 minute and then mix with the cauliflower on the baking sheet. Toss the vegetables with pepper to taste.
½ cup breadcrumbs	
1 tablespoon butter, cut into small cubes	**4** Spoon the Béchamel sauce over the vegetables. Top with the cheese and breadcrumbs. Dot the breadcrumbs with butter pieces and bake for 20 minutes.
	5 Increase the oven temperature to broil and broil and cook for an additional 3 to 5 minutes or until golden.

Per serving: Calories 173 (From Fat 85); Fat 9g (Saturated 6g); Cholesterol 25mg; Sodium 306mg; Carbohydrate 17g (Dietary Fiber 2g); Protein 7g.

Tip: You can find the Béchamel recipe in Chapter 9.

Note: Chicken base is similar to bouillon but uses chicken meat and chicken juices along with spices. If you can't find chicken base in your local grocery store, you can replace it with the equivalent amount of bouillon.

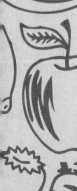

Sautéed Eggplant with Tomatoes and Black Olives

Prep time: 10 min • **Cook time:** 30 min • **Yield:** 6 servings

Ingredients	*Directions*
2 tablespoons olive oil	*1* In a heavy skillet, heat the olive oil over medium heat. Add the garlic, eggplant, and oregano and sauté for 10 minutes.
3 cloves garlic, chopped	
1 large eggplant, unpeeled, cut into ½-inch cubes (see Figure 12-1)	
1 tablespoon dried oregano	*2* Add the tomatoes, olives, tomato paste, and red wine vinegar and reduce the heat to medium-low. Cover and cook until the eggplant softens, stirring often, about 15 minutes. If needed, occasionally add 1 tablespoon of water to the pan to help the eggplant soften and cook.
One 28-ounce can no-salt-added diced tomatoes	
¼ cup kalamata or black olives	
¼ cup tomato paste	*3* Stir in the basil and simmer for 3 to 5 minutes. Season with salt and pepper to taste. Place into a serving dish, dollop with spoonfuls of the ricotta, and serve.
2 tablespoons red wine vinegar	
1 to 3 tablespoons water	
1 cup fresh basil, sliced thinly	
Salt and pepper to taste	
¼ cup ricotta cheese	

Per serving: *Calories 118 (From Fat 61); Fat 7g (Saturated 2g); Cholesterol 5mg; Sodium 164mg; Carbohydrate 13g (Dietary Fiber 5g); Protein 4g.*

Tip: Figure 12-1 shows how to cube an eggplant.

CUBING AN EGGPLANT

Figure 12-1: When cubing an eggplant, keep the cubes at ½ inch.

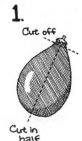

1. Cut off / Cut in half

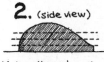

2. (side view) Make slices lengthwise, parallel to the cutting board

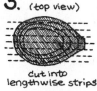

3. (top view) cut into lengthwise strips

4. Cubed

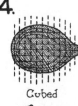

Helping Yourself to Hearty Winter Vegetables

The winter months, December through February, are often the time when you're less active, which makes it one of the most important times of the year to ramp up your vegetable intake. The extra fiber and roughage help you feel full and satisfied as you expend less energy through activity and exercise. Potatoes, broccoli, and cauliflower are great winter choices. Turn on your stovetop and heat up your oven; this section provides some amazing recipes for the winter harvest.

Perusing potato possibilities

Mediterranean cooking uses many varieties of potato, and which potato you choose to work with largely just depends on the flavor you enjoy. Your best choices for roasting are Yukon gold, fingerling, and new potatoes. Use Idaho baking or russet potatoes for baking and red, purple, and white potatoes for pan-frying. Idaho, Yukon gold, and red potatoes work beautifully in soups and stews. Take a look at the potato options in this figure.

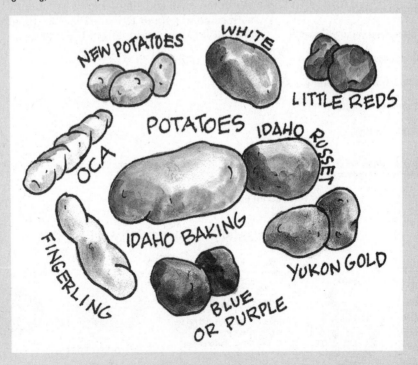

Garlic and Lemon Roasted Potatoes

Prep time: 6 min • **Cook time:** 35 min • **Yield:** 6 servings

Ingredients	Directions
1½ pounds fingerling or new potatoes	*1* Preheat the oven to 425 degrees. Slice the potatoes in half (for fingerling) or quarters (for new) and place them on a baking sheet or roasting pan.
3 tablespoons olive oil	
3 cloves garlic, minced	*2* Drizzle the potatoes with the olive oil, garlic, and oregano and toss to coat. Bake the potatoes for 20 minutes; gently stir. Continue cooking for an additional 15 minutes or until golden brown. Remove from the oven and place into a serving bowl.
½ teaspoon dried oregano	
½ teaspoon pepper	
Zest of 1 lemon (about 1 tablespoon)	
¼ teaspoon sea salt	*3* Toss the warm potatoes with the pepper, zest, and sea salt to serve.

Per serving: *Calories 139 (From Fat 62); Fat 7g (Saturated 1g); Cholesterol 0mg; Sodium 104mg; Carbohydrate 18g (Dietary Fiber 2g); Protein 2g.*

Tip: If you have small or two-inch new potatoes, cut them only in half.

Note: Flip to the color insert for a photo of this recipe.

Finding fun ways to get daily exercise

Formalized exercise wasn't exactly a traditional part of life on the Mediterranean coast — we doubt that the old folks in Crete spent much time in a gym 50 years ago. Rather, work and fun were the main sources of physical activity. You can also look to incorporate exercise into your daily life to increase your level of physical activity.

Make a list of all the physical activities you enjoy — pastimes such as gardening, swimming, hiking, jogging, bike riding, skateboarding, or skiing — and make more time to partake in those hobbies. If you love hitting the gym, by all means, add that to your list. Incorporating one fun activity each day, even if it's just a simple walk, goes a long way for your health.

Meri's Italian grandmother had this down. She walked nearly every day, except for the winter months, to get out and get some fresh air. She also loved swimming and gardening and was on a bowling league. She may never have hit the gym, but she loved life, enjoyed many forms of physical activity, and managed her weight for a lifetime.

For maximum benefit, you still need to focus on getting some sort of strength training exercise (unless your fun activity is lifting weights). Work on strength training, such as walking, lifting weights, or using resistance bands, three to four times per week.

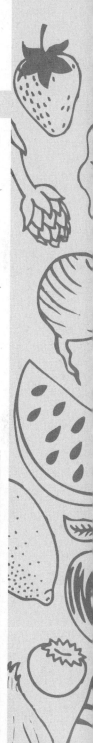

Sautéed Broccoli Rabe

Prep time: 6 min • **Cook time:** 14 min • **Yield:** 6 servings

Ingredients	*Directions*
2 pounds broccoli rabe	*1* Remove the leaves on the broccoli rabe stem and set them aside. Cut the stalk into 3-inch pieces.
2 tablespoons olive oil	
4 cloves garlic, sliced	*2* In a skillet, heat the olive oil over medium high heat. Sauté the broccoli rabe stalks and leaves and the garlic for 3 minutes.
½ cup chicken stock	
¼ teaspoon red pepper flakes	
	3 Add the chicken stock and red pepper flakes and bring to a simmer. Cover and cook for 10 minutes. Serve.

Per serving: Calories 76 (From Fat 48); Fat 5g (Saturated 1g); Cholesterol 0mg; Sodium 114mg; Carbohydrate 4g (Dietary Fiber 4g); Protein 5g.

Note: Figure 12-2 shows an example of broccoli rabe.

Note: If your broccoli rabe has thick stalks, peel the outer layer of the stem with a vegetable peeler before cutting the stalks in Step 1.

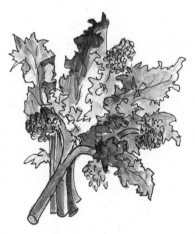

Figure 12-2:
A broccoli rabe may be labeled as broccoli rapini in your grocery store.

Lemony Broccoli and Olives

Prep time: 8 min • **Cook time:** 9 min • **Yield:** 6 servings

Ingredients	*Directions*
½ **teaspoon salt**	*1* Fill a 6-quart pot with water and the salt and bring to a boil. Meanwhile, cut the broccoli florets from the stalks; with a vegetable peeler, remove the outer skin from the stalks and cut the stalks into 1-inch cubes.
1½ **pounds broccoli**	
2 **tablespoons olive oil**	
¼ **cup black olives, pitted and halved**	*2* Add the stalks to the boiling water and blanch for 2 minutes; add the florets and blanch for 1 more minute. Drain all the broccoli pieces and run under cold water.
2 **cloves garlic, thinly sliced**	
Zest and juice of 1 lemon	
	3 Heat the olive oil in a nonstick skillet over medium-high heat until hot. Add the broccoli, olives, and garlic and sauté for 4 minutes or until they reach the desired tenderness. Add the lemon zest and juice, toss, and serve.

Per serving: Calories 84 (From Fat 49); Fat 5g (Saturated 1g); Cholesterol 0mg; Sodium 281mg; Carbohydrate 8g (Dietary Fiber 3g); Protein 3g.

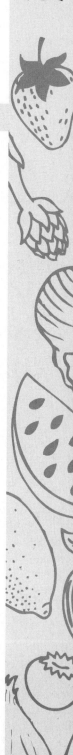

Curry-Roasted Cauliflower

Prep time: 6 min • **Cook time:** 35 min • **Yield:** 6 servings

Ingredients	Directions
1 head cauliflower	*1* Preheat the oven to 425 degrees.
¼ cup olive oil	
½ cup red wine vinegar	*2* Cut the cauliflower (including the stalk and leaves) into bite-sized pieces and place in a medium bowl.
1 teaspoon ground coriander	
1 teaspoon ground cumin	*3* In a small bowl, whisk the remaining ingredients. Pour over the cauliflower and toss to coat.
1 tablespoon curry powder	
1 tablespoon paprika	*4* Pour the cauliflower and sauce onto a baking sheet and bake for 35 minutes, stirring every 5 minutes. Serve.
1 teaspoon salt	

Per serving: Calories 118 (From Fat 85); Fat 9g (Saturated 1g); Cholesterol 0mg; Sodium 431mg; Carbohydrate 7g (Dietary Fiber 3g); Protein 3g.

Springing into Spring

Springtime in the Mediterranean (March through May) brings warm weather and new crops such as brightly colored, pencil-thin asparagus; dark leafy greens; and artichokes. Nothing is quite like seeing these welcoming veggies lined up in the produce aisle or at the farmers' market after a long, cold winter. This section shows you some simple Mediterranean-inspired veggie dishes to go along perfectly with a spring meal.

Featuring fennel

Fennel is a tall bulbous plant that has a flavor similar to licorice. The bulb contains layers similar to cabbage or Brussels sprouts, but is firm and hard. When buying fennel, look for a bright green top with no wilting or sprouting flowers. The appearance of flowers or buds indicates that the plant is past its maturity, and the taste will be compromised. Look for a pale green or white bulb with no slashes or marks. Figure 12-3 later in the chapter gives you a glimpse of a fennel bulb.

You don't see fennel used a lot in traditional American cuisine, but Mediterranean cooking often utilizes fennel, and this veggie can easily become a delicious part of your meal. You can use it raw in salads, or you can grill or braise the bulb until it's warm and soft and the flavors pop out. However you use it, wash the bulb thoroughly to remove any dirt and debris, and make sure to slice it very thinly for best flavor. Check out the Grilled Fennel recipe in this chapter and the Grilled Tuna with Braised Fennel recipe in Chapter 18.

Lemon Asparagus with Parmesan

Prep time: 8 min • **Cook time:** 3 min • **Yield:** 6 servings

Ingredients	*Directions*
½ teaspoon salt	**1** Fill a 6-quart pot with water and a ½ teaspoon of salt. Bring the water to a boil.
1¼ pounds asparagus	
Zest and juice of 1 lemon	**2** Meanwhile, trim tops of the asparagus and remove the outer skin of the bottom of the stalks (about 2 inches from the bottom) with a vegetable peeler. Cut the stalks into 3-inch pieces.
1 clove garlic, minced	
¼ cup parsley, chopped	
2 tablespoons olive oil	
1 tablespoon butter, melted	**3** Add the asparagus to the boiling water and boil for 3 minutes; strain. Immediately place asparagus into a large bowl of ice water for 1 minute. Strain again and place in a serving bowl.
¼ teaspoon salt	
2 ounces Parmesan cheese	
	4 Combine the lemon zest and juice, garlic, olive oil, melted butter, and salt. Pour the mixture over the asparagus and toss. Peel long strands of Parmesan over the top of the asparagus and serve.

Per serving: Calories 116 (From Fat 83); Fat 9g (Saturated 4g); Cholesterol 13mg; Sodium 451mg; Carbohydrate 4g (Dietary Fiber 2g); Protein 6g.

Braised Artichokes

Prep time: 25 min • **Cook time:** 23 min • **Yield:** 6 servings

Ingredients	Directions
4 small artichokes	*1* Using a sharp knife, cut off the tip of the artichoke stems and remove the artichokes' tough outer leaves. Cut a ½-inch off the top of each artichoke and trim any remaining thorns on the tips. Cut the artichokes in half.
1 lemon	
¼ cup olive oil	
1 leek	
4 cloves garlic, sliced	*2* Place all the halves in a large bowl of water. To prevent browning, slice the lemon in half, squeeze the juice into the water, and place the lemon halves in the water as well.
¼ cup mint or basil, chopped	
1½ cups chicken stock	
½ cup white wine	*3* Using a spoon or paring knife, cut out the purple choke (not to be confused with the heart) in the center of the artichoke. Slice each artichoke half into 4 to 6 wedges and return them to the lemon water.
Salt to taste	
	4 In a Dutch oven, heat the olive oil over medium heat. Cut the leek into ¼-inch slices, separate the rings, and rinse well to remove any sand. Add the leeks and garlic to the heated olive oil and sauté for 6 minutes.
	5 Drain the artichokes and pat dry. Add the mint and artichokes to the pan and continue to cook over low heat for 2 to 3 minutes. Pour in the stock.
	6 Bring the pot to a boil, reduce the heat to a simmer, and cover for 10 minutes. Stir in the white wine and simmer uncovered for 5 to 10 minutes or until tender. Season with salt and serve.

Per serving: Calories 152 (From Fat 85); Fat 9g (Saturated 1g); Cholesterol 1mg; Sodium 113mg; Carbohydrate 12g (Dietary Fiber 5g); Protein 4g.

Tip: You can save time by using frozen artichoke hearts rather than cutting them fresh. Just thaw them out and skip to Step 3.

Note: Leeks are grown in sandy soil, so rinsing fresh leeks well and separating the rings to remove all sandy debris is important.

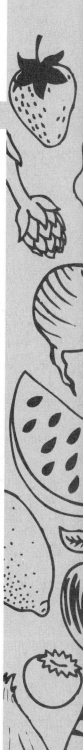

Grilled Fennel

Prep time: 5 min • **Cook time:** 8 min • **Yield:** 4 servings

Ingredients	Directions
2 fennel bulbs	**1** Heat a grill over medium-high heat. Cut the fennel bulbs in half, drizzle them with 1 tablespoon of the olive oil, and season with the salt and red pepper flakes. Grill the fennel for 4 to 6 minutes on each side.
1 tablespoon plus 1 tablespoon olive oil	
⅛ teaspoon salt	**2** Using a sharp knife, cut the skin away from the orange, removing the white outer portion. Cut the orange in half, break it into segments.
⅛ teaspoon red pepper flakes	
1 orange	
¼ cup raw almonds, chopped	**3** Toast the almonds in a skillet over medium heat for 3 to 4 minutes, stirring or tossing constantly to avoid burning. Sprinkle the almonds over the orange slices.
	4 Thinly slice the fennel and toss it with the orange slices and almonds. Drizzle with the remaining olive oil and serve.

Per serving: Calories 169 (From Fat 103); Fat 11g (Saturated 1g); Cholesterol 0mg; Sodium 235mg; Carbohydrate 16g (Dietary Fiber 6g); Protein 4g.

Note: You can see how to cut fennel for this recipe in Figure 12-3. Head to the sidebar "Featuring fennel" earlier in this chapter for more on this vegetable.

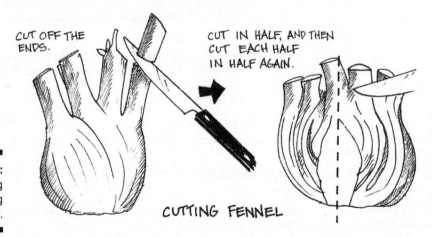

Figure 12-3: Cleaning and cutting fennel.

CUT OFF THE ENDS.

CUT IN HALF, AND THEN CUT EACH HALF IN HALF AGAIN.

CUTTING FENNEL

Loving Light, Fresh Summer Classics

You can find an abundance of fresh fruits and vegetables in the summer — a perfect fit for great summer activities such as grilling or sharing a tasty meal with friends and family on the back porch. Enjoying summer's bounty is what living the Mediterranean lifestyle means. Fresh tomatoes, green beans, eggplant, and cucumbers are in full bloom and, as the recipes in this section demonstrate, you can be prepare them in many different ways. Find some new favorite recipes for those long summer days.

Secrets to perfectly grilled vegetables

If you haven't tried your hand at grilling vegetables, doing so can be a fast and easy way to bring amazing flavor to your meal. Vegetables are a lot more sensitive than meats (to heat, at least; no word on which one cries more at sad movies), so here are a few tips to get great veggie grilling results:

✔ For a robust flavor, marinate your vegetables in your favorite concoction for 20 minutes to an hour in the refrigerator. The veggies will soak up that great flavor.

✔ Always scrub your grill before grilling vegetables. The last thing you want is your grill's old charred meat flavor ruining your light, fresh veggies.

✔ Be sure to oil your clean grill or spray nonstick cooking spray on the racks prior to heating to make sure your vegetables don't stick.

✔ Heat your grill to medium-high heat. You don't want huge flames because vegetables are so delicate. You're not going for that charred-marshmallow look, which is what you'll get if your heat's too high.

✔ Keep a small bowl of oil or your marinade handy to brush your veggies with if they begin to dry out on the grill.

✔ Stand by your vegetables the entire time. Vegetables need to be turned often, and they cook quickly, so you don't want to shut the grill lid and walk away. Keep it open and baste, flip, and remove the veggies as needed.

✔ When you see the vegetables begin to blister, take them off the grill. They continue to cook a little from the residual heat after you pull them, so timing is important. Let them cool slightly, and you're ready to serve.

Chilled Cucumbers with Dill Sauce

Prep time: 1 hr, 30 min • **Yield:** 4 servings

Ingredients	Directions
3 cucumbers	**1** Cut the ends off the cucumbers, slice the cucumbers in half lengthwise, and remove the seeds like in Figure 12-4.
½ teaspoon salt	
1 cup nonfat Greek yogurt	
2 tablespoons fresh dill, chopped	**2** Cut the cucumbers in ½-inch half moons and place them into a small bowl. Sprinkle them with the salt and allow them to sit for 20 minutes.
2 cloves garlic, minced	
¼ cup green onions, chopped	**3** Rinse the cucumbers with cold water in a colander and pat dry. In a small bowl, combine the Greek yogurt, dill, garlic, green onions, and lemon zest. Mix in the cucumbers and chill for at least 1 hour prior to serving.
1 tablespoon lemon zest	

Per serving: Calories 66 (From Fat 2); Fat 0g (Saturated 0g); Cholesterol 0mg; Sodium 321mg; Carbohydrate 11g (Dietary Fiber 1g); Protein 7g.

Tip: Figure 12-4 shows the way to remove the seeds from a cucumber.

HOW TO SEED A CUCUMBER

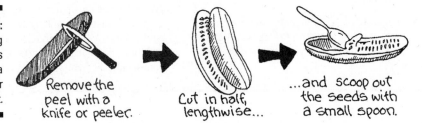

Figure 12-4:
Removing the seeds from a cucumber isn't difficult.

Remove the peel with a knife or peeler.

Cut in half, lengthwise...

...and scoop out the seeds with a small spoon.

Grilled Eggplant and Zucchini

Prep time: 45 min • **Cook time:** 8 min • **Yield:** 6 servings

Ingredients	Directions
1 large eggplant, or 2 Japanese eggplants	**1** Peel the eggplant with a vegetable peeler and cut it into ½-inch-thick rounds.
1 teaspoon sea salt	
3 medium zucchinis	**2** To extract the eggplant's bitterness, layer several paper towels on a large plate. Place a generous amount of sea salt (around ½ teaspoon) on the towels and stack the eggplant rounds in a single layer.
¼ cup olive oil	
1 clove garlic, minced	
1 cup parsley, finely chopped	**3** Sprinkle the remaining sea salt on top of the eggplant slices. Layer more paper towels on top and top with a weighted plate. Allow the eggplant to sit for 20 to 30 minutes. Rinse the eggplant well under cold water and pat dry.
3 tablespoons balsamic or red wine vinegar	
¼ teaspoon red pepper flakes	
¼ teaspoon salt	**4** Slice the zucchinis into three ½-inch slices lengthwise. Rinse under cold water and pat dry.
¼ teaspoon pepper	
	5 Oil the grill or grill pan and heat it over medium-high heat. Grill the eggplant for about 8 minutes per side and the zucchini for 4 minutes per side or until they reach the desired tenderness.
	6 Combine the olive oil, garlic, parsley, vinegar, red pepper flakes, salt, and pepper. Pull the vegetables off the grill and dip the ends of each piece into dressing. Pour the remaining dressing over the top to taste and serve.

Per serving: Calories 129 (From Fat 86); Fat 10g (Saturated 1g); Cholesterol 0mg; Sodium 502mg; Carbohydrate 10g (Dietary Fiber 4g); Protein 2g.

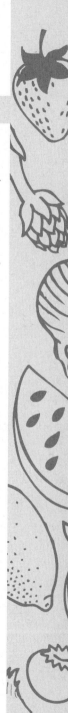

Rice-Stuffed Tomatoes

Prep time: 15 min • **Cook time:** 1 hr • **Yield:** 6 servings

Ingredients	Directions
6 medium tomatoes	*1* Cut ½-inch caps off the tops of the tomatoes and set aside. Carefully scoop out the tomato pulp and put it into a medium saucepan. Put the hollowed tomatoes upright into an 8-x-8-inch baking dish.
1 cup white rice	
1½ cups chicken stock	
¼ cup plus 1 cup white wine	*2* Heat the saucepan over medium high-heat, add the rice to the tomato pulp, and cook for 1 minute. Add the stock, ¼ cup of the wine, the bay leaf, and the olive oil and bring to a boil.
1 bay leaf	
1 teaspoon olive oil	
⅓ cup plus 6 teaspoons grated Parmesan cheese	*3* Reduce the heat to a simmer and cover for 20 to 25 minutes or until the liquid is absorbed. Discard the bay leaf. Remove the pot from the heat and allow the rice mixture to cool for 10 minutes.
¼ cup green onions, chopped	
¼ cup fresh basil leaves, chopped	*4* Preheat the oven to 350 degrees. Stir in ⅓ cup of the Parmesan, the green onions, and basil to the cooled rice. Fill the tomatoes with rice mixture.
	5 Top each tomato with 1 teaspoon of Parmesan cheese. Place the top onto each tomato and lightly cover the pan with foil.
	4 Bake the tomatoes for 20 minutes. Remove the foil, pour the remaining wine over the tomatoes, and continue baking for 10 minutes. Let cool for 5 minutes and serve with the wine drippings over the top.

Per serving: Calories 236 (From Fat 36); Fat 4g (Saturated 2g); Cholesterol 8mg; Sodium 197mg; Carbohydrate 34g (Dietary Fiber 2g); Protein 8g.

Tip: Look for flat-bottomed tomatoes so they stand up easily in the baking dish. If necessary, you can slice a small sliver off the bottom of the tomato to create a flat surface.

Chapter 13

Rediscovering Whole Grains

If you're tired of the same old boring plain white rice and potatoes with your meals, you've come to the right chapter. You can add some flavorful and interesting grain side dishes to your table with the Mediterranean diet. If you're convinced eating grains is worse than eating cardboard, banish the thought. Grain side dishes can be not only healthy but also incredibly flavorful, with added Mediterranean staples such as olive oil, beans, and fresh herbs. And don't forget about incorporating fresh produce; that's another great Mediterranean trick for ratcheting up a dish's health benefits.

Popular grains used in the Mediterranean include rice; wheat products such as bulgur wheat and couscous; and polenta, which is made from cornmeal. If you haven't cooked with some of these grains, we're confident you can find some new favorites that add more variety to the whole grains that you consume.

Whole grains provide carbohydrates for energy along with fiber, vitamins, and minerals to keep you at your best.

The good news is many of these products are as easy to cook as rice and potatoes, so you don't have to worry about being in the kitchen all day. (Flip to Chapter 6 for general information on cooking grains.) In this chapter, we show you some amazing side dishes, including some of the most traditional recipes on the Mediterranean coast.

Exploring Rice and Couscous

Rice and couscous are always great staples to have on hand to make great, easy side dishes. Although brown rice provides more fiber, you can still enjoy other types of rice (such as long-grain) and give them an extra punch of nutrients by adding healthy ingredients. *Couscous* is made from semolina wheat and is a popular dish all along the Mediterranean coast. It's one of the quickest and easiest grains to cook with, and you can find it in any major grocery store.

You can find both regular and whole-wheat varieties of couscous at your local grocery store. The whole-wheat version gives you more fiber, vitamins, and minerals.

If you're ready to put that sad-looking buttered white rice on the side of your plate to rest, get ready for some amazing flavor! This section provides some fabulous rice and couscous recipes for everyday eating or your next dinner party.

Keeping your recipes fresh: Cooking with lemons

As you cook recipes from this book, you may start to notice that your shopping cart is full of lemons each week. Lemon trees grow well in the Mediterranean climate, and the people of the Mediterranean coast are experts at using their abundant crops in their cooking. Lemon juice provides a nice, light citrus flavor and can also enhance the overall flavor of a meal.

By using lemons, you can use much less salt and fewer added fats without sacrificing flavor. And that's not to mention the health benefits: Lemons are high in vitamin C and other phytonutrients, which both act as antioxidants to help prevent damage to your cells. Here are a few tips for using lemons in your cooking:

- Juice lemons at room temperature instead of cold to yield more juice.

- Roll your lemons firmly on the counter before juicing to break up the pulp and give you more juice.

- When making a recipe that calls for lemon juice, go the extra mile and fill an ice cube tray with lemon juice so that you can freeze portions for easy use in later recipes.

- Use a few squeezes of lemon juice on your salad and use a third to half less salad dressing to save some fat and calories. (This tip only works with vinaigrettes, and specifically those that aren't lemon-based; using the juice with already-lemony dressings creates an overwhelming lemon flavor.)

- Add lemon juice to sliced apples and pears to keep them from browning.

- Use lemon juice to tenderize meats.

- Add lemon juice to cooked rice to make it fluffier and enhance the flavor.

Golden Pilaf

Prep time: 10 min • **Cook time:** 25 min • **Yield:** 6 servings

Ingredients	Directions
2 teaspoons olive oil	**1** In a 2-quart saucepan, heat the olive oil over medium-high heat. Add the onions and raisins and sauté for 3 minutes.
1 medium onion, chopped	
¼ cup golden raisins	
1 cup long-grain rice	**2** Stir in the rice, turmeric, cinnamon, and cardamom and sauté for 1 minute. Add the stock, bring the mixture to a boil, and cover.
½ teaspoon turmeric	
⅛ teaspoon cinnamon	
⅛ teaspoon cardamom	**3** Reduce the heat to a simmer for 15 to 18 minutes or until the liquid is fully absorbed. Meanwhile, toast the pistachios in small nonstick skillet for 1 minute or until fragrant. Add the pistachios and parsley to the cooked rice and serve.
2 cups low-sodium chicken or vegetable stock	
¼ cup pistachios, chopped	
¼ cup parsley, chopped	

Per serving: Calories 205 (From Fat 43); Fat 5g (Saturated 1g); Cholesterol 0mg; Sodium 48mg; Carbohydrate 36g (Dietary Fiber 2g); Protein 6g.

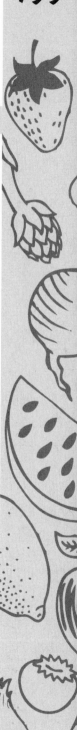

Wild Rice Pilaf

Prep time: 12 min • **Yield:** 8 servings

Ingredients	Directions
2 cups wild rice, cooked	**1** In a large bowl, combine the rice, orzo, spinach, olives, dill, and olive oil. Toss to coat.
2 cups orzo, cooked	
2 cups baby spinach leaves, chopped	**2** Add the lemon juice and gently stir in the tomatoes and parsley. Season with salt and pepper to taste. Top with the cheese and serve.
¼ cup kalamata olives, pitted	
¼ cup fresh dill, chopped	
¼ cup fresh parsley, chopped	
¼ cup olive oil	
Juice of 1 lemon	
1 cup grape tomatoes, halved lengthwise	
Salt and pepper to taste	
2 ounces feta cheese, crumbled	

Per serving: Calories 186 (From Fat 83); Fat 9g (Saturated 2g); Cholesterol 6mg; Sodium 211mg; Carbohydrate 21g (Dietary Fiber 2g); Protein 5g.

Moroccan Couscous

Prep time: 5 min • **Cook time:** 15 min • **Yield:** 8 servings

Ingredients	*Directions*
1½ cups vegetable stock	*1* In a medium saucepan, bring the stock to a boil. Add the orange juice and zest, dates, apricots, raisins, spices, and couscous.
Zest and juice of 1 orange	
⅓ cup chopped dates	
⅓ cup chopped dried apricots	*2* Cover and remove the pan from the heat. Allow the couscous to absorb the liquid, about 15 minutes. If your couscous is too dry, add a bit of water, cover, and wait 5 minutes; repeat until the couscous is the desired consistency.
⅓ cup golden raisins	
¼ teaspoon ground cinnamon	
½ teaspoon ground cumin	
¼ teaspoon coriander	
½ teaspoon ground ginger	*3* Uncover, add the butter, and mix well. Stir in the almonds and mint and season with salt to taste before serving.
½ teaspoon turmeric	
2 cups dry plain or whole-wheat couscous	
1 tablespoon butter	
½ cup slivered almonds, toasted	
¼ cup mint, chopped	
Salt to taste	

Per serving: Calories 264 (From Fat 46); Fat 5g (Saturated 1g); Cholesterol 4mg; Sodium 124mg; Carbohydrate 48g (Dietary Fiber 4g); Protein 8g.

Vary It! For a spicier version, add ¼ teaspoon of cayenne pepper when you add the spices.

Note: Check out the color insert for a photo of this recipe.

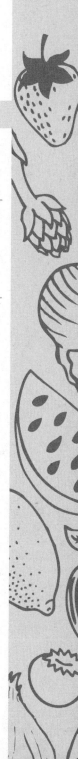

Couscous with Tomatoes and Cucumbers

Prep time: 2 hours, plus chilling time • **Cook time:** 5 min • **Yield:** 6 servings

Ingredients	Directions
2 cups water	*1* In a medium saucepan, bring the water to a boil. Stir in the couscous and coriander, cover, and remove from the heat. Allow the couscous to absorb the liquid completely, about 15 minutes.
1 cup whole-wheat couscous	
½ teaspoon coriander	
2 Roma or plum tomatoes, chopped	*2* Combine the cooked couscous with the tomatoes, cucumber, onions, chickpeas, and mint in a large bowl. Whisk together the lemon juice and olive oil, pour the mixture over the couscous salad, and stir well.
1 small cucumber, seeded and chopped	
½ medium red onion, chopped	
One 14.5-ounce can chickpeas, drained and rinsed	*3* Cover and refrigerate for at least 2 hours. Serve.
½ cup fresh mint, chopped	
⅓ cup lemon juice	
1 tablespoon olive oil	
Salt and pepper to taste	

Per serving: Calories 222 (From Fat 33); Fat 4g (Saturated 0g); Cholesterol 0mg; Sodium 102mg; Carbohydrate 40g (Dietary Fiber 6g); Protein 8g.

From Mush to Gold: Making Polenta

Polenta is cooked cornmeal, which historically was used in the Mediterranean by the peasants as mush. Now, however, many upscale restaurants all along the Mediterranean coast (not to mention in the United States) use it, which we're sure would surprise many peasants. Polenta provides a great whole grain that has a sweet flavor and works in a lot of applications.

This section celebrates all things polenta. After you create your basic polenta recipe, you can use it in a variety of simple and delicious side dishes. Don't take our word for it; try some of these recipes with your next meal.

If you don't want to make your own polenta from scratch, you can buy it prepared in any major grocery store. However, the flavor is always best when you make your polenta from scratch.

Using dried fruits

Dried fruits have been used in the Mediterranean region for thousands of years and are a main staple in Mediterranean pantries. Traditionally, fruits such as raisins, dates, prunes, figs, apricots, and apples were dehydrated in the sun, but today, special dryers and dehydrators do the job. Regardless of the process, the result is a highly sweetened fruit with a long shelf life.

Just like regular fruit, dried fruits are loaded in healthy vitamins, minerals, phytochemicals, and antioxidants, making them yet another healthy addition to the Mediterranean diet. When you're buying dried fruits, be aware that many commercial offerings contain added sugars, which aren't necessary; actually, these products are often considered fruit candy rather than a traditional dried fruit.

Note: If you have allergies or sensitivities to sulfites, avoid dried fruits because they're often used as preservatives in dried fruits.

Dried fruit is the perfect vehicle to add a strong punch of flavor to grain dishes, salads, and desserts. Check out the Golden Pilaf and Moroccan Couscous recipes in this chapter to see how adding sweet fruit to the nutty, earthy flavor of grains is an amazing duo!

Basic Polenta

Prep time: 5 minutes, plus chilling time 1 hour • **Cook time:** 20 min • **Yield:** 8 servings

Ingredients	Directions
Nonstick cooking spray **6 cups water** **1 teaspoon salt** **1¾ cups instant polenta** **1 tablespoon butter**	*1* Coat an 8-x-11-inch glass baking pan with nonstick cooking spray.
	2 In a 4-quart saucepan, bring the water to a boil. Add in 1 teaspoon of salt and gradually whisk in the polenta. Reduce the heat to low.
	3 Whisking continuously, cook the polenta until thickened, about 15 minutes. Remove from the heat and stir in the butter until melted.
	4 Pour the polenta into the baking pan and level with a straight-edged spatula. Place the polenta into the refrigerator for at least one hour to cool before using in another recipe or baking/frying to eat on its own.

Per serving: Calories 204 (From Fat 21); Fat 2g (Saturated 1g); Cholesterol 4mg; Sodium 741mg; Carbohydrate 41g (Dietary Fiber 2g); Protein 4g.

Tip: You can serve this basic polenta recipe with sautéed veggies or different types of cheese. You can also smother baked polenta with sauces such as the Marinara, Pesto, or Chickpea Sauce in Chapter 9.

Tip: Be sure to get instant polenta; otherwise, you may be stirring for 45 minutes.

Tip: Lower your calories and fat by omitting the butter all together.

Grilled Polenta with Gorgonzola

Prep time: 5 min • **Cook time:** 14 min • **Yield:** 8 servings

Ingredients	Directions
1 batch Basic Polenta	*1* With a sharp knife score, the polenta into triangle wedges.
2 tablespoons olive oil, or olive oil cooking spray	
½ cup Gorgonzola cheese, crumbled	*2* Heat a grill pan until it's smoking or heat a grill to medium-high heat. Brush one side of the polenta wedge with olive oil or lightly spray with olive oil cooking spray.
	3 Grill the polenta in batches, leaving it alone until it has grill marks, about 5 minutes.
	4 Drop the heat to medium, carefully flip the polenta, and continue to grill for 8 minutes. Transfer to a warm platter, top with the cheese crumbles, and serve.

Per serving: Calories 289 (From Fat 99); Fat 11g (Saturated 5g); Cholesterol 18mg; Sodium 890mg; Carbohydrate 41g (Dietary Fiber 2g); Protein 6g.

Vary It! You can replace the Gorgonzola with another blue cheese, goat cheese, or feta, depending on what type of flavor you enjoy. You can also try topping the grilled polenta with Parmesan or mozzarella and broiling them for 4 minutes to melt the cheese.

Tip: Check out the Basic Polenta recipe earlier in this chapter.

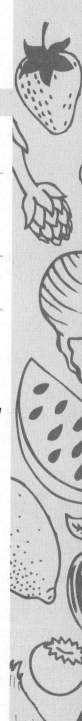

Pan-Fried Polenta with Prosciutto and Parmesan

Prep time: 10 min • **Cook time:** 30 min • **Yield:** 8 servings

Ingredients	Directions
1 batch Basic Polenta	**1** Heat the oven to broil. With a sharp knife, score the polenta into triangle wedges.
½ cup flour	
⅓ cup grapeseed or canola oil	**2** In a large skillet, heat the oil over medium-high heat. Lightly dust each polenta wedge with flour and fry for 6 minutes on each side or until lightly browned.
½ pound prosciutto, thinly sliced	
½ cup grated Parmesan cheese	**3** Immediately drain the fried polenta on paper towels to absorb the excess oil. Place the drained polenta onto a baking sheet.
	4 Top each polenta wedge polenta with prosciutto and 1 teaspoon of the cheese. Broil them in the oven for 4 minutes or until the cheese is slightly browned. Serve immediately.

Per serving: Calories 413 (From Fat 159); Fat 18g (Saturated 5g); Cholesterol 37mg; Sodium 1632mg; Carbohydrate 47g (Dietary Fiber 2g); Protein 15g.

Tip: You know your oil is ready when it fries a one-inch cube of bread. If the bread sinks and takes in oil, your oil isn't hot enough.

Tip: If the flour doesn't stick well to your polenta, sprinkle a little water on the polenta first to help the flour adhere better. Check out the Basic Polenta recipe earlier in this chapter.

Creating Amazing Sides with Bulgur Wheat

Side dishes prepared with bulgur wheat are very common along the Mediterranean coast; many of the region's most celebrated, classic recipes use this grain. *Bulgur* combines several different wheat species with the bran partially removed. Using this wheat is a great way to add more whole grains in your diet, and compared to white rice, bulgur offers more fiber, protein, minerals, and vitamins. Plus, it's a *low-glycemic* grain (creating a low blood sugar spike) and boasts a great nutty flavor. You can find bulgur wheat in any major grocery store.

This section shows you some traditional ways to cook with bulgur for some tasty side dishes. If you've never tried tabbouleh or kibbeh, now is the time. Nothing celebrates the Mediterranean coast like the classics.

Bulgur, the perfect quick grain

Bulgur is created by parboiling wheat and grinding it into smaller particles. The process of creating bulgur wheat originated in the Mediterranean, and the result has been a Middle Eastern diet staple for thousands of years; it's even touted as being the first processed food.

Although the grinding process partially removes some of the bran, bulgur remains a high-fiber, high-nutrient cereal grain. Bulgur has a great nutty flavor and can be used like rice in dishes.

The good news is that bulgur has more vitamins, minerals, and protein and lower glycemic index level (a measure of how a food affects blood sugar levels) than white rice, so it's a great replacement.

Even more good news is that bulgur is simple to cook with because it's partially processed. All you do is add boiling water or broth, remove the bulgur from the heat, and let it stand covered for 10 to 15 minutes. Then you can add any seasonings you enjoy for a quick, healthy side dish.

Bulgur Salad with White Beans and Spinach

Prep time: 20 minutes, plus 30 minutes chilling time • **Cook time:** 5 minutes • **Yield:** 8 servings

Ingredients	*Directions*
¾ cup bulgur	*1* In a 2-quart saucepan, boil the water. Pour in the bulgur, cover, and remove from the heat. Allow the bulgur to sit for 20 minutes.
2 cups water	
1 pound baby spinach, chopped	*2* Meanwhile, toss together the spinach, parsley, mint, sun-dried tomatoes, and beans. In a small bowl, whisk the lemon juice and zest, olive oil, cumin, coriander, garlic, salt, and pepper.
¼ cup fresh parsley, chopped	
¼ cup fresh mint, chopped	
¼ cup sundried tomatoes (packed in oil), finely chopped	*3* Add the spinach mixture to the bulgur and toss with a fork. Whisk the dressing and pour over the top of the bulgur/spinach mixture, stirring to mix. Cover and chill for 30 minutes to 1 hour prior to serving.
One 14.5-ounce can cannellini beans, drained and rinsed	
Zest and juice of 2 lemons	
¼ cup olive oil	
½ teaspoon ground cumin	
¼ teaspoon coriander	
1 clove garlic, crushed	
½ teaspoon sea salt	
½ teaspoon pepper	

Per serving: Calories 174 (From Fat 71); Fat 8g (Saturated 1g); Cholesterol 0mg; Sodium 394mg; Carbohydrate 22g (Dietary Fiber 6g); Protein 7g.

Tabbouleh

Prep time: 15 min, plus chilling time • **Cook time:** 5 min • **Yield:** 6 servings

Ingredients	*Directions*
1 cup water	*1* Boil the water in a medium saucepan. Add the bulgur, cover, and remove from the heat. Allow the bulgur to absorb liquid for at least 15 minutes
½ cup bulgur	
¼ cup olive oil	
Juice of 1 to 2 lemons	*2* Whisk the olive oil and lemon juice in a serving bowl. Toss the vegetables and herbs into the bowl and stir. Season the mixture with salt.
½ cup chopped green onions	
4 cups chopped fresh parsley	
¼ cup chopped fresh mint	*3* Add the bulgur, stir, and refrigerate for at least 30 minutes before serving.
1 large tomato, diced small	
1 English cucumber, diced small	
½ teaspoon salt	

Per serving: Calories 150 (From Fat 87); Fat 10g (Saturated 1g); Cholesterol 0mg; Sodium 224mg; Carbohydrate 15g (Dietary Fiber 4g); Protein 3g.

VaryIt! You can use couscous as an alternative to bulgur.

Finding that community spirit

A hallmark of Mediterranean life is time spent with family and friends. In fact, many families in the Mediterranean have dinner parties once or twice a week rather than the once or twice a year many Americans do. The idea is to get together for a meal, spend time together, and celebrate nothing more than the week to provide a much-needed sense of community.

Don't wait until the next birthday party or graduation. Call up your family, friends, and neighbors and invite them over for grill night or the big football game. If you're new to an area, what better way to get to know people than to invite your neighbors for an open house? Find that sense of community wherever you live.

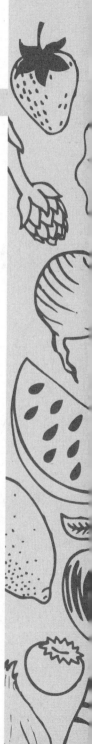

Stuffed Kibbeh

Prep time: 30 min • **Cook time:** 20 min • **Yield:** 6 servings

Ingredients	*Directions*
½ **pound plus ½ pound lean ground beef or lamb**	*1* Preheat the oven to 400 degrees. In a heavy skillet, cook half the meat and half the onion over medium heat until browned, about 10 minutes.
1 medium onion, finely chopped, divided	
¼ **teaspoon plus ¼ teaspoon salt**	*2* Add half the salt, the pine nuts, cumin, coriander, and allspice and cook for 3 minutes. Remove from the heat, stir in the chopped cilantro, and set aside. Soak the bulgur in cold water for 10 minutes and squeeze out the moisture.
¼ **cup pine nuts**	
1 teaspoon ground cumin	
½ **teaspoon coriander**	*3* Blend the bulgur; the remaining meat, onion, and salt; the pepper; and the cayenne in a food processor for 1 minute or until it forms a paste.
¼ **teaspoon allspice**	
½ **cup cilantro, chopped**	
1½ **cups bulgur**	*4* Shape about 3 tablespoons of the bulgur mixture into a ½-inch-thick pancake with your hands. Place 1 tablespoon of the meat filling in the center and close up all four sides. Repeat with the remaining bulgur mixture and filling, evenly dividing the filling among the pancakes.
1 teaspoon pepper	
⅛ **teaspoon cayenne pepper**	
Nonstick cooking spray	
6 lemon wedges	
	5 With wet fingers, shape the kibbeh into ovals and place onto a baking sheet. Spray the kibbeh with the cooking spray and bake for 20 minutes. Serve on a platter with the lemon wedges.

Per serving: Calories 338 (From Fat 141); Fat 16g (Saturated 5g); Cholesterol 51mg; Sodium 255mg; Carbohydrate 32g (Dietary Fiber 7g); Protein 20g.

Tip: You can freeze the cooked kibbeh up to 1 month. Simply microwave to reheat.

Tip: Serve kibbeh as a side dish with your meal or eat one as a snack — try it with the Cucumber Yogurt Sauce in Chapter 9. Because the kibbeh have protein, you can combine them with a light bean dish or salad for a great meal.

Bulgur-Stuffed Zucchini

Prep time: 20 min • **Cook time:** 28 min • **Yield:** 6 servings

Ingredients	*Directions*
1 cup water	*1* Preheat the oven to 350 degrees. In a medium sauce-pan, bring the water to a boil. Add the bulgur, cover, and remove from the heat. Allow the bulgur to sit for 15 minutes.
½ cup bulgur	
3 medium zucchinis	
⅛ plus ¼ teaspoon salt	*2* Slice the zucchinis in half lengthwise. Using a spoon, scoop out each zucchini's pulp, leaving about ¼-inch of the flesh to retain the zucchini's shape; chop the pulp and set aside. Season the zucchini with ⅛ tea-spoon of the salt and the pepper.
⅛ teaspoon pepper	
1 tablespoon olive oil	
½ medium onion, finely chopped	
1 teaspoon coriander	*3* In a skillet, heat the olive oil over medium-high heat. Add the onion, coriander, and cumin and cook for 3 minutes. Add the tomatoes, reduce the heat to medium-low, and allow the mixture to cook for 5 minutes.
1 teaspoon ground cumin	
One 28-ounce can chopped no-salt-added tomatoes	
1 cup plus ¼ cup parsley, chopped	*4* Add the chopped zucchini pulp, 1 cup of the parsley, and the remaining salt to the bulgur and mix well. Place the zucchini halves faceup in an 8-x-8-inch glass baking dish. Fill the zucchini halves with the bulgur mixture.
3 Roma or plum tomatoes, thinly sliced	
1 lemon, thinly sliced	
	5 Pour the tomato sauce over the zucchini. Top with the sliced tomatoes and then the lemon slices. Bake for 20 minutes. Garnish with the remaining parsley and serve.

Per serving: *Calories 96 (From Fat 26); Fat 3g (Saturated 0g); Cholesterol 0mg; Sodium 137mg; Carbohydrate 16g (Dietary Fiber 4g); Protein 3g.*

Tip: Depending on the size of your zucchinis, you may end up with extra filling. If so, simply place it in a small glass dish and bake it alongside the zucchinis. The filling still makes a tasty side dish!

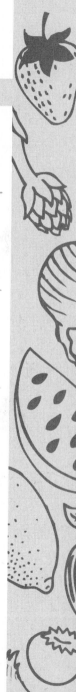

Fat or fluid? The scale can't tell

Stepping on the scale can be your greatest win for the day if you lost a few pounds or destroy your day if the number goes up a few ticks. You can easily forget that when you weigh yourself, you aren't just weighing fat; you're also weighing muscle, water, organs, tissue, and other bodily fluids. When the scale shifts a few pounds, you may assume the culprit must be that stubborn fat you're trying to lose, but the reality is that your body can shift weight a few pounds from morning to night because of fluid.

Water fluctuations can occur for many reasons, including eating a high-sodium meal, spending time in the hot sun, following a low-carbohydrate/high-protein diet, taking certain medications, or experiencing hormonal shifts. This consideration is especially true if the drastic weight gain happens overnight. You have to take in or burn 3,500 calories to gain or lose one pound of body fat. So if you gained three pounds in one day, you can chalk that gain up to fluid weight; otherwise, you'd have had to consume 10,500 extra calories that day, which isn't likely! True body fat gain and loss happen gradually.

Check your weight once a week and look for overall trends if your weight continues to go up without bouncing back down. Give yourself a break! Your body is just shifting fluid weight in a natural way.

Part IV
Main Entrees and Desserts

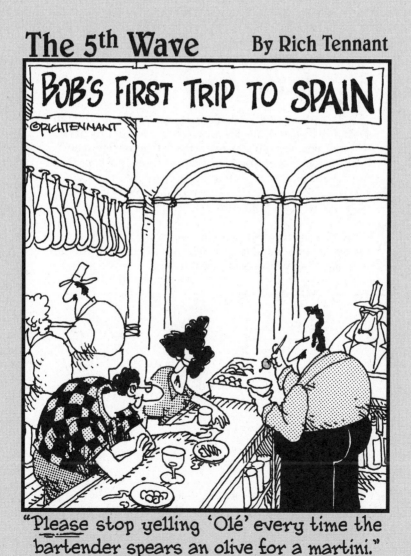

The 5th Wave   By Rich Tennant

BOB'S FIRST TRIP TO SPAIN

"Please stop yelling 'Olé' every time the bartender spears an olive for a martini."

In this part . . .

No matter what kind of mood you're in, you can find full-flavored entrees for any occasion in this part, whether you want to go vegetarian with some lentil and bean recipes; fix up some seafood, chicken, pork, or beef; or perhaps kick back with pizza or pasta. We show you easy-to-make recipes for every day and some classic dishes perfect for your next celebration.

But save room for dessert! This part also includes recipes for weekly treats and large celebrations, showing you how to include tasty sweets in a healthy way.

Chapter 14

Enjoying Legumes the Mediterranean Way

....

In This Chapter

▶ Discovering new ways to cook with lentils

▶ Exploring common bean dishes of the Mediterranean

....

*E*ating a plant-based diet is one of the funda-
mentals of Mediterranean cuisine and one of
the major reasons for the health benefits found
in the Mediterranean diet. Eating ample amounts
of fruits and vegetables isn't the only way to
incorporate plant foods; people who live on the
Mediterranean coast also consume a good amount
of *legumes,* otherwise known as lentils and beans,
which are chock-full of fiber, vitamins, and minerals and are a good source of protein. (They also
contain trace amounts of fats.)

Many people consume lentils and beans only
occasionally, such as when they have a burrito or
lentil soup. Others may enjoy them more often on
salads or with side dishes. No matter what camp
you fall in, this chapter shows you different ways
to cook lentils and beans for amazing side dishes to add to your next meal.

The bottom line is simple: The more nutrients you eat from your foods, the
better health you experience. Part of the goal with eating the Mediterranean
way is to decrease animal protein and increase plant-based proteins. So
instead of eating a steak and potatoes with a salad at your next meal, eat less
meat and add a bean or lentil side for more healthy nutrients and better long-
term health.

Looking at legumes' protein power

The amount of protein in a legume varies depending on the legume variety, but it averages around 8 grams for a half-cup serving size, making legumes a good animal-protein replacement or partial replacement (depending on how much meat you're looking to cut out of your diet).

The bean with the most protein is the soybean (about 15 grams *per serving*), followed by the Mediterranean favorite, the fava bean (about 12 grams *per serving*). You don't have to just stick to the bean side of the legume family, though; lentils provide about 9 grams of protein *per serving*. Most beans and lentils (soybeans excluded) don't provide all the essential amino acids needed to make up a complete protein, but you can easily find the remainder of those amino acids in other foods, such as grains, you eat during the day.

Letting in Lentils

Lentils are small, round legumes that make a healthy choice for any meal. They're a great source of plant-based protein, fiber, and vitamins and minerals such as folate and iron. Lentils are great to cook with because they take on flavors well from other ingredients such as herbs, spices, or broths. If you think the only way to eat lentils is lentil soup, read on; this section shows some simple ways to cook with lentils for delicious, hearty side dishes.

Picking the best lentils for your dish

If you look hard enough, you can find a variety of different types of lentils, all with their own unique flavor, color, and texture. Some types are better for soups, while others are great as a standalone side dish. Use this guide to help you select the perfect type of lentil for your next dish:

✔ *Brown lentils* are the most common type of lentil found in major grocery stores. They range in color from light brown to dark black and have an earthy, nutty flavor. Brown lentils can turn soft quickly if you don't watch your cooking time. The mild flavor works well for many dishes, such as soups and salads, and these lentils are also good for purees because they're easily mashed.

✔ *Green lentils* are often glossy-looking, with a pale green/brown mix of colors. They have a strong flavor and take a little longer to cook than other lentils. The plus about green lentils, other than their taste, is the fact that they retain their texture and shape, well making them perfect for side salads.

✔ *Red lentils* range from gold to red and have a sweet, nutty flavor. Like brown lentils, they run the risk of turning mushy from overcooking. You see red lentils most often in Indian dal or curry dishes. Red lentils are also fabulous in soups.

Mediterranean Lentil Salad

Prep time: 8 min • **Cook time:** 30 min • **Yield:** 6 servings

Ingredients	Directions
2 cups water	*1* In a 2-quart stockpot, bring the water and lentils to a boil on high heat; reduce the heat to low and simmer for 30 minutes or until tender. Drain any excess liquid.
½ cup dry brown or red lentils	
One 14.5-ounce can chickpeas, drained and rinsed	
3 Roma or plum tomatoes, chopped, or one 14.5-ounce can chopped tomatoes, drained	*2* In a serving bowl, mix the cooked lentils, chickpeas, tomatoes, bell peppers, and carrot. Whisk together the lemon juice and olive oil.
½ yellow bell pepper, chopped	*3* Stir the lemon vinaigrette into the salad, top with the cilantro, season with salt to taste, and serve.
1 red bell pepper, chopped	
1 carrot, grated	
Juice of 1 lemon	
2 tablespoons olive oil	
½ cup chopped fresh cilantro	
Salt to taste	

Per serving: Calories 194 (From Fat 50); Fat 6g (Saturated 1g); Cholesterol 0mg; Sodium 101mg; Carbohydrate 30g (Dietary Fiber 9g); Protein 8g.

Tip: Figure 14-1 shows how to prepare a bell pepper for this recipe.

Note: This dish is excellent served chilled or at room temperature. Check out the color insert for a photo of this recipe.

Figure 14-1:
Coring, seeding, slicing, and chopping a bell pepper is easy.

HOW TO CORE, SEED, AND CHOP A PEPPER

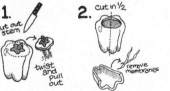
1. cut out stem / twist and pull out

2. cut in ½ / remove membranes

3. Cut into lengthwise strips

4. For cubes, hold strips together and cut crosswise

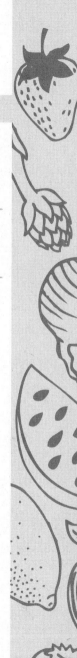

Spanish Lentils with Vegetables

Prep time: 15 min • **Cook time:** 45 min • **Yield:** 8 servings

Ingredients	Directions
3 tablespoons olive oil 1 medium onion, diced	*1* In a 4-quart saucepan, heat the olive oil over medium heat. Add the onion and garlic and sauté for 2 minutes.
3 cloves garlic, mashed 4 ounces Spanish chorizo or Portuguese sausage (linguiça)	*2* Add the sausage and cook for 5 minutes. Add the dried lentils, chopped tomatoes, carrots, and potatoes and sauté for 3 minutes.
2 cups dried red lentils 1 medium tomato, diced 2 medium carrots, sliced in ½-inch rounds 1 large potato, cut in 1-inch cubes 4 cups low-sodium chicken stock ½ teaspoon ground cumin 1 teaspoon sweet paprika 1 bay leaf Salt to taste	*3* Pour the stock over the vegetable mixture, season with the cumin, paprika, and bay leaf, and bring mixture to a boil. Drop the temperature to medium-low and simmer the lentil mixture for 30 minutes or until tender. Season with salt to taste, remove the bay leaf, and serve.

Per serving: Calories 353 (From Fat 112); Fat 12g (Saturated 3g); Cholesterol 12mg; Sodium 234mg; Carbohydrate 43g (Dietary Fiber 7g); Protein 19g.

Spinach and Lentils with Feta

Prep time: 5 min • **Cook time:** 45 min • **Yield:** 6 servings

Ingredients	*Directions*
½ cup brown lentils	**1** In a 2-quart stockpot, bring the stock and lentils to a boil over medium-high heat. Reduce the heat to a simmer and cook for 30 minutes or until tender.
2 cups low-sodium vegetable stock	
2 tablespoons olive oil	**2** In a medium skillet, heat the olive oil over medium-high heat for 1 minute; add the onions and sauté for 5 minutes.
½ a medium onion, sliced	
16 ounces frozen spinach, defrosted	**3** Meanwhile, drain and squeeze the spinach dry over a colander. Add the spinach to the onions and continue sautéing for 3 minutes. Add the cooked lentils, garlic, curry, and paprika and cook for 5 minutes. Serve with crumbled feta over top.
2 cloves garlic, chopped	
1 teaspoon curry powder	
¼ teaspoon paprika	
¼ cup feta, crumbled	

Per serving: Calories 153 (From Fat 59); Fat 7g (Saturated 2g); Cholesterol 6mg; Sodium 238mg; Carbohydrate 16g (Dietary Fiber 4g); Protein 8g.

Vary It! For a spicier version, add ¼ teaspoon of cayenne pepper when you add the spices.

Putting the car keys away for a healthy stroll

Getting in your car to run every errand isn't a way of life on the Mediterranean coast. Walking to the corner market or bakery is more common practice (much like a New Yorker's experience). If you live within walking distance of shops or restaurants, give it a try. For example, if you want to go to a restaurant a few blocks away, walk to it and enjoy the activity as part of the experience. Or perhaps your child's school is within walking distance. Stroll to or from school each day with your child. You can enjoy each other's company and talk about the day, and you teach him or her the importance of a good walk each day.

If you live in an area where forgoing your car for errands is impossible (such as a rural area or a city where walking isn't conducive), you can still incorporate walking into your daily life. No matter what type of city, town, burg, or hamlet you live in, try your best to take a stroll every day. Walking can help with weight management, bone health, heart health, and your mood and energy.

Simple Lentils and Spiced Rice

Prep time: 10 min • **Cook time:** 45 min • **Yield:** 8 servings

Ingredients	*Directions*
1 cup dried lentils, or 2 cups canned lentils, rinsed and drained	*1* In a 2-quart stockpot, bring the dried lentils and 2 cups of the water to a boil over medium-high heat. Reduce the heat to a simmer and cook for 30 minutes or until tender.
2 cups plus 1½ cups water	
½ cup basmati rice	*2* Rinse the rice in a colander at least three times to remove excess starch.
1 tablespoon olive oil	
1 onion, chopped	*3* In a saucepan, heat the olive oil over medium heat; add the onion and sauté for 5 minutes.
½ teaspoon ground cumin	
¼ teaspoon cinnamon	*4* Add the rice to the onion mixture and sauté for 1 minute. Add the remaining water, cumin, cinnamon, and turmeric and bring the mixture to a boil. Cover, reduce the heat, and allow the mixture to simmer for 30 minutes or until the rice is tender.
¼ teaspoon turmeric	
½ cup cilantro, chopped	
½ teaspoon salt	
	5 Mix the rice, lentils, cilantro, and salt before serving.

Per serving: Calories 153 (From Fat 21); Fat 2g (Saturated 0g); Cholesterol 27mg; Sodium 151mg; Carbohydrate 27g (Dietary Fiber 3g); Protein 7g.

Note: If you're using canned lentils, you can skip Step 1.

Lentil Loaf

Prep time: 15 min • **Cook time:** 1 hr, 25 min, plus resting time • **Yield:** 8 servings

Ingredients	*Directions*
1 cup dried lentils 2 cups water Nonstick cooking spray 1 tablespoon plus 1 tablespoon olive oil ½ medium onion, chopped	*1* Combine the lentils and water in a medium stockpot and bring to a boil over medium-high heat. Reduce the heat, and simmer until tender, about 30 minutes. Drain excess liquid and gently mash the lentils together.
1 carrot, grated	*2* Preheat the oven to 400 degrees. Grease a 9-x-5-inch loaf pan with cooking spray.
2 cloves garlic, minced ½ cup breadcrumbs	*3* In a small skillet, heat 1 tablespoon of the olive oil over medium heat. Sauté the onion, carrot, and garlic for 3 minutes.
2 eggs 1 cup low-sodium vegetable stock 2 tablespoons tomato paste	*4* In a large bowl, combine 2 cups of the mashed lentils, the breadcrumbs, eggs, stock, tomato paste, coriander, pepper, parsley, the remaining olive oil, and the onion mixture. Press this lentil mixture into the prepared loaf pan.
½ teaspoon coriander ½ teaspoon pepper ½ cup parsley, chopped ¼ cup grated Parmesan cheese	*5* Bake for 40 minutes. Sprinkle the top with the Parmesan cheese and continue baking another 10 minutes. Allow the lentil loaf to rest for 10 minutes before removing from pan and serving.

Per serving: Calories 179 (From Fat 48); Fat 5g (Saturated 1g); Cholesterol 3mg; Sodium 312mg; Carbohydrate 24g (Dietary Fiber 4g); Protein 10g.

Tip: To shorten the cook time, use 2 cups of canned lentils and skip to Step 2.

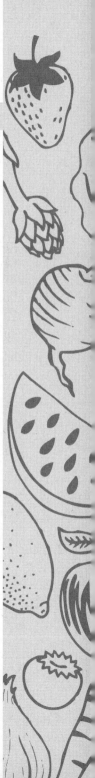

Bringing Beans to the Table

Beans are such a great food because they add delicious plant-based protein, tons of vitamins and minerals, fiber, and phytochemicals (which help prevent chronic diseases). Plus, they're economical, tasty, and satisfying, which means you'll be less likely to snack on junk a couple of hours after eating a meal. You can't go wrong with all those benefits. Chickpeas (also known as garbanzo beans) and fava beans are two of the most common beans in Mediterranean cooking, but you also see other varieties, such as black beans and kidney beans (see the nearby sidebar "Finding the perfect bean" for more info). This section shows some ways to bring beans to your diet.

When adding beans to your diet, do so gradually, because they can be a little gas-forming if your body isn't used to them. Don't love the texture of beans? Try using the bean-featuring recipes in Chapters 8 and 11, where the beans are mashed into dips, soups, and stews.

Finding the perfect bean

The wide variety of available beans can be confusing and intimidating, so here's a breakdown of various kinds of beans with their distinct flavors and common uses:

- ✔ *Black beans* taste slightly sweet and are a great addition to salads, casseroles, soups, burritos, and dips.

- ✔ *Cannellini beans* offer a mild flavor and are common in Italian cooking. They work well in soups, stews, and casseroles and are in Pasta Fagioli — see the recipe in Chapter 11.

- ✔ *Chickpeas* have a nutty flavor and a tougher texture than other beans. They're great in casseroles and stews or with couscous or hummus. Chapter 8 has a hummus recipe.

- ✔ *Fava beans* have a nutty flavor and are often seen in stews and side dishes. They're also used as a breakfast food in many regions, and Chapter 7 has a great recipe for incorporating fava beans into breakfast.

- ✔ *Great Northern beans* are large, white beans with a mild flavor. Soups, stews, and casseroles are where you find them most often.

- ✔ *Lima beans* are green-colored beans that offer a mild, earthy flavor. They're great alone, warmed up as a side dish, or in soups and stews.

- ✔ *Pinto beans* are brown/orange beans with a rich, earthy flavor. You find pintos in foods like refried beans, burritos, or rice and beans.

- ✔ Red kidney beans are — you guessed it — red, kidney-shaped beans with a meaty flavor that are perfect tossed on a salad or in soups or stews.

- ✔ Soybeans are full-flavored, and they're great as a warm side dish or used in soups.

Black Beans with Tomatoes and Feta

Prep time: 10 min • **Yield:** 8 servings

Ingredients	*Directions*
4 Roma or plum tomatoes, diced	*1* In a serving bowl toss together everything but the feta and salt. Top with the feta and season with salt to taste before serving.
Two 14.5-ounce cans black beans, drained and rinsed	
½ red onion, sliced	
¼ cup fresh dill, chopped	
Juice of 1 lemon	
2 tablespoons extra-virgin olive oil	
¼ cup crumbled feta cheese	
Salt to taste	

Per serving: Calories 121 (From Fat 42); Fat 5g (Saturated 1g); Cholesterol 4mg; Sodium 173mg; Carbohydrate 15g (Dietary Fiber 5g); Protein 6g.

Vary It! You can substitute fresh basil for the dill for a sweet flavor.

Taking some time to smell the roses

People on the Mediterranean coast enjoy all aspects of life including food, art, music, and nature. They fill their senses with great appreciation. When was the last time you listened to music or sat in a garden admiring the flowers? These small things can make a big impact on your health because taking in things that are beautiful to you is a significant part of relaxation and stress management.

Make time to enjoy these small moments. Go to your local museum, take a hike in the woods, sit on your front porch with a cup of tea, or go do some fishing along a brook. Taking some time to smell the roses may just be the best-kept health secret.

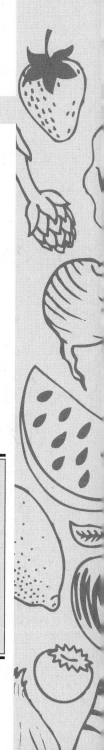

Chickpeas with Sun-Dried Tomatoes and Roasted Red Peppers

Prep time: 25 min • **Cook time:** 22 min • **Yield:** 6 servings

Ingredients	Directions
1 red bell pepper	**1** Slice the red bell pepper in half lengthwise. Place it skin side up on a baking sheet and broil (about 5 inches from the broiler) for 5 to 8 minutes, or until it's slightly blackened and the skin is bubbled.
2 cups water	
4 sun-dried tomatoes	
¼ cup red wine vinegar	**2** Place the charred bell pepper halves into a brown paper bag and roll the bag down to seal it. Allow the pepper to steam for 10 minutes. Then remove the pepper, pull off the charred skin, and cut the peppers into thin strips.
2 cloves garlic, chopped	
2 tablespoons extra-virgin olive oil	
Two 14.5-ounce cans chickpeas, drained and rinsed	**3** Meanwhile, microwave 2 cups of water in a microwave-safe bowl for 4 minutes or until boiling. Add the sun-dried tomatoes and allow them to reconstitute for 10 minutes. Drain the tomatoes and thinly slice them into strips.
½ cup parsley, chopped	
Salt to taste	
	4 In a serving bowl, whisk together the red wine vinegar, garlic, and olive oil. Toss in the chickpeas, roasted red bell pepper strips, sun-dried tomato strips, and parsley. Season the mixture with salt to taste and serve.

Per serving: Calories 195 (From Fat 65); Fat 7g (Saturated 1g); Cholesterol 0mg; Sodium 198mg; Carbohydrate 26g (Dietary Fiber 8g); Protein 8g.

Tip: You can buy red peppers already roasted in your local grocery store for a quick version of this recipe.

Beet and Kidney Bean Salad

Prep time: 12 min • **Cook time:** 15 min • **Yield:** 4 servings

Ingredients	*Directions*
4 beets, scrubbed and stems removed	*1* Fill a 2-quart stockpot with water and add the beets. Bring the water to a boil and reduce the heat to a simmer until the beets are fork tender (about 10 minutes). Strain in a colander and immediately put the beets in ice water to halt cooking.
One 14.5-ounce can kidney beans, drained and rinsed	
4 green onions, chopped	
Juice of 1 lemon	*2* Allow the beets to chill for 3 minutes. Remove the skins of the beets (they should peel easily without the need for a paring knife). Cut the beets into thin half-moon shapes and set aside.
2 tablespoons olive oil	
1 tablespoon pomegranate syrup or juice	
Salt and pepper to taste	*3* In a serving dish, toss together the kidney beans, green onions, lemon juice, olive oil, and pomegranate syrup and toss gently to mix. Add the beets, season with salt and pepper to taste, and serve.

Per serving: Calories 175 (From Fat 67); Fat 7g (Saturated 1g); Cholesterol 0mg; Sodium 200mg; Carbohydrate 22g (Dietary Fiber 7g); Protein 6g.

Note: You can serve this bean salad at room temperature or chilled.

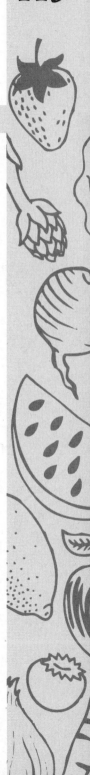

Warm Fava Beans with Feta

Prep time: 8 min • **Cook Time:** 8 min • **Yield:** 4 servings

Ingredients	Directions
Nonstick cooking spray	**1** Spray a medium skillet with cooking spray. Add the onions and garlic and sauté the vegetables for 1 minute over medium heat.
¼ of an onion, chopped	
2 cloves garlic, minced	
14.5 ounces can fava beans, rinsed and drained, or frozen fava beans, thawed	**2** Add the fava beans and tomatoes and sauté for 5 minutes. Stir in the chopped parsley and top with feta before serving.
One 14.5-ounce can no-salt-added tomatoes	
¼ cup fresh parsley, chopped	
¼ cup feta cheese, crumbled	

Per serving: Calories 144 (From Fat 23); Fat 3g (Saturated 1g); Cholesterol 8mg; Sodium 341mg; Carbohydrate 22g (Dietary Fiber 6g); Protein 9g.

Vary It! It goes without saying, if you have fresh fava beans on hand all shucked and ready to go, use them for best quality and flavor. Fresh fava beans may require 5 to 10 more minutes of cooking time, so be sure to taste a bean to see whether it's tender prior to serving. (See the nearby sidebar "Working with the fava bean" for more on shucking fresh fava beans.)

Working with the fava bean

Fava beans, also known as *broad beans,* are a common crop in the Mediterranean that's popular for breakfast and in side dishes. They were one of the only beans eaten in Europe before the discovery of America and all the new beans it had to offer. In many regions, this little bean represents good luck. Not a bad thing to add to your dinner every now and then!

In America, fava beans haven't quite caught on, possibly because preparing them requires some time. Most often, fava beans come in their pod, which means you have to take on the labor-intensive task of shelling them yourself. You can find fava beans canned or frozen in many stores, but they don't have the same flavor as fresh.

Shucking fava beans is a great way to dive into the Mediterranean lifestyle. Take some time on a weekend, grab a bowl for your beans, and open the windows or go outside (if weather permits). Pour yourself a nice, cold drink and get to work! Simply open up the pod, remove the white waxy coating that covers the bean, and place the small green beans in a bowl. Then you can make great recipes such as the Warm Fava Beans with Feta in this chapter. You'll enjoy the dish even more after shucking your own beans. Enjoying the process of preparing the beans all the way up to eating them at the table is a great example of taking time to prepare and cook your food, a hallmark of the Mediterranean philosophy.

Chickpeas with Spinach

Prep time: 5 min • **Cook time:** 8 min • **Yield:** 4 servings

Ingredients	*Directions*
1 tablespoon extra-virgin olive oil	*1* Heat the olive oil in a skillet over medium-low heat. Cook the onion and garlic in the oil until translucent, about 5 minutes.
½ onion, sliced	
4 cloves garlic, minced	*2* Stir in the spinach, chickpeas, cumin, paprika, and salt. Use your stirring spoon to lightly mash the beans as the mixture cooks. Allow to cook until thoroughly heated. Remove from the heat and serve.
16 ounces frozen chopped spinach, thawed	
One 14.5-ounce can chickpeas, drained	
½ teaspoon ground cumin	
¼ teaspoon paprika	
½ teaspoon salt	

Per serving: *Calories 178 (From Fat 52); Fat 6g (Saturated 1g); Cholesterol 0mg; Sodium 541mg; Carbohydrate 25g (Dietary Fiber 8g); Protein 10g.*

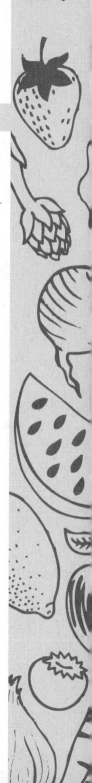

Falafel

Prep time: 12 min • **Cook time:** 35 min • **Yield:** 6 servings

Ingredients	*Directions*
Two 14.5-ounce cans chickpeas, drained and rinsed ½ a large onion, roughly chopped (about 1 cup) 2 tablespoons finely chopped fresh parsley 2 tablespoons finely chopped fresh cilantro ½ teaspoon salt ½ to 1 teaspoon red pepper flakes 4 cloves garlic, minced 1 teaspoon ground cumin 1 teaspoon baking powder ¼ cup flour 2 tablespoons olive oil Cucumber Yogurt Sauce for serving	*1* In a food processor, pulse the chickpeas, onion, parsley, cilantro, salt, red pepper flakes, garlic, and cumin for 3 minutes, stopping every 30 seconds to stir the mixture for even mixing. *2* Combine the baking powder and flour in a small bowl. Remove the chickpea mixture from the food processor, stir in the flour mixture, and form the bean dough into twelve 3-inch patties. *3* Heat a skillet over medium-high heat for 1 minute or until hot. Add the patties, being careful not to crowd the pan. Pan-fry the patties for 3 to 4 minutes on each side or until a golden crust is formed. *4* Serve hot or at room temperature. Serve with 1 to 2 tablespoons of tzatziki sauce.

Per serving: Calories 207 (From Fat 62); Fat 7g (Saturated 1g); Cholesterol 0mg; Sodium 465mg; Carbohydrate 29g (Dietary Fiber 7g); Protein 8g.

Tip: Try the Cucumber Yogurt Sauce recipe (often called tzatziki) in Chapter 9.

Chapter 15

Pasta, Pasta, Pasta!

In This Chapter

▶ Enjoying pasta without going overboard

▶ Creating delicious vegetarian pasta dishes

▶ Adding seafood to your next pasta dish

▶ Beefing up your pasta entrees by adding meat

Many regions in the Mediterranean enjoy pasta, but it's the crown jewel of Italian cooking in particular. You may have picked up this book in the first place because the idea of Mediterranean cooking conjures up delicious bowls of pasta served with wine. Yum!

Pasta can be part of your meal in myriad ways, from a small side dish of orzo to a large entree such as meat-filled lasagne. This chapter demonstrates exceptional dishes for all your pasta needs.

Note: The pasta in this chapter's recipes is dry pasta unless otherwise noted.

Eating Pasta Responsibly

Pasta is one of those foods that can be part of a healthy diet or can become a not-so-healthy problem. People in the United States and Canada typically eat pasta in large portion sizes and with high-calorie sauces, which can contribute to weight gain. Keeping pasta healthy is a fine line, but if you stick to the following tips, you can enjoy your pasta, keep your figure, and stay in good health:

✔ **Watch your portion sizes closely.** Pasta is most commonly a side dish in the Mediterranean. Keep your portion sizes at between ½ cup and 1 cup to avoid eating too many calories and to keep your blood sugar stable. This strategy helps you stay trim and keeps your heart healthy.

✔ **Avoid eating heavy entrees with heavy side dishes.** If you're eating pasta with a heavier, higher-fat and -calorie sauce (such as a béchamel sauce), make sure the rest of your meal is on the light side, like a simple salad.

✔ **Add a little protein.** If you're eating an entree that includes pasta, make sure you have some protein as well. This addition may mean including seafood or meat in your pasta or having nuts and beans in a side salad. Adding protein provides a more balanced meal and helps maintain stable blood sugar.

✔ **Don't fill up on just pasta.** You don't want to eat a large amount of pasta at once. Instead, load up your small portion of pasta with proteins and lots of fresh vegetables so that you still feel like you have a hearty entree. Imagine ½ cup of pasta with tomato sauce on a plate compared to ½ cup of pasta mixed with broccoli, carrots, and chicken. The latter makes a larger volume of food without filling up an entire dish with pasta.

✔ **Don't overcook your pasta.** In Italy, pasta is always cooked *al dente*, firm to the teeth but tender for chewing. Cooking your pasta al dente is actually a healthier way to eat because doing so makes the pasta have a lower glycemic index (the pasta doesn't spike your blood sugar as quickly). Check out the sidebar "Cooking pasta to perfection" in this chapter for information on cooking pasta.

Going Vegetarian

Although including protein with your pasta is a good idea (see the preceding section), not all pasta dishes have to be laden with meatballs and meaty sauce. Residents of the Mediterranean often eat pasta as a side dish with simple sauces and fresh vegetables, herbs, and spices. You can also find vegetarian pastas as main entrees, often with cheese and beans for protein. In this section, you can find some amazing vegetarian pasta dishes for your next meal or get-together with friends.

Puttanesca

Prep time: 8 min • **Cook time:** 23 min • **Yield:** 6 servings

Ingredients	Directions
One 12-ounce box penne	*1* Bring 4 quarts of water to a boil. Cook the pasta according to the package directions (8 to 12 minutes). Drain the pasta, reserving 1 cup of pasta water.
½ cup extra-virgin olive oil	
3 cloves garlic, chopped	
1 teaspoon red pepper flakes	*2* Meanwhile, heat the olive oil in a saucepan over medium heat. Add the garlic and red pepper flakes and cook for 30 seconds. Stir in the tomatoes, oregano, olives, capers, and tomato paste; increase the heat to medium-high and cook for 10 minutes.
One 28-ounce can Italian plum tomatoes	
1½ teaspoons dried oregano	
½ cup pitted kalamata olives, chopped	*3* Add the cooked pasta to the sauce and toss. If the sauce is too thick, add the reserved pasta water ¼ cup at a time until you reach the desired consistency.
3 tablespoons capers, drained and rinsed	
2 tablespoons tomato paste	*4* Top with chopped parsley and grated Parmesan and serve.
¼ cup fresh Italian parsley, chopped	
¼ cup finely grated Parmesan cheese	

Per serving: Calories 428 (From Fat 192); Fat 21g (Saturated 4g); Cholesterol 4mg; Sodium 528mg; Carbohydrate 50g (Dietary Fiber 4g); Protein 11g.

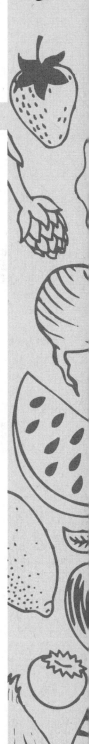

Vegetarian Lasagne

Prep time: 14 min • **Cook time:** 53 min • **Yield:** 6 servings

Ingredients	Directions
1 tablespoon plus 1 tablespoon olive oil	**1** Preheat the oven to 350 degrees. Drizzle 1 tablespoon of the olive oil on the bottom of a 7-x-11-inch glass baking pan.
2 cups mushrooms, sliced	**2** Heat a nonstick skillet with the remaining olive oil over medium heat. Add the mushrooms and cook for 5 minutes. Add half the garlic and the tomatoes and allow the sauce to simmer while you prepare the remaining ingredients, about 6 minutes. Sprinkle ½ teaspoon of the oregano into the sauce.
3 cloves plus 3 cloves garlic, chopped	
Two 14.5-ounce cans no-salt-added diced tomatoes	
½ teaspoon plus ½ teaspoon dried oregano	**3** In a microwave-safe bowl, microwave the spinach and 2 tablespoons of water for 2 minutes. Drain the liquid, squeezing the spinach to remove excess liquid. Mix the spinach with the cottage cheese and the remaining garlic and oregano.
One 6-ounce bag baby spinach	
8 ounces lowfat cottage cheese	**4** Lay the zucchini along the bottom of your baking pan widthwise. Sprinkle with the salt. Lay 3 lasagna noodles over the top widthwise.
2 medium zucchinis, sliced ¼ inch lengthwise	
½ teaspoon salt	**5** Carefully spread the cottage cheese and spinach mixture on top of the lasagna noodles. Top with another layer of 3 lasagna noodles.
9 no-boil lasagna noodles	**6** Pour half of the mushroom-tomato sauce onto the noodles and add a final layer of 3 noodles. Top with the remaining tomato sauce, covering any exposed noodle. Sprinkle with the shredded cheese.
1½ cups shredded lowfat mozzarella cheese	
	7 Cover with foil and bake for 35 minutes. Uncover and broil for 5 minutes to brown the top and get bubbly. Allow the lasagne to rest for 5 minutes before slicing and serving.

Per serving: Calories 333 (From Fat 107); Fat 12g (Saturated 4g); Cholesterol 17mg; Sodium 731mg; Carbohydrate 38g (Dietary Fiber 4g); Protein 20g.

Note: No-boil lasagna noodles are precooked and then dried, making it easy to layer your lasagne without having to deal with wet, cooked noodles. You can find no-boil noodles at any major grocery store chain in the pasta section.

Tortellini with Vegetables and Pesto

Prep time: 5 min • **Cook time:** 15 min • **Yield:** 6 servings

Ingredients	*Directions*
1 red bell pepper, julienned **½ pound asparagus, ends trimmed and cut into 1-inch pieces** **1 small zucchini, cut in half moons**	*1* Bring a 2-quart saucepan of water to a boil and prepare an ice bath (large bowl with ice water). Boil the red bell pepper, asparagus, and zucchini for 3 minutes.
One 13-ounce package fresh cheese tortellini **1 teaspoon olive oil**	*2* Drain the vegetables and transfer them to the ice bath to chill for 2 minutes. Drain the vegetables and pat dry.
8 cherry or grape tomatoes, cut in half **½ cup pesto**	*3* Meanwhile, bring 4 quarts of water to a boil in a large stockpot. Cook the tortellini according to package directions (4 to 8 minutes).
	4 In a medium skillet, heat the olive oil over medium-high heat. Add the blanched vegetables and tomatoes and sauté until heated (about 3 minutes). Add the cooked pasta and toss.
	5 Pour the tortellini into a serving bowl and toss with the pesto.

Per serving: Calories 272 (From Fat 128); Fat 14g (Saturated 4g); Cholesterol 23mg; Sodium 261mg; Carbohydrate 28g (Dietary Fiber 3g); Protein 10g.

Tip: Try the Pesto from Chapter 9 in this recipe.

Note: Check out the color insert for a photo of this recipe.

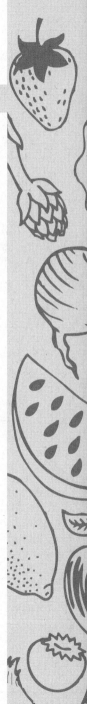

Lemon Orzo Pasta

Prep time: 15 min, plus chilling time • **Cook time:** 10 to 12 min • **Yield:** 8 servings

Ingredients	*Directions*
½ **pound orzo**	*1* Bring 4 quarts of water to a boil in a large pot, add the orzo, and cook according to package instructions (10 to 12 minutes). Drain the pasta and run it under cold water to cool.
4 green onions (scallions), chopped	
4 Roma or plum tomatoes, diced	*2* Meanwhile, place the vegetables into a serving bowl. In a small bowl, whisk the lemon juice and zest, olive oil, and salt.
1 cucumber, seeded and chopped	
Zest and juice of 1 lemon	*3* Mix the pasta with the vegetables, pour the lemon sauce over the mixture, and stir. Chill for at least 1 hour and serve with crumbled feta over top.
¼ **cup olive oil**	
¼ **teaspoon salt**	
¼ **cup feta cheese**	

Per serving: Calories 131 (From Fat 73); Fat 8g (Saturated 2g); Cholesterol 4mg; Sodium 194mg; Carbohydrate 12g (Dietary Fiber 1g); Protein 3g.

Note: Avoid adding more salt until the pasta has cooled and you have mixed in the feta, which is salty.

Tip: Drain the pasta in a colander with small openings so none of the small pasta escapes.

Pecorino Pasta

Prep time: 5 min • **Cook time:** 12 min • **Yield:** 8 servings

Ingredients	Directions
1 pound spaghetti 1 cup pecorino cheese, finely grated 1 cup parsley, chopped 2 tablespoons olive oil 1 tablespoon pepper	**1** Bring 4 quarts of water to a boil, add the spaghetti, and cook according to package instructions (9 to 12 minutes).
	2 Meanwhile, combine the cheese, parsley, olive oil, and pepper in a serving bowl. Drain the cooked pasta and transfer it to the serving bowl, reserving ¼ cup of the cooking liquid.
	3 Toss the pasta to coat with the cheese mixture, adding 1 to 2 tablespoons of the cooking liquid as necessary if the dish seems dry. Serve immediately.

Per serving: Calories 297 (From Fat 71); Fat 8g (Saturated 3g); Cholesterol 11mg; Sodium 199mg; Carbohydrate 43g (Dietary Fiber 2g); Protein 12g.Making time for rest

Making time for rest

Sleep is a basic, fundamental need that is now getting pushed aside by busy schedules. The average amount of sleep Americans get is now 2 hours less than it was 50 years ago. Sleep is crucial for proper health, and a lack of sleep can affect you in many ways, including decreasing your cognitive thinking like problem solving and increasing your risk of heart disease, high blood pressure, stroke, weight gain, and skin aging. For health purposes, doctors recommend you get eight hours of sleep each night. A Mediterranean lifestyle promotes rest time, including basic downtime and sleep. An afternoon siesta isn't all that uncommon.

Slow down and give your body the basic support it needs. To help you relax, turn off the television and computer screen because the light can turn on your body's "awake" signals. Spend some time relaxing before bed or curl up with a good book on the couch.

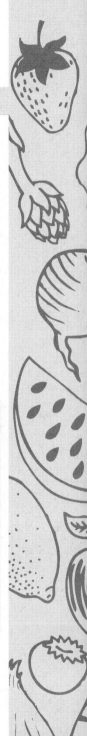

Pasta a Funghi (with Mushrooms)

Prep time: 10 min • **Cook time:** 25 min • **Yield:** 6 servings

Ingredients	*Directions*
1 pound angel hair pasta	*1* Boil 4 quarts of water. Add the pasta and cook according to package instructions, about 4 minutes.
2 tablespoons extra-virgin olive oil	
½ a medium onion, thinly sliced	*2* In a heavy saucepan, heat the olive oil over medium-high heat for 1 minute. Add the onions and garlic and sauté for 5 minutes, reducing the heat if the garlic begins to brown.
4 cloves garlic, sliced	
1 pound cremini mushrooms, sliced	*3* Add the mushrooms and continue to sauté for 10 minutes, allowing mushrooms to get golden. Whisk in the butter and flour and allow the mixture to get golden in color, about 4 minutes.
4 tablespoons butter	
4 tablespoons flour	
1 cup dry white wine	*4* Combine the wine and stock and add ¼ cup of the mixture to the mushrooms at a time, whisking for a minute in between each addition to allow the flour to get evenly dispersed in the sauce.
1 cup vegetable stock	
Salt and pepper to taste	
½ cup fresh parsley, finely chopped	*5* When you've added all the liquid, season the sauce with the salt, pepper, and herbs.
1 tablespoon fresh thyme leaves, finely chopped	
¼ cup Romano cheese, finely grated	*6* Drain the pasta and toss it with the sauce in the saucepan. Transfer to a serving dish and top with the cheese to serve.

Per serving: Calories 545 (From Fat 167); Fat 19g (Saturated 9g); Cholesterol 40mg; Sodium 393mg; Carbohydrate 69g (Dietary Fiber 3g); Protein 19g.

Spinach Gnocchi

Prep time: 40 min • **Cook time:** 9 min • **Yield:** 6 servings

Ingredients	Directions
One 9-ounce box frozen spinach, defrosted, drained, and squeezed dry	*1* Pulse the spinach, potatoes, egg, ¼ cup of the Parmesan cheese, the pepper, and salt in a food processor with a dough blade attachment until combined, about 1 to 2 minutes.
2½ pounds Yukon gold or Russet potatoes	
1 egg	*2* Place the dough onto a floured surface. Sprinkle in the flour and mix by hand for 1 minute. Pat the dough into a circular mound and cut into 4 roughly equal parts. Roll each portion into long, thin ropes about ½-inch thick, being careful not to overwork.
¼ cup plus ½ cup grated Parmesan cheese	
1 teaspoon pepper	
¼ teaspoon salt, plus more to taste	*3* Cut each rope into 1-inch pieces. Use a fork to gently press an indent into each gnocchi.
⅓ cup flour, plus more for dusting	*4* Bring 3 quarts of water to a boil. Working in batches, cook the gnocchi for 3 to 5 minutes or until the dumplings float to the surface. Using a strainer, remove the cooked gnocchi and then cook the next batch.
¼ cup olive oil	
2 cloves garlic, sliced	
¼ teaspoon red pepper flakes	*5* Heat the olive oil in a heavy skillet over medium-low heat. Add the garlic and red pepper flakes. Place the drained gnocchi in the skillet while the remaining batches cook. Gently toss the gnocchi in the sauce quickly and transfer to a serving bowl.
	6 Sprinkle with the remaining cheese and season with salt if needed. Serve.

Per serving: Calories 322 (From Fat 118); Fat 13g (Saturated 3g); Cholesterol 11mg; Sodium 342mg; Carbohydrate 41g (Dietary Fiber 4g); Protein 12g.

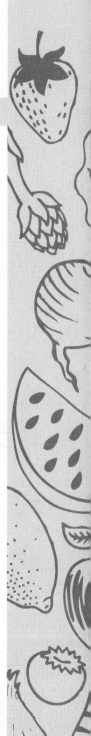

Baked Eggplant Parmesan with Linguini

Prep time: 30 min • **Cook time:** 15 min • **Yield:** 8 servings

Ingredients	Directions
1 cup flour	**1** Preheat the oven to 400 degrees. Combine the flour, salt, and pepper in a medium bowl. Whisk together the eggs and water in another medium bowl, and combine the panko and oregano in a third.
1 teaspoon salt	
1 teaspoon pepper	
2 eggs	**2** Remove the stem and bottom of the eggplant and cut ½-inch thick slices lengthwise. Rub the cut portion of the eggplant with the lemon wedge to stop browning.
¼ cup water	
1 teaspoon dried oregano	
3 cups panko breadcrumbs	**3** Dip the eggplant in the flour and dust off the excess; dip the floured eggplant into the egg mixture and then the panko. Set aside on a large plate and repeat with the remaining eggplant.
2 medium eggplants	
½ a lemon	
¼ cup olive oil	**4** Meanwhile, heat 1 tablespoon of the olive oil in a heavy cast-iron Dutch oven or skillet on medium-high heat. Working in batches, brown the breaded eggplants for about 3 minutes on each side, being careful not to crowd the pan.
4 ounces fresh mozzarella	
1 pound linguini	
4 cups roasted red pepper sauce or Marinara	**5** Transfer to a baking sheet. Repeat with the remaining eggplant, using 1 tablespoon of olive oil for each batch. Top each eggplant with a thin slice of fresh mozzarella and bake for 15 minutes.
	6 Bring 3 quarts of water to a boil. Cook the linguini according to the package instructions and drain. Divide the linguini evenly on 8 serving plates, cover with ½ cup of heated sauce and top with the eggplant Parmesan. Serve.

Per serving: Calories 550 (From Fat 140); Fat 16g (Saturated 4g); Cholesterol 12mg; Sodium 1350mg; Carbohydrate 84g (Dietary Fiber 11g); Protein 18g.

Tip: Check out the Marinara recipe in Chapter 9.

Diving into Noodles with Seafood

This section exemplifies the coming together of two of Mediterranean cooking's star players: pasta and seafood. The Mediterranean coast definitely has no shortage of seafood, so you often see seafood served in many pasta dishes or as a stand-alone entree. Clams, shrimp, and fish are all popular additions to pasta, and such combinations make a delicious, healthy meal. Coming from an Italian family, Meri was the only kid on the block whose family had cod in spaghetti alongside the roast for Christmas dinner. The following recipes help you try out some pasta-seafood combos.

Cooking pasta to perfection

Pasta has been a main staple in Italy for centuries. Making pasta in the home was common once upon a time, but now pasta is readily available in all grocery stores. Dried pasta comes in something like 350 different shapes today, from your basic spaghetti noodle to shell-shaped pastas to pastas with complex shapes or ridges to help them hold on to sauce.

The key to cooking pasta is to make sure it's cooked al dente and not overly soft. Although cooking pasta al dente isn't common in the United States and Canada, we suggest you give it a try because it makes all the difference in your meal. If your pasta breaks apart when you mix it in your sauce, it's too soft. Soft pasta not only creates an undesirable texture and flavor but also has a higher glycemic index, making it less healthy, as we note earlier in the chapter. (Check out Meri's *The Glycemic Index Diet For Dummies* [John Wiley & Sons, Inc] for more on this topic.)

Here are some tips for cooking great, healthy pasta:

- ✔ **Be sure to use a large pot with a good amount of water so that the pasta cooks evenly and doesn't stick together.** If you cook your pasta in enough water, usually at least 3 quarts, you shouldn't have to use any oil in the water to keep the pasta from sticking. In fact, adding oil to the water can make your pasta slippery, causing your sauce to not adhere as well.

- ✔ **Stir the cooking pasta occasionally to make sure it doesn't stick to the bottom of the pot.**

- ✔ **For more flavor, add salt to your pasta water while it's boiling.**

- ✔ **After you drain your pasta, toss it directly with the sauce without rinsing.** Rinsing pasta decreases the flavor and makes the pasta less sticky, causing the sauce to slip off rather than hold. For noodles (such as manicotti or lasagna) that you're going to stuff or layer, however, you want to go ahead and rinse so that you can handle them more easily and so that you halt any further cooking.

Now it's time to eat! Remember these tips as you enjoy the recipes from this chapter.

Shrimp Pasta with Kalamata Olives and Feta Cheese

Prep time: 4 min • **Cook time:** 14 min • **Yield:** 4 servings

Ingredients	*Directions*
Nonstick cooking spray 2 teaspoons olive oil 3 cloves garlic, minced ½ teaspoon red pepper flakes 2 cups frozen baby artichoke hearts, quartered ½ cup chopped pitted kalamata olives 1 cup white wine 1 pound medium shrimp, peeled and deveined ½ pound angel hair pasta ¼ cup fresh basil, cut into long strips ¼ cup crumbled feta cheese	**1** Bring 3 quarts of water to a boil. Meanwhile, coat a nonstick skillet with cooking spray and heat the olive oil over medium heat. Add the garlic and red pepper flakes and sauté for 1 minute. **2** Add the artichoke hearts and olives and sauté for 3 minutes. Add the wine and shrimp and continue to cook until the shrimp is no longer translucent (about 4 minutes). Add the pasta to the water. **3** Cook the pasta according to package instructions (2 to 5 minutes). Drain the pasta and gently toss with the shrimp sauce in a large serving bowl until well coated. Top with the basil and feta to serve.

Per serving: Calories 500 (From Fat 78); Fat 9g (Saturated 2g); Cholesterol 181mg; Sodium 431mg; Carbohydrate 60g (Dietary Fiber 4g); Protein 34g.

Note: For best flavor, always cook with a wine you're willing to drink and avoid using cooking wines.

Tiger Prawns with Vegetable Medley and Tagliatelle

Prep time: 15 min • **Cook time:** 18 min • **Yield:** 6 servings

Ingredients	Directions
1 pound tagliatelle 2 tablespoons olive oil 2 shallots, chopped ½ cup julienned zucchini ½ cup julienned yellow squash ½ cup julienned carrots 18 large tiger prawns, shelled and deveined ¼ cup dry white wine 1½ cups chicken broth ½ cup heavy cream 1 teaspoon curry powder 1 teaspoon butter 1 cup fresh spinach, julienned Salt and pepper to taste	**1** Bring 4 quarts of water to a boil in a large saucepan, add the pasta, and cook according to package instructions (9 to 12 minutes). Drain. **2** Meanwhile, heat the olive oil in a large skillet over medium heat. Add the shallots, zucchini, yellow squash, and carrots and cook for 2 minutes. Add the prawns and cook on each side for 1 minute. Add the wine and cook for 2 minutes. **3** Whisk in the broth, cream, and curry. Reduce the temperature to medium-low heat and cook for 5 minutes. Whisk in the butter. **4** Add the cooked pasta to the pan and toss. Pour into serving bowl and toss with fresh spinach. Season with salt and pepper to taste prior to serving.

Per serving: Calories 459 (From Fat 132); Fat 15g (Saturated 6g); Cholesterol 65mg; Sodium 530mg; Carbohydrate 61g (Dietary Fiber 3g); Protein 18g.

Tip: If you can't find tagliatelle, you can replace it with linguini.

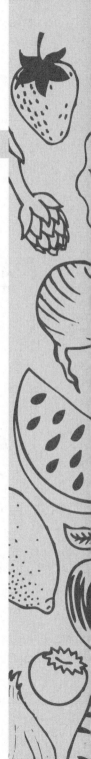

Spaghetti and Clams

Prep time: 40 min • **Cook time:** 18 min • **Yield:** 8 servings

Ingredients	*Directions*
24 littleneck clams	**1** In a bowl, cover the clams with cold water and 1 tablespoon of salt. Allow the clams to sit for 30 minutes and then drain and rinse under cold, running water and set aside.
1 tablespoon salt, plus more to taste	
¼ cup olive oil	
8 cloves garlic, sliced	**2** Heat the olive oil in a large saucepan over medium heat; add the garlic and clams and cook for 1 minute. Stir in the tomatoes, wine, pepper, and oregano; cover and simmer for 12 minutes or until the clams open. Slice open any clams that don't open (refer to Figure 15-1 for how to open the clams).
4 Roma or plum tomatoes, cut into ¼-inch cubes	
1 cup dry white wine	
½ teaspoon pepper	
1 teaspoon dried oregano	**3** Meanwhile, bring 4 quarts of water to a boil. Add the spaghetti and cook according to package instructions (9 to 12 minutes). Drain the pasta and toss with the clam sauce. Fold in the basil and season with salt if needed. Serve.
1 pound spaghetti	
½ cup basil, julienned	

Per serving: Calories 324 (From Fat 72); Fat 8g (Saturated 1g); Cholesterol 9mg; Sodium 22mg; Carbohydrate 46g (Dietary Fiber2g); Protein 11g.

HOW TO CUT AND OPEN CLAMS

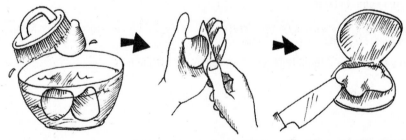

Figure 15-1:
How to open clams.

1. SCRUB THE CLAMS.

2. HOLD THE CLAM FIRMLY. CAREFULLY SLICE THROUGH THE CENTER WITH A KNIFE.

3. OPEN UP THE SHELL AND DETACH THE CLAM WITH THE KNIFE.

Salmon with Spinach and Rigatoni

Prep time: 12 min • **Cook time:** 29 min • **Yield:** 6 servings

Ingredients	*Directions*
1 pound salmon, skin on	*1* Heat a grill or grill pan to medium-high heat. Bring the salmon to room temperature and drizzle with 1 teaspoon of the olive oil. Sprinkle the salt, lemon zest, and crushed garlic over the top.
1 teaspoon plus 2 tablespoons olive oil	
¼ teaspoon salt	
Zest of 1 lemon	*2* Bring 4 quarts of water to a boil and cook the rigatoni according to package instructions (9 to 12 minutes). Drain and set aside.
2 cloves garlic, crushed	
2 cloves garlic, sliced	
1 pound rigatoni	*3* Grill the salmon, skin side first, for 4 minutes on each side. Remove from the heat and cover with foil.
8 cups baby spinach leaves	
1 cup white wine	*4* In a large skillet, heat the remaining olive oil over medium-high heat. Add the sliced garlic and sauté for 2 minutes. Add the spinach and cook for 3 minutes, tossing frequently to evenly heat spinach until lightly wilted.
1 cup basil, thinly sliced	
¼ teaspoon red pepper flakes	
½ a lemon	
¼ cup crumbled feta cheese	*5* Flake the salmon and add it to the spinach; toss this mixture with the pasta and place in serving dish. In the spinach pan, heat the wine over medium-high heat and cook for 4 minutes or until the wine begins to reduce. Add the basil and red pepper flakes and pour over the pasta. Juice the lemon over the top and serve with crumbled feta and salt and pepper to taste.
Salt and pepper to taste	

Per serving: Calories 295 (From Fat 70); Fat 8g (Saturated 2g); Cholesterol 45mg; Sodium 427mg; Carbohydrate 27g (Dietary Fiber 2g); Protein 22g.

Note: You don't need to completely cook the salmon on the grill; it'll finish cooking in the sauce.

Adding Meat to Pasta

A great way to make a one-pot meal is to add some type of meat, such as chicken, pork, or beef, to your pasta. Add some vegetables and a fresh sauce, and you have a complete meal. Using meat is a good way to add more volume to your pasta so that you don't overdo the carbohydrate portion of the meal. Although not all the recipes in this section require only one pot, you can still enjoy these hearty pasta meals with friends and family.

The history of meat sauce

You may be surprised to hear that meat sauce isn't a very traditional part of the Mediterranean diet, but it's true. So how did the classic meat sauce or Bolognese sauce come about? The traditional recipe was registered in 1982 by the Bolognese Delegation of Accademia Italiana Della Cucina to include beef, pancetta, onions, tomato paste, meat broth, white wine, and milk or cream. However, these ingredients aren't necessarily what were used in rural southern Italy where Mediterranean diet research has taken place (or, for that matter, in all recipes from Bologna).

Because of the high cost of meat in southern Italy, cooks there more commonly used left-over scraps such as beef neck, chicken, rabbit, goose liver, or even pig's feet. Of course, using these ingredients evolved into using beef, sausage, pancetta, salami, and prosciutto, the more common meats you find in sauces today. Don't worry; we aren't going to make you eat pig's feet or goose liver sauce (unless you want to). Nor do we ask you to try to master a true Bolognese sauce. Instead, you can enjoy a simple and modern version of meat sauce, using ground beef, found in Chapter 9.

Classic Meat Lasagne

Prep time: 12 min • **Cook time:** 1 hr • **Yield:** 12 servings

Ingredients	Directions
1 pound lean ground beef	*1* Preheat the oven to 350 degrees.
½ pound pork sausage	
5 cups tomato sauce	*2* Cook the beef and sausage in a large nonstick skillet over medium heat until browned. Drain the meat, return it to the pan, and add the tomato sauce. Cook over medium heat for 5 minutes.
2 cloves garlic, minced	
3 cups lowfat ricotta cheese	
One 9-ounce package frozen spinach, defrosted and squeezed dry	*3* In a large bowl, combine the garlic, ricotta, spinach, Parmesan, parsley, oregano, and pepper.
¼ cup Parmesan cheese, finely grated	*4* Pour 2 cups of the meat sauce in the bottom of a 9-x-13-inch baking pan and top with 4 lasagna noodles (breaking a few to fit as necessary). Spread half the ricotta mixture over the noodles. Repeat the layers, topping the second ricotta layer with sauce.
½ cup parsley, chopped	
1 tablespoon oregano	
½ teaspoon pepper	
8 lasagna noodles	*5* Sprinkle the mozzarella over the top. Cover with foil and bake for 45 minutes. Remove the foil and continue baking for 15 minutes. Allow the dish to cool for 10 minutes before serving.
1 cup mozzarella cheese, grated	

Per serving: Calories 337 (From Fat 151); Fat 17g (Saturated 8g); Cholesterol 64mg; Sodium 943mg; Carbohydrate 22g (Dietary Fiber 3g); Protein 25g.

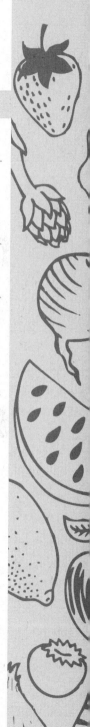

Spaghetti and Meatballs

Prep time: 12 min • **Cook time:** 45 min • **Yield:** 8 servings

Ingredients	*Directions*
Nonstick cooking spray	**1** Heat the oven to 350 degrees. Spray a large cookie sheet with nonstick cooking spray and set aside.
1 pound lean ground beef	
½ to ¾ cup breadcrumbs	**2** In a large bowl, combine the ground beef, ½ of the breadcrumbs, the egg, parsley, basil, oregano garlic powder, and salt and mix well. If the mixture seems loose and wet, add ¼ cup more bread crumbs.
1 egg, lightly beaten	
1 tablespoon dried parsley	
1 teaspoon dried basil	
1 teaspoon dried oregano	**3** Roll meatballs about the size of a golf ball and set them about one inch apart on the prepared cookie sheet. Bake for 35 minutes.
½ teaspoon garlic powder	
¼ teaspoon salt	**4** Meanwhile, warm up the tomato sauce in a large saucepan over low heat, stirring frequently so that it doesn't stick to the bottom.
6 cups tomato sauce	
1 pound spaghetti	
	5 Boil 4 quarts of water in a large pot. Cook the spaghetti according to package directions (10 to 12 minutes). Drain.
	6 Using tongs, transfer the cooked meatballs into the saucepan and mix into the sauce. Let the meatballs simmer in the sauce for 10 minutes. Top the spaghetti with the meatballs and sauce and serve.

Per serving: Calories 396 (From Fat 67); Fat 7g (Saturated 3g); Cholesterol 37mg; Sodium 1157mg; Carbohydrate 60g (Dietary Fiber 5g); Protein 23g.

Tip: Use the Marinara from Chapter 9 as the tomato sauce in this recipe.

Penne with Chicken, Sun-Dried Tomatoes, and Green Beans

Prep time: 15 min • **Cook time:** 16 min • **Yield:** 8 servings

Ingredients	Directions
1 tablespoon olive oil	*1* In a medium skillet, heat the olive oil over medium-high heat. Add the chicken, sprinkle with salt and pepper to taste, and sauté until the chicken is cooked through, about 4 minutes.
3 boneless, skinless chicken breasts, cut into 1-inch chunks	
Salt and pepper to taste	
1 pound penne	*2* Boil 4 quarts of water in a large pot and cook the penne according to package directions (9 to 12 minutes). Drain.
1 cup fresh green beans, trimmed and cut into 1-inch pieces	*3* Meanwhile, steam the green beans in a small pot until just tender, about 3 minutes. Drain and run under cool water to stop the cooking.
¾ cup oil-packed sun-dried tomatoes, drained and sliced	
4 ounces basil pesto	*4* In a large serving bowl, combine the pasta, chicken, green beans, sun-dried tomatoes, and pesto until well blended. Fold in the pine nuts.
⅓ cup pine nuts, lightly toasted	
8 tablespoons grated Parmesan cheese	*5* Divide the pasta among 8 plates, top each with 1 tablespoon of the cheese, and serve.

Per serving: Calories 470 (From Fat 164); Fat 18g (Saturated 4g); Cholesterol 54mg; Sodium 462mg; Carbohydrate 47g (Dietary Fiber 3g); Protein 29g.

Note: You can serve this dish hot or at room temperature, making it great for parties.

Tip: Use the Pesto recipe in Chapter 9 for this recipe.

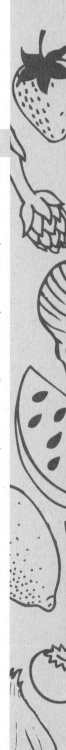

Chicken-and-Broccoli-Stuffed Manicotti

Prep time: 25 min • **Cook time:** 45 min • **Yield:** 6 servings

Ingredients	*Directions*
12 manicotti shells Nonstick cooking spray 3 chicken breasts, diced 16 ounces frozen broccoli ¼ cup onion, chopped 8 ounce Neufchâtel cheese 1 cup milk 2 tablespoons chives ¼ cup plus ½ cup Parmesan cheese ½ teaspoon paprika	*1* Bring 5 quarts of water to a boil and cook the manicotti for 7 minutes. Drain and rinse with cool water. *2* In a large nonstick skillet sprayed with nonstick cooking spray, cook the chicken breast over medium heat until cooked and browned. Add the frozen broccoli and onions and cook for 5 minutes. Remove from the heat. *3* Meanwhile, heat the Neufchâtel in a saucepan over medium-low heat, stirring constantly until melted. Whisk in the milk ¼ cup at a time until you have a thin sauce. *4* Continue whisking; add the chives and ¼ cup of the Parmesan. Whisk over the heat until smooth. *5* Pour half of the cheese sauce over the chicken and broccoli mixture just to coat, and stir until combined. Let it cool for about 10 minutes. Using your hands, fill each manicotti with about ¼ cup of the broccoli mixture. *6* Lay the manicotti side-by-side in a 9-x-13-inch baking pan. Pour the remaining sauce over the top and sprinkle with the remaining Parmesan and the paprika. *7* Cover the dish with foil and bake for 30 minutes. Remove the foil and bake for 5 minutes. Allow the manicotti to cool for 5 minutes before serving.

Per serving: Calories 385 (From Fat 124); Fat 14g (Saturated 7g); Cholesterol 107mg; Sodium 856mg; Carbohydrate 24g (Dietary Fiber 3g); Protein 41g.

Tip: Avoid overcooking the pasta or the shells will be too flimsy to work with.

Chicken and Vodka Sauce over Linguini

Prep time: 8 min • **Cook time:** 16 min • **Yield:** 4 servings

Ingredients	*Directions*
3 boneless, skinless chicken breasts **Salt and pepper to taste** **½ pound linguini**	*1* Heat a grill or grill pan to medium-high heat. Sprinkle the chicken breasts with salt and pepper to taste and grill on each side for 10 minutes or until the internal temperature reaches 165 degrees.
1 tablespoon olive oil **6 cloves garlic, chopped**	*2* Allow the chicken breasts to rest for 5 minutes prior to slicing. Slice the chicken breast on an angle in ½-inch-thick slices.
Two 14.5-ounce cans diced tomatoes **¼ teaspoon red pepper flakes**	*3* Bring 4 quarts of water to a boil in a large pot. Cook the pasta according to package directions (about 7 to 8 minutes). Drain.
⅓ cup vodka **½ cup half and half or whipping cream** **¼ cup parsley or basil, chopped**	*4* In a large skillet, heat the olive oil over medium heat and add the garlic. Sauté for 3 minutes, stir in the tomatoes and pepper flakes, and cook for 3 minutes. Add the vodka and cook for 2 minutes.
	5 Reduce the heat to medium low and stir in the cream. Use a blender or stick blender to mix the sauce until smooth.
	6 In the pan, add the fresh herbs to the sauce and season with salt. Toss the sauce with the pasta. Divide the pasta evenly onto 4 plates and top with the chicken. Serve.

Per serving: Calories 386 (From Fat 100); Fat 11g (Saturated 4g); Cholesterol 91mg; Sodium 533mg; Carbohydrate 25g (Dietary Fiber 3g); Protein 35+g.

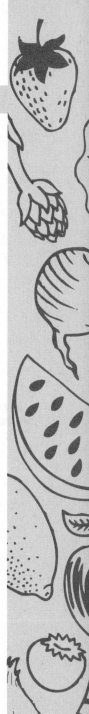

Working to live rather than living to work

In many areas, especially the Mediterranean region, working is a way to live life to the fullest rather than the main focus of life. Many people in the United States and Canada are working longer and longer days, and competition makes the daily grind feel like an unending battle to reach your career goals. Although the traditional workday is 8 hours, 10-to-12-hour days seem to have become the norm. If this description sounds like you, work may be consuming more than its fair share of your life.

In order to live more like the people in the Mediterranean, make sure to give yourself the much needed time for rest, friends, family, exercise, and fun. Life is a balancing act, and each of these factors is equally important.

If you are working long hours and want to slow down, you can talk to your boss about a flexible schedule; perhaps you work a few longer days in order to have some shorter workdays. You can also set up clear boundaries about your time when you start a new job. You also want to work smarter and not harder, finding ways to decrease any wasted time during the workday so you can still get your work done, manage your competition, and have a life outside of work! Get tips for making a flexible schedule work for you at `www.workoptions.com/about.htm`.

Chapter 16

From Pizza to Pitas: Mastering Mediterranean Fast Food

In This Chapter

▶ Creating homemade pizzas the Mediterranean way

▶ Putting together classic gyros and pitas

▶ Making sandwiches with all the flavors of the Mediterranean

*E*very culture has its version of fast food. However, the fast food we're talking about isn't greasy drive-through restaurants; it's quick, easy-to-pull-together foods. Pizzas, pitas, gyros, and sandwiches are all popular forms of quick meals on the Mediterranean coast.

Although the food in this chapter does often require cooking, many of the items are dishes you can quickly throw together from ingredients readily on hand in the kitchen. And you can make even faster food by simply planning and prepping a little ahead like people in the Mediterranean do. For example, folks in Italy may make extra pizza dough so that it's ready to go when they want to throw on some favorite items for a quick meal later. Greek cooks often make gyro meat ahead of time for easy-to-prepare gyros.

The casual foods in this chapter are always nice for lunches or a laid-back dinner. Pairing these items with a combination of vegetables, side salads (see Chapter 10), or fruit gives you a balanced and delicious meal.

Tossing Up Pizza Night

The simple idea of melting cheese on a crispy crust is so tempting to the palate that most people can't resist it! Pizza is a great way to feed your family when you don't feel like slaving in the kitchen. You can also whip up a couple of pies for a small party or to watch the big game. Making your own pizza like the people in the Mediterranean do has never been easier and more fun.

Although pizza is loved throughout many countries, it's one of those food items that can become very unhealthy quickly. The classic Italian pizza isn't the fat, calorie, and sodium bomb that many American versions are; Italians use just a whisper of sauce or oil, a small sprinkling of cheese, and only one layer of meat (if any at all). The bread, not the toppings, is the highlight of Mediterranean pizzas.

These slight variations in pizza-making philosophy make all the difference in your health. This section shows you some unique pizza combinations with a classic flatbread style of crust. Use these recipes or simply make the pizza dough and come up with some of your own creations. (*Note:* The pizza recipes in this section all call for the Pizza Dough recipe we feature here.) If you're short on time, you can also use store-bought dough; just bake it according to the package instructions.

From Naples to U.S tables: A pizza history

Thanks to the folks in Naples Italy for coming up with the concept of pizza as early as 500 B.C., making it an even older food tradition than pasta for Italians. What started as a simple flatbread cooked in wood-fired ovens was only eaten by the poor and sold by street vendors. Next came the tomato sauce, and before long, pizza spread throughout Italy, with each region creating special versions all its own.

The addition of meats, herbs, and vegetables added more and more variety. Even Queen Margherita had a pizza pie named for her; the classic Pizza Margherita consists of basil, cheese, and tomatoes to represent the Italian flag. It was also the first pizza to include cheese. (See our recipe in this chapter for this classic.)

In the 19th century, Italian immigrants brought pizza to the United States, where street vendors in large cities like New York and San Francisco sold it in keeping with the Italian tradition. Pizzerias later began sprouting throughout the United States, but the dish didn't start to gain widespread popularity until after World War II, when the troops who were stationed in Italy took their appreciation home and let their families in on the secret of this great new food. Now pizza is a staple in American culture, with pizzerias and take-out and delivery options available for all to enjoy.

Pizza Dough

Prep time: 25 min • **Yield:** 1 pizza, 10 servings

Ingredients	Directions
One ¼-ounce package active dry yeast 2 teaspoons honey 1¼ cups warm water (about 110 to 120 degrees) 2 tablespoons olive oil 1 teaspoon sea salt 3 cups flour	*1* Combine the yeast, honey, and warm water in a large mixer or food processor with a dough attachment. Let the mixture rest for 5 minutes to be sure that the yeast is alive (look for bubbles on the surface). *2* Add the olive oil and salt and blend for 30 seconds. Begin to slowly add 3 cups of the flour, about ½ cup at a time, mixing for 2 minutes between additions. *3* Allow the mixture to knead in the mixer for 10 minutes, sprinkling with flour if needed to keep the dough from sticking to the bowl, until elastic and smooth. *4* Remove the dough from the bowl and allow it to rest for 15 minutes under a warm, moist towel. Follow the pizza recipe for baking instructions.

Per serving: *Calories 167 (From Fat 28); Fat 3g (Saturated 0g); Cholesterol 0mg; Sodium 234mg; Carbohydrate 30g (Dietary Fiber 1g); Protein 4g.*

Note: You can freeze this pizza dough for 1 month. Form the dough into a ball and cover it with plastic wrap before placing it into a freezer-safe container.

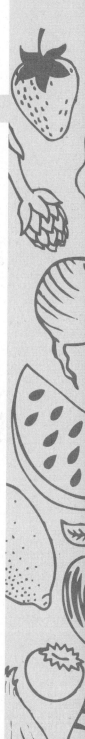

Margherita Pizza

Prep time: 15 min • **Cook time:** 20 min • **Yield:** 10 servings

Ingredients	*Directions*
1 batch Pizza Dough	**1** Preheat the oven to 450 degrees. Roll out the dough to ½-inch thick, dusting the pizza dough with flour as needed. See Figure 16-1 for how to roll out pizza dough.
¼ cup flour as needed for rolling	
2 tablespoons olive oil	**2** Poke holes in the pizza dough with a fork (to prevent crust bubbling) and bake it on a baking sheet or pizza stone for 5 minutes. Remove the pan and drizzle the crust with the olive oil and crushed tomatoes.
½ cup crushed canned tomatoes	
3 Roma or plum tomatoes, sliced ¼-inch thick	**3** Top the pizza with the tomato slices and season with the salt. Blot the mozzarella slices dry with a paper towel and lay them on top of the pizza in no exact pattern. Top the pizza with the basil.
½ teaspoon sea salt	
6 ounces fresh or block mozzarella, cut into ¼-inch slices	
½ cup fresh basil leaves, thinly sliced	**4** Bake the pizza for 15 minutes or until the cheese is bubbling. To brown the cheese, place the pizza under the broiler for 2 to 3 minutes if desired. Allow the pizza to cool for 5 minutes before slicing.

Per serving: Calories 251 (From Fat 76); Fat 8g (Saturated 2g); Cholesterol 11mg; Sodium 474mg; Carbohydrate 34g (Dietary Fiber 1g); Protein 9g.

ROLLING OUT PIZZA DOUGH

Figure 16-1:
You don't
need to
work in a
pizza parlor
to roll out
pizza dough.

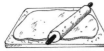

1. ROLL THE DOUGH OUT ON A WELL-FLOURED SURFACE, EVENLY, ABOUT ¼" THICK. DON'T WORRY ABOUT MAKING A PERFECTLY ROUND SHAPE.

2. CAREFULLY, LOOSEN THE DOUGH WITH A LONG SPATULA. PLACE ON A COOKIE SHEET OR DRAPE OVER A ROLLING PIN.

3. PLACE ON PIZZA TRAY.

IF YOU DON'T GET IT RIGHT THE 1ST TIME, RESHAPE THE DOUGH INTO A BALL AND ROLL AGAIN. YOU CAN MAKE 3 OR 4 PIES INSTEAD OF 1 BIG ONE!

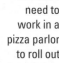

Potato and Pesto Pizza

Prep time: 20 min • **Cook time:** 18 min • **Yield:** 10 servings

Ingredients	*Directions*
4 red potatoes, sliced into ⅛-inch rounds	*1* Preheat the oven to 450 degrees.
1 batch Pizza Dough	*2* Blanch the potato slices in 2 quarts of boiling water for 2 minutes. Drain the slices and allow them to cool slightly before drying them with paper towels.
¼ cup flour as needed for rolling	
½ cup pesto	*3* Roll out the pizza dough about ½-inch thick into your desired shape and place it onto a lightly floured baking sheet. Spread the pesto onto the dough all the way to the edges and sprinkle with ½ cup of the cheese.
1 cup grated part-skim mozzarella cheese	
1 tablespoon olive oil	
¼ teaspoon dried rosemary, minced	*4* Lay the potatoes on the pizza, overlapping them slightly in a circular fashion. Brush the potatoes with the olive oil and sprinkle with rosemary, oregano, salt, and pepper. Top with the remaining cheese and sprinkle with the red pepper flakes (if desired).
¼ teaspoon dried oregano	
¼ teaspoon sea salt	
½ teaspoon pepper	
¼ teaspoon red pepper flakes (optional)	*5* Bake the pizza for 10 to 15 minutes or until the potatoes are golden. Allow the pizza to rest for 5 minutes before slicing and serving.

Per serving: Calories 341 (From Fat 113); Fat 13g (Saturated 2g); Cholesterol 8mg; Sodium 462mg; Carbohydrate 47g (Dietary Fiber 3g); Protein 10g.

Tip: Try the homemade Pesto from Chapter 9 in this recipe.

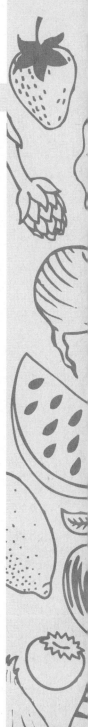

Chicken and Arugula Pizza

Prep time: 12 min • **Cook time:** 35 min • **Yield:** 10 servings

Ingredients	*Directions*
1 batch Pizza Dough	*1* Preheat the oven to 450 degrees. Roll out the pizza dough about ½-inch thick into your desired shape and place it onto a parchment paper-lined baking sheet.
¼ cup flour as needed for rolling	
1 tablespoon plus ⅓ cup olive oil	*2* Heat 1 tablespoon of the olive oil in a nonstick skillet over medium-high heat. Add the chicken and cook for 3 to 5 minutes on each side or until no longer pink.
8 ounces chicken breast, thinly sliced	
Juice of 1 lemon	*3* Meanwhile, whisk together the remaining olive oil, the lemon juice, garlic, thyme, pepper, and red pepper flakes.
2 cloves garlic, crushed	
1 teaspoon dried thyme, or 1 tablespoon fresh thyme	
½ teaspoon pepper	*4* Brush the pizza crust with 3 tablespoons of the olive oil mixture. Place the sautéed chicken onto the crust and top with the cheeses.
¼ teaspoon red pepper flakes	
8 ounces grated fontina cheese	*5* Bake the pizza for 15 minutes or until the cheese is browned. Remove from the oven and cool for 5 minutes. Meanwhile, toss the arugula with the remaining dressing and top the cooled pizza with the arugula.
4 ounces goat cheese, crumbled	
8 ounces baby arugula	

Per serving: Calories 426 (From Fat 205); Fat 23g (Saturated 8g); Cholesterol 54mg; Sodium 558mg; Carbohydrate 34g (Dietary Fiber 1g); Protein 20g.

Sausage and Pepper Pizza

Prep time: 15 min • **Cook time:** 25 min • **Yield:** 10 servings

Ingredients	*Directions*
1 batch Pizza Dough **¼ cup flour as needed for rolling**	*1* Preheat the oven to 450 degrees. Roll out the pizza dough about ½-inch thick into your desired shape and place it onto a parchment paper-lined baking sheet.
1 tablespoon olive oil **1 onion, thinly sliced** **1 green bell pepper, julienned** **½ teaspoon sea salt**	*2* Heat the olive oil in a nonstick skillet over medium-high heat. Add the onions and peppers and cook for 5 minutes. Remove from the heat and season with ½ teaspoon of sea salt.
1 cup Pizza Sauce **½ pound Italian sausage, casing removed** **½ pound cremini mushrooms, quartered**	*3* Spread the pizza sauce onto the pizza dough and top with the pepper and onion mixture. Form ½-inch balls with the sausage and add them and the mushrooms to the pizza. Top the pizza with the cheese and sprinkle with the dried oregano.
8 ounces fontina cheese, grated **½ teaspoon dried oregano**	*4* Bake the pizza for 15 to 20 minutes or until the cheese is browned. Remove the pizza from the oven and let it cool for 5 minutes before serving.

Per serving: Calories 389 (From Fat 171); Fat 19g (Saturated 7g); Cholesterol 44mg; Sodium 748mg; Carbohydrate 39g (Dietary Fiber 2g); Protein 15g.

Note: You can find the Pizza Sauce recipe in Chapter 9.

Note: Be sure to make form the sausage into small ½-inch balls to ensure even and complete cooking time. Test your sausage prior to serving to make sure it's cooked through. If it's not, place the pizza back in the oven and continue cooking until the sausage is no longer pink.

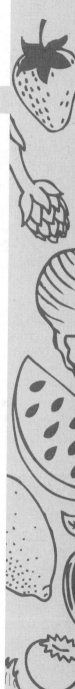

Spanish Chorizo and Manchego Pizza

Prep time: 10 min • **Cook time:** 20 min • **Yield:** 10 servings

Ingredients	*Directions*
1 batch Pizza Dough ¼ cup flour as needed for rolling 1 cup Pizza Sauce	*1* Preheat the oven to 450 degrees. Roll out the pizza dough about ½-inch thick into your desired shape and place it onto a parchment paper-lined baking sheet. Bake the crust for 5 minutes.
6 ounces Spanish chorizo, sliced ¼-inch thick on the bias 10 green olives, sliced 1 cup manchego cheese, grated ½ a red onion, thinly sliced	*2* Top the crust with the remaining ingredients. Bake for an additional 15 to 20 minutes or until the cheese is golden. Remove the pizza from the oven and let it cool for 5 minutes before serving.

Per serving: Calories 319 (From Fat 120); Fat 13g (Saturated 4g); Cholesterol 25mg; Sodium 704mg; Carbohydrate 36g (Dietary Fiber 2g); Protein 13g.

Note: You can find the Pizza Sauce recipe in Chapter 9.

Note: Spanish chorizo isn't the same as Mexican chorizo; rather, it's a dry, cured sausage you don't need to cook. If you get Mexican chorizo, be sure it's cooked before you use it in the recipe.

Tip: If you can't find Spanish chorizo in your grocery store, you can substitute a hard smoked sausage. You can also replace the manchego with grated Romano cheese.

Gearing Up for Classic Gyros and Pitas

Gyros and pita sandwiches are common casual foods in the Mediterranean. Just like pizza and other Mediterranean sandwiches, many different versions of pita sandwiches and gyros exist today, and this section provides some classic sandwiches along with original combinations to make a great casual meal for your family.

Pitas are round breads with a pouch in the center created by steam. You can cut them in half and fill them with any type of sandwich fixings or use them whole as a wrap. *Gyros,* popular in Greece and Cyprus, refer to a specific pita-style sandwich with lamb, chicken, or veal broiled on a vertical spit. The gyro meat is then wrapped in the pita with tomatoes, onion, and tzatziki sauce. Because most people don't have a vertical spit lying around, the recipes here show you different ways to cook your gyro meats.

The secrets of gyro meat

Cooking gyro meat in a traditional way is a little more complicated than you may expect, but the end result provides amazing flavor. Boneless cuts of lamb, beef, chicken, veal, or pork are seasoned and then wrapped around a vertical, cone-shaped spit that rotates in front of an electric broiler or other heat source. The larger cuts of meats are wrapped at the top so that when they drip, the lower cuts of meats soak up all the moisture and flavor. When the meat starts to dry out, extra fat is added to keep it moist.

After the meat is cooked and ready to serve, it is shaved into thin slices, with both the top and bottom parts used for each serving to provide a delicious, well-rounded flavor. We know mimicking this cooking method at home is difficult, so we encourage you to try traditionally cooked gyros at a Greek restaurant to experience the unique flavor and texture of the meats.

Char-Grilled Pork Loin Pita with Tomatoes and Onions

Prep time: 15 min, plus marinating time • **Cook time:** 25 min • **Yield:** 6 servings

Ingredients	Directions
8 cloves garlic, chopped	*1* Combine the garlic, lemon zest and juice, olive oil, cumin, coriander, and oregano in a bowl and add the pork. Cover and chill the mixture in the refrigerator for 1 hour and then remove it from the refrigerator and marinate 15 minutes more.
Zest and juice of 1 lemon	
¼ cup olive oil	
1 teaspoon ground cumin	
½ teaspoon coriander	*2* Heat the grill to medium-high for 10 minutes. Cook the tenderloin for 15 to 20 minutes or until the meat reaches 145 degrees as measured by a meat thermometer.
½ teaspoon dried oregano	
1 pound pork tenderloin	
6 pita pockets or flatbreads	*3* Remove the meat from the grill, cover it with foil, and allow it to rest for 15 minutes. Slice the meat in ½-inch slices.
3 Roma or plum tomatoes, diced	
½ red onion, thinly sliced	*4* Heat the pitas or flatbreads on a hot griddle or in a cast-iron skillet for 3 to 5 minutes or until hot.
½ cup feta cheese, crumbled	
6 lemon wedges	*5* Fill each sandwich with 2 to 3 ounces of meat and top with the tomatoes, red onion, and crumbled feta. Serve each pita with a lemon wedge to be squeezed over the filling before enjoying.

Per serving: Calories 334 (From Fat 125); Fat 14g (Saturated 4g); Cholesterol 60mg; Sodium 424mg; Carbohydrate 29g (Dietary Fiber 2g); Protein 22g.

Roasted Vegetables with Feta Cheese Pita

Prep time: 15 min • **Cook time:** 5 min • **Yield:** 4 servings

Ingredients	Directions
1 red bell pepper, cut into 1-inch pieces	**1** In a broiler-safe baking dish, toss together the peppers, tomatoes, and chickpeas. Drizzle with the olive oil and broil 5 to 7 inches from the heating element for 5 to 8 minutes or until slightly blackened.
1 yellow bell pepper, cut into 1-inch pieces	
1 green bell pepper, cut into 1-inch pieces	**2** Meanwhile, in a large bowl, combine the lemon juice, garlic, parsley, cumin, and salt. After the veggies are broiled, immediately toss them in the vinaigrette.
1 large tomato, cut into ½-inch wedges	
One 14.5-ounce can chickpeas, drained and rinsed	**3** Heat the pitas or flatbreads on a hot griddle or in a cast-iron skillet for 3 to 5 minutes or until hot. Fill each sandwich with vegetables and top with 2 tablespoons of feta. Serve immediately.
¼ cup olive oil	
Juice of 1 lemon	
2 cloves garlic, minced	
½ cup parsley, chopped	
¼ teaspoon ground cumin	
½ teaspoon salt	
4 pita pockets or flatbreads	
½ cup feta cheese, crumbled	

Per serving: Calories 397 (From Fat 175); Fat 19g (Saturated 5g); Cholesterol 17mg; Sodium 841mg; Carbohydrate 46g (Dietary Fiber 7g); Protein 12g.

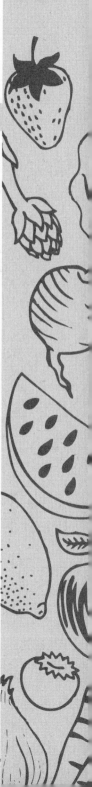

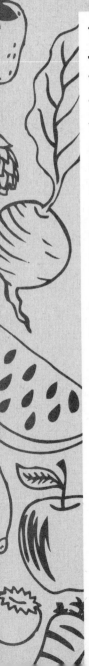

Beef Gyros

Prep time: 8 min, plus marinating time • **Cook time:** 20 min • **Yield:** 6 servings

Ingredients	*Directions*
1 cup red wine vinegar Juice of 1 lemon, divided 1 teaspoon allspice 1 teaspoon paprika ⅛ teaspoon cardamom 1 tablespoon plus 1 clove garlic, minced ½ teaspoon sea salt 2 pounds sirloin steak ½ cup fresh parsley ½ red onion, chopped 1 tablespoon tahini sauce ½ cup Greek yogurt 6 pita pockets or flatbreads	**1** In a large bowl, whisk the vinegar, half the lemon juice, the allspice, paprika, cardamom, 1 tablespoon of the garlic, and the sea salt. Add the meat to the mixture and toss to coat. Cover and refrigerate for at least 8 hours or overnight. **2** Preheat the oven to 350 degrees. Combine the parsley, onion, tahini, yogurt, and the remaining lemon juice and garlic in a small bowl. **3** Place the meat on a baking sheet and bake for 15 to 20 minutes, or until well done (170 degrees). Allow the meat to rest for 5 minutes and then slice into ½-inch slices against the grain. **4** Heat the pitas or flatbreads on a hot griddle or in a cast-iron skillet for 3 to 5 minutes or until hot. Evenly divide the meat among the 6 sandwiches and serve with the yogurt sauce.

Per serving: Calories 547 (From Fat 197); Fat 22g (Saturated 8g); Cholesterol 101mg; Sodium 565mg; Carbohydrate 29g (Dietary Fiber 2g); Protein 54g.

Chicken-Style Gyros

Prep time: 10 min, plus marinating time • **Cook time:** 10 min • **Yield:** 4 servings

Ingredients	Directions
¼ cup red wine vinegar Juice of 1 lemon 1 tablespoon dried oregano ½ teaspoon coriander 4 cloves garlic, chopped ¼ teaspoon sea salt 1 pound chicken breast, cut into 1-inch pieces 4 pita pockets or flatbreads ¼ red onion, sliced ½ cup Cucumber Yogurt Sauce	*1* In a large bowl, combine the vinegar, lemon juice, oregano, coriander, garlic, and sea salt and then add the chicken. Marinate the chicken in the refrigerator for at least 1 hour and no more than 4 hours. *2* Drain the chicken from the marinade, discard the marinade, and sauté the chicken over medium-high heat in a nonstick skillet until cooked through, about 5 to 6 minutes. *3* Heat the pitas or flatbreads on a hot griddle or in a cast-iron skillet for 3 to 5 minutes or until hot. Fill each sandwich with the onion, meat, and 2 tablespoons of the tzatziki sauce.

Per serving: *Calories 250 (From Fat 23); Fat 3g (Saturated 1g); Cholesterol 30mg; Sodium 482mg; Carbohydrate 30g (Dietary Fiber 1g); Protein 26g.*

Note: You can find the Cucumber Yogurt Sauce recipe in Chapter 9.

Creating a life where fun is a priority

Enjoying life, having a good laugh, and making time for fun is a priority in certain regions of the Mediterranean coast. Fun is unique to you. Perhaps it means spending time with family, watching a funny movie, doing something active like skiing, or simply playing cards. No matter what you find fun, do more of it! Fun activities help you combat stress, not to mention make memories.

Live your life to the fullest so that you have plenty of fun memories to look back on instead of only remembering the day-to-day grind. If you can't remember the last time you had some fun, schedule one pronto!

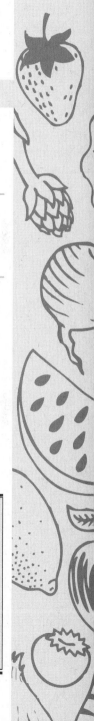

Munching Sensational Sandwiches

Different styles of sandwiches are popular in many countries, especially on the Mediterranean coast, as a quick, casual food. Pairing bread with a variety of meats, cheeses, and vegetables makes using foods you have on hand (and cleaning up those leftovers) easy.

Italians in particular love their bread, and you see it used in many different ways throughout their cooking. *Paninis* are a popular style of Italian sandwich that involves smashing the final sandwich between hot irons similar to a waffle iron. Of course, big crusty bread topped with local favorites like vegetables and seafood is another common choice. So throw out those boring old peanut butter and jelly sandwiches and try some of this section's Mediterranean-inspired twists.

Creating healthy sandwiches with a punch

Here are some tips to make a boring sandwich sensational while keeping it sensible:

✔ **Beginning with the right breads:** Some breads are healthier than others. Choose whole-grain breads, sourdough bread, and whole-wheat pitas for more fiber for digestive and heart health. Fiber also helps you feel fuller longer.

✔ **Meating in the middle:** Go for lean meats like turkey or chicken breast; if you can't resist the higher-calorie and -fat meats like beef, layer them lightly.

✔ **Making your cheese count:** Use a small amount of a strong-flavored cheese such as feta or goat cheese to maximize taste without going overboard on fat and calories. And go easy on melting layers of cheese on your sandwiches; add tomatoes and basil leaves instead.

✔ **Adding vegetables:** Piling on simple vegetables such as dark leafy greens, tomatoes, and cucumbers can pack plenty of flavor and nutrients. Try adding cooked veggies to your sandwich as well.

✔ **Give fresh herbs a chance.** Fresh herbs like basil leaves can add big flavor to your next sandwich, and they contain important nutrients and phytochemicals to help you stay healthy and combat diseases. Use fresh dill with fish sandwiches or sprinkle a little fresh cilantro on a turkey sandwich.

✔ **Balancing light with heavy:** Combine heavy foods with light foods for better balance. If you're eating a beef sandwich at a restaurant, opt for a salad or soup rather than the French fries or potato chips or get just half a sandwich.

✔ **Spreading the health:** Try some healthier and tastier spreads: Brush olive oil on your bread in place of butter when making a hot sandwich. Spread hummus, pesto, or avocado on a cold sandwich. These swaps add more nutrients and help you switch to healthy fats.

Grilled Chicken and Roasted Pepper Panini

Prep time: 30 min, plus marinating time • **Cook time:** 40 min • **Yield:** 4 servings

Ingredients	Directions
1 pound chicken breast	*1* In a bowl, top the chicken with the balsamic vinegar, rosemary, half of the garlic, the sugar, red pepper flakes, and 1 tablespoon of the olive oil. Toss to coat. Marinate in the refrigerator for 30 minutes to 2 hours.
¼ cup balsamic vinegar	
½ teaspoon rosemary, minced	
1 clove plus 1 clove garlic, minced	*2* Preheat the oven to 350 degrees. Bake the chicken for 20 minutes or until no longer pink on the inside.
1 teaspoon sugar	
¼ teaspoon red pepper flakes	*3* Allow the chicken to rest for 5 minutes and then slice into ½-inch slices. Combine the mayonnaise and remaining garlic in a bowl and spread ½ tablespoon of the mixture on the unoiled side of 4 slices of bread.
1 tablespoon olive oil	
Eight ½-inch slices French or sourdough bread	
2 tablespoons mayonnaise	*4* On top of the mayonnaise, layer 1 slice of the cheese, 2 tablespoons of the roasted peppers, 2 basil leaves, a quarter of the chicken breast slices, and another slice of cheese. Top each sandwich with another piece of bread (oiled side showing).
Eight ½-ounce slices fresh mozzarella or fontina cheese	
½ cup roasted red bell peppers, jarred or fresh	
8 leaves basil	*5* Heat a grill pan over medium-high heat. Place one or two sandwiches in the pan and top with something heavy (such as a tea kettle filled with water) for 5 minutes on each side. Repeat with remaining sandwiches and serve.

Per serving: Calories 438 (From Fat 122); Fat 14g (Saturated 5g); Cholesterol 67mg; Sodium 970mg; Carbohydrate 45g (Dietary Fiber 2g); Protein 32g.

Tip: If you have a panini press or a tabletop grill, simply cook each sandwich in the press with the top closed for about 5 minutes. To save time, you can cook your chicken on the same press or grill as well.

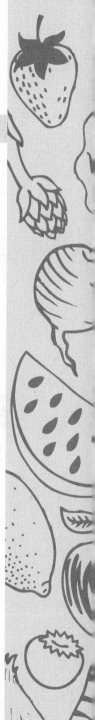

Oven-Fried Fish Sandwich with Fresh Spring Mix

Prep time: 15 min • **Cook time:** 20 min • **Yield:** 6 servings

Ingredients	Directions
½ cup flour	**1** Preheat the oven to 425 degrees.
½ teaspoon garlic powder	
¼ teaspoon paprika	**2** In a medium bowl, combine the flour, garlic powder, paprika, and salt. In another bowl, combine the egg and Greek yogurt; place the bread crumbs in a third bowl.
⅛ teaspoon salt	
1 egg	
½ cup Greek yogurt	**3** Dredge the fish in the flour mixture and shake off any excess. Dip the floured fish into the yogurt mixture and then coat it with the breadcrumbs. Place the breaded fish onto a baking sheet.
1 cup panko breadcrumbs	
Four 6-ounce fillets flounder or other white fish	
¼ cup grated Parmesan cheese	**4** Bake the fish for 20 minutes or until golden. Immediately upon removing from the oven, top each fillet with 1 tablespoon of Parmesan cheese.
1 French bread baguette	
2 cups spring mix lettuce	**5** Cut the baguette in half lengthwise and top it with the cooked fish. In a medium bowl, toss the greens with the lemon juice and olive oil to coat; season to taste with salt and pepper.
Juice of 1 lemon	
2 tablespoons extra-virgin olive oil	
Salt and pepper to taste	**6** Place the greens over the fish, cut the sandwich into 4 servings, and serve.

Per serving: Calories 424 (From Fat 82); Fat 9g (Saturated 2g); Cholesterol 58mg; Sodium 706mg; Carbohydrate 49g (Dietary Fiber 2g); Protein 35g.

Grilled Vegetarian Sandwich with Hummus

Prep time: 45 min • **Cook time:** 8 min • **Yield:** 4 servings

Ingredients	*Directions*
1 large eggplant, or 2 Japanese eggplants 3 medium zucchinis	*1* Prepare and grill the vegetables according to directions in Chapter 12's Grilled Eggplant and Zucchini recipe.
1 rosemary and garlic foccacia or ciabatta bread 1 large tomato, sliced into ½-inch slices ½ cup hummus ½ cup feta cheese, crumbled	*2* Cut the bread into four pieces and then slice each piece in half to make 8 bread slices. Add 2 tablespoons of hummus to each sandwich; layer with the grilled vegetables, tomato, and 2 tablespoons of feta and serve.

Per serving: Calories 301 (From Fat 72); Fat 8g (Saturated 4g); Cholesterol 17mg; Sodium 579mg; Carbohydrate 48g (Dietary Fiber 9g); Protein 13g.

Tip: Try the Hummus recipe from Chapter 9 in this recipe.

Mediterranean diet quiz: Rate your plate

You may already be on board with many of the principles of a Mediterranean diet. Take this quiz to see where you fall and what changes you can focus on toward adopting a Mediterranean diet.

Answer the questions below; the numbers in parentheses are point totals, but you don't have to worry about those until after you take the quiz.

1. How many total fruits and vegetable servings do you eat each day?

    a. Five to nine (2)

    b. Three to four (1)

    c. Fewer than three (0)

2. How often do you eat fish or seafood?

    a. Several times a week (2)

    b. Once or twice a month (1)

    c. Once or twice a year (0)

(continued)

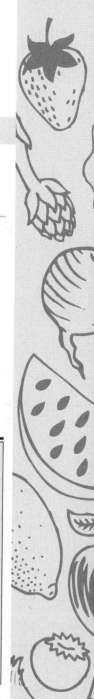

(continued)

3. How often do you use fresh herbs with cooking?

   a. At least four times a week (2)

   b. Three to four times a month (1)

   c. Once or twice a year (0)

4. On average, how often do you eat beef?

   a. Two to three times a week (0)

   b. Three to four times a month (1)

   c. Once or twice a month at most (2)

5. How often do you eat beans and lentils, including those found in soups and stews or dips (such as hummus)?

   a. At least four times a week (2)

   b. Several times a month (1)

   c. Several times a year (0)

6. When you eat beef or poultry, what serving size do you most often eat?

   a. Six to eight ounces (0)

   b. Four to five ounces (1)

   c. Two to three ounces (2)

7. How often do you use olive oil for cooking or in salad dressings and spreads?

   a. Daily (2)

   b. Two to three times a week (1)

   c. Two to three times a month (0)

8. How often do you eat nuts or nut butter?

   a. At least four times a week (2)

   b. Two to three times a month (1)

   c. Two to three times a year (0)

Now figure out your score by adding up the points to the right of your answers and comparing the total to these ranges:

13–16: Great job! You're right on track with a Mediterranean way of life. Use the recipes in this book to inspire you to stick with this dietary pattern.

8–12: You're almost there! Many of your habits are right on track, but others could use some small changes. Focus on areas where you scored less than two points and see whether you can improve those dietary habits. This book offers lots of tips, suggestions, and delicious recipes to get you inspired.

Less than 8: You've got some dietary changes to focus on to master the Mediterranean diet. Focus on areas where you scored less than two 1 points and use this book for inspiration to make small changes that better align your habits with a Mediterranean style of eating.

Chapter 17

Preparing Classic Chicken Entrees

• •

In This Chapter

▶ Cooking chicken the Italian way

▶ Taking some tips from Crete

▶ Spicing it up with Moroccan and Spanish flavors

• •

Chicken is a popular dish served throughout the Mediterranean. Maybe that popularity comes because chicken is so versatile: With a variety of cooking methods (such as grilling, sautéing, and roasting) and Mediterranean-inspired herbs and spices, you can banish those plain old baked chicken breasts.

Although boneless, skinless chicken breasts are a lean source of protein, the dark meat of the legs, thighs, and wings are slightly higher in fat content. However, as long as you watch your portion size, you can enjoy all types of chicken meat. In the Mediterranean, poultry is most often a small, supporting part of the meal rather than the main dish. This smaller serving means individuals in the Mediterranean consume less animal fat. They fill that extra plate space with plant-based proteins such as beans and lentils. This way of eating may seem a bit odd, but give it a try. You'll notice the health benefits after a short while.

This chapter shows you some delicious ways to cook chicken so that you're never bored. Plus, the smaller portion sizes help you make chicken the star supporting act.

Chicken can carry *salmonella,* a type of bacteria that can cause food-borne illness. Always cook your chicken through — to 165 degrees — so that no pink is left in the center. Verify the temperature by placing a kitchen thermometer into the thickest part of the meat so that it isn't touching any bones. Be certain to wash your hands and work surfaces thoroughly with antibacterial soap. Don't forget to always discard marinades after using.

Crafting Some Chicken Classics from Southern Italy

Chicken is widely popular in Italy, including in some of those classic, much-loved dishes such as chicken cacciatore and chicken piccata. Most Italian cooking uses the whole chicken, but in this section, we provide some simplified versions that use chicken breasts or pre-cooked rotisserie chicken to make cooking these recipes easier. If you love Italian food, check out these delicious classics.

Uncovering the truth about chicken and fat

You've likely heard the message that chicken is a great source of lean protein to include in your weekly meal plan. However, we want to uncover a few myths about chicken to help you get the most flavor from your chicken and make the best choices.

✔ **Myth 1: All chicken meat is lean.** Actually, each part of the chicken contains varying degrees of fat. The white meat from the breast is the leanest cut, followed by the thigh (as long as the skin is removed). The wings and legs are higher in fat and have about as much fat as some cuts of beef.

✔ **Myth 2: You have to remove the skin prior to cooking to eliminate the fat.** Although removing the skin can lower the fat content,

you can do so after cooking to create a juicier and tastier poultry dish that is still considered lowfat.

✔ **Myth 3: The majority of fat found in chicken is saturated or "bad" fat.** In reality, chicken fat consists of mostly good-for-you mono-unsaturated and polyunsaturated fats. One tablespoon of chicken fat contains about 4 grams of saturated fat, 6 grams monounsaturated fats, and 3 grams polyunsaturated fats. Limiting your saturated fat intake on a daily basis is still important, but eating some dark chicken meat once in awhile isn't as harmful to your health as you may have thought. Just watch your portion size (2 to 3 ounces) and don't deep fry it.

Chicken Cacciatore

Prep time: 12 min • **Cook time:** 50 min • **Yield:** 6 servings

Ingredients	Directions
1½ pounds boneless, skin-on chicken breasts	**1** Season the chicken with the salt and pepper. In a large plastic freezer bag, combine the flour, 1 teaspoon of the oregano, and the red pepper flakes. Add the chicken, seal the bag, and shake to coat.
½ teaspoon sea salt, plus more to taste	
¼ teaspoon pepper, plus more to taste	
⅓ cup flour	**2** In a large Dutch oven or an electric skillet, heat the olive oil over medium-high heat. Add the chicken, skin side down, and cook for 5 minutes on each side. Remove the chicken from the pan and set aside.
1 teaspoon plus 1 teaspoon dried oregano	
½ teaspoon red pepper flakes	
2 tablespoons olive oil	**3** Add the bell peppers, onions, and garlic to the pan and sauté for 3 minutes, scraping the bottom to pick up the browned bits. Add the wine and sauté the vegetables for 5 minutes.
1 large red bell pepper, chopped	
1 large green bell pepper, chopped	
1 onion, chopped	**4** Add the tomatoes (with the liquid), chicken stock, capers, and remaining oregano and return the chicken to the pan. Bring the mixture to a boil, cover, reduce the heat to a simmer, and cook for 30 minutes.
6 cloves garlic, finely chopped	
½ cup dry white wine	
One 28-ounce can diced tomatoes	
1 cup chicken stock	**5** Stir in the parsley and season with salt and pepper to taste. Remove the chicken to a cutting board and let it sit for a few minutes prior to cutting. Using a sharp knife, cut each breast if necessary to ensure six servings.
¼ cup capers, drained and rinsed	
¼ cup fresh parsley, chopped	
½ cup fresh basil, thinly sliced	**6** Place the chicken onto a serving platter, ladle the sauce over the top, and top with the basil and Parmesan prior to serving.
¼ cup Parmesan cheese, grated	

Per serving: Calories 399 (From Fat 139); Fat 15g (Saturated 4g); Cholesterol 99mg; Sodium 1129mg; Carbohydrate 22g (Dietary Fiber 4g); Protein 39g.

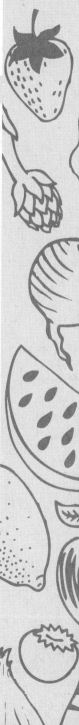

Chicken Piccata

Prep time: 12 min • **Cook time:** 18 min • **Yield:** 4 servings

Ingredients	Directions
Four 4-ounce boneless, skinless chicken breasts	**1** Preheat the oven to 425 degrees.
¼ cup plus ½ cup flour	**2** Using a meat mallet or heavy pan, pound the chicken into ½-inch-thick pieces.
½ teaspoon garlic power	
¼ teaspoon salt	**3** In a shallow bowl, combine ¼ cup of the flour, the garlic powder, salt, and paprika. In another bowl, combine the egg and 1 tablespoon of the water; place the remaining flour in a third bowl.
¼ teaspoon paprika	
1 egg, lightly beaten	
1 tablespoon plus 1 cup water	
¼ cup olive oil	**4** Dredge the chicken in the flour-garlic mixture and shake off any excess. Dip the chicken into the egg mixture and then coat with the plain flour and place onto a baking sheet.
2 teaspoons chicken bouillon or base	
1 cup water	**5** Heat the olive oil in a heavy skillet over medium heat. Add the chicken pieces and brown on each side (3 to 4 minutes per side). Return the chicken to the baking sheet and bake for 5 minutes.
¼ cup lemon juice	
1 teaspoon cornstarch	
¼ cup fresh parsley, chopped	
	6 Meanwhile, add the bouillon and the remaining water to the skillet. Scrape up any browned bits into the sauce. Bring the mixture to a boil and then reduce to a simmer.
	7 Whisk together the lemon juice and cornstarch in a small bowl and add to the sauce. Add the parsley. Transfer the cooked chicken to a serving dish and top with the sauce prior to serving.

Per serving: Calories 405 (From Fat 161); Fat 18g (Saturated 3g); Cholesterol 95mg; Sodium 797mg; Carbohydrate 20g (Dietary Fiber 1g); Protein 39g.

Note: You can purchase either bouillon cubes or chicken base, which is more of a paste.

Chicken Carbonara with Petit Peas

Prep time: 10 min • **Cook time:** 20 min • **Yield:** 8 servings

Ingredients	Directions
1 pound farfalle	*1* Bring 4 quarts of water to a boil. Add the pasta and cook according to package directions (about 9 to 12 minutes) or until al dente.
2 teaspoons olive oil	
2 ounces pancetta, chopped	*2* While you wait for the water to boil, heat the olive oil over medium heat in a Dutch oven. Add the pancetta and cook for 5 minutes. Add the garlic and cook for 5 minutes.
4 cloves garlic, sliced	
½ cup whipping cream	
½ cup milk	*3* Meanwhile, whisk together the whipping cream, milk, cheese, egg yolks, and parsley.
½ cup grated Parmesan cheese	
4 egg yolks	*4* Add the shredded chicken to the skillet to reheat, about 2 minutes. Add the cooked pasta and the peas and pour the sauce over the top.
½ cup fresh parsley, chopped	
4 cups cooked white and/or dark chicken, shredded	
2 cups petit peas, fresh or thawed frozen	*5* Cook the mixture over low for 5 minutes, tossing to mix as the sauce heats. Season the mixture with salt and pepper. Transfer to a serving dish, top with chopped walnuts, and serve.
Salt and pepper to taste	
¼ cup walnuts, finely chopped	

Per serving: Calories 560 (From Fat 206); Fat 23g (Saturated 9g); Cholesterol 195mg; Sodium 228mg; Carbohydrate 51g (Dietary Fiber 4g); Protein 36g.

Note: Although adding green peas isn't traditional, we prefer to keep them for a pop of color and flavor!

Tip: In place of the shredded chicken, you can use the meat from 1 rotisserie chicken.

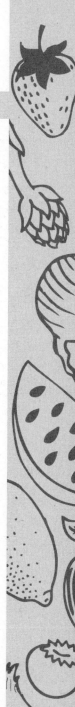

Lemon Chicken Scaloppine

Prep time: 12 min • **Cook time:** 24 min • **Yield:** 8 servings

Ingredients	*Directions*
Four 6-ounce boneless, skinless chicken breasts	*1* Preheat the oven to 300 degrees.
¼ cup plus ¼ cup flour	*2* Cut each chicken breast in half lengthwise to create thin chicken breasts fillets.
¼ teaspoon salt	
¼ teaspoon pepper	*3* In a shallow bowl, combine ¼ cup of the flour and the salt and pepper. In another bowl, combine the eggs and water. Mix the panko and the remaining flour in a third bowl.
2 eggs, lightly beaten	
2 tablespoons water	
1 cup panko breadcrumbs	
¼ cup olive oil	*4* Dredge chicken in the flour-salt mixture and shake off any excess. Dip the chicken into the egg mixture and then coat with the panko mixture and place onto a baking sheet.
Juice of 1 lemon	
	5 Heat the olive oil in a heavy skillet over medium-high heat. Add the chicken pieces in batches and brown on each side (6 to 8 minutes per side).
	6 Keep the chicken warm in the oven on an ovenproof serving platter until you cook all the pieces. Drizzle the lemon juice over the cooked chicken and serve.

Per serving: Calories 271 (From Fat 95); Fat 11g (Saturated 2g); Cholesterol 71mg; Sodium 522mg; Carbohydrate 13g (Dietary Fiber 1g); Protein 29g.

Creating Amazing Cretan Chicken Dishes

Grilling and braising are the most popular ways to cook meats in Crete; combined with fresh herbs and spices and traditional foods such as yogurt, cheese, and olives, these techniques create chicken dishes with a whole lot of flavor. This section provides some easy-to-make, Cretan-inspired meals that your family and friends will love.

Deciphering poultry label claims

With more and more terms like "organic" and "free-range" showing up in the meat section, reading food labels is becoming more challenging each year. So which products do you buy? The answer isn't clear cut — it's largely a personal choice. Here are some of the USDA definitions behind the claims you find on poultry labels to help you make the best choices for you and your family:

✔ *Certified* means that the poultry has been evaluated for class or grade by the USDA's Food Safety and Inspection Service and the Agriculture Marketing Service.

✔ *Free-range or free-roaming* indicates that the chickens have access to the outdoors instead of being cooped up (pun intended) in chicken coops. Keep in mind that these designations don't necessarily guarantee that the chickens actually decided to wander, so a given chicken labeled free-range/free-roaming may or may not be any different than one without the label.

✔ *Fresh* poultry means that the whole chicken and cuts have never been frozen.

✔ *Natural* is used when the poultry doesn't contain any artificial ingredients and has undergone minimal processing.

✔ The phrase *no hormones* can't be used by itself on a label because hormones aren't allowed in raising poultry (that is, no poultry should contain added hormones, so producers can't advertise as though other poultry might). To include this statement on packaging, it must be followed with the clarification "Federal regulations prohibit the use of hormones."

✔ The phrase *no antibiotics* can be used on a package if the manufacturer can provide sufficient evidence to back it up.

✔ *Organic* means the chicken can't contain artificial ingredients, hormones, or antibiotics.

Sautéed Chicken Breasts in Red Wine Tomato Sauce

Prep time: 10 min • **Cook time:** 45 min • **Yield:** 4 servings

Ingredients	Directions
Four 4-ounce bone-in, skin-on chicken breasts	**1** Preheat the oven to 350 degrees. Rub the chicken with 2 tablespoons oil and season with the salt and pepper.
2 tablespoons plus 2 tablespoons olive oil	
¼ teaspoon salt	**2** Heat the remaining olive oil in a heavy ovenproof (preferably cast-iron) Dutch oven over medium-high heat. Brown the chicken on each side for 4 minutes and remove them from the pan and set aside.
½ teaspoon pepper	
1 tablespoon fennel seeds	
2 celery stalks, chopped	**3** Add the fennel seeds, celery, onion, and garlic and cook for 3 minutes, stirring frequently. Add the red pepper flakes and olives, cook for 1 minute, and return the chicken to the pan. Add the tomatoes and stir in the wine.
½ a medium onion, chopped	
4 cloves garlic, sliced	
1 teaspoon red pepper flakes	
¼ cup black kalamata olives, pitted	**4** Bake for 30 minutes. Top the chicken with the parsley and mint and serve.
One 14.8-ounce can tomatoes, chopped	
1 cup spicy red wine, such as a red Zinfandel	
2 tablespoons parsley, chopped	
2 tablespoons mint, chopped	

Per serving: Calories 343 (From Fat 175); Fat 19g (Saturated 3g); Cholesterol 50mg; Sodium 649mg; Carbohydrate 12g (Dietary Fiber 3g); Protein 20g.

Roasted Rice-Stuffed Chicken

Prep time: 30 min • **Cook time:** 2 hr • **Yield:** 10 servings

Ingredients	Directions
¼ **cup pine nuts**	*1* Preheat the oven to 350 degrees.
1 medium onion, chopped	
2 cups chicken stock	*2* In a 2-quart saucepan, toast the pine nuts over medium heat for 1 minute; add the onions and cook for 3 minutes, stirring frequently. Add the chicken stock and scrape the bottom of the pan.
¼ **cup green olives**	
1 cup wild rice	
One 5- pound whole skinless chicken, giblets removed	*3* Bring the mixture to a boil over medium-high heat. Add the olives and rice, cover, and reduce the heat to a simmer for 40 minutes or until the rice absorbs the liquid.
2 tablespoons plus 1 tablespoon olive oil	
Zest of 1 lemon	*4* Meanwhile, place the chicken onto a roast rack. Rub the inside cavity with 2 tablespoons of the olive oil. Combine the lemon zest, salt, pepper, and paprika. Rub the chicken with the spice mixture and brush with the remaining olive oil.
½ **teaspoon salt**	
1 teaspoon pepper	
1 teaspoon paprika	
2 cups dry white wine	*5* Stuff the chicken with the rice mixture and pour the wine over the chicken.
	6 Bake uncovered for 1½ hours until both the chicken and the rice reach an internal temperature of 165 degrees (begin checking the internal temperature at 1 hour) and the juices run clear from the breast. Baste the chicken every 20 minutes.
	7 Allow the chicken to rest for 10 minutes prior to cutting into the meat. Remove the rice from the cavity and place into a serving bowl. Serve 2 to 3 ounces of chicken over ½ cup of rice.

Per serving: Calories 305 (From Fat 97); Fat 11g (Saturated 2g); Cholesterol 70mg; Sodium 324mg; Carbohydrate 18g (Dietary Fiber 2g); Protein 25g.

Note: If rice doesn't completely fit into the cavity, bake the extra in a heat-proof baking dish next to the chicken during the last 20 minutes of baking.

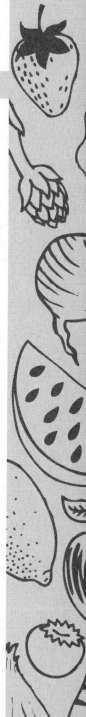

Chicken Wrapped in Phyllo

Prep time: 24 min • **Cook time:** 45 min • **Yield:** 8 servings

Ingredients	Directions
½ cup French or Greek feta cheese, crumbled	**1** Preheat the oven to 350 degrees. In a small bowl, combine the feta, egg, garlic, green onions, parsley, mint, red pepper flakes, and lemon zest.
1 egg	
4 cloves garlic, minced	**2** Using a heavy pan or mallet, flatten the chicken to a ½-inch thickness. Cut each breast into half to make 8 pieces. Evenly divide the herb mixture among the chicken pieces, placing the mixture across the entire piece.
½ cup chopped green onion	
½ cup chopped fresh parsley	
½ cup chopped fresh mint	
½ teaspoon red pepper flakes	**3** Brush 1 phyllo sheet with some of the olive oil. Place a piece of the chicken at one end of the sheet, fold the sides over, brush with more olive oil, and roll up.
1 lemon, zested and sliced into wedges	
4 6-ounce boneless, skinless chicken breasts	**4** Brush the roll with olive oil and sprinkle with sea salt. Repeat with the remaining chicken. Bake on a baking sheet for 35 to 45 minutes or until golden and crisp. Serve with the lemon wedges.
8 sheets phyllo pastry	
½ cup olive oil	
Coarse sea salt or kosher salt	

Per serving: Calories 309 (From Fat 171); Fat 19g (Saturated 4g); Cholesterol 63mg; Sodium 309mg; Carbohydrate 13g (Dietary Fiber 1g); Protein 22g.

Tip: Work with one piece of phyllo at a time, and be certain to cover the remaining phyllo with a moist cloth or towel to prevent cracking or drying out.

Grilled Yogurt Chicken with Mint

Prep time: 30 min, plus marinating time • **Cook time:** 10 min • **Yield:** 6 servings

Ingredients	Directions
1 5-pound whole chicken, butterflied	*1* Place the butterflied chicken into a glass baking pan. Combine the remaining ingredients and pour the mixture over the chicken to coat both sides. Marinate the chicken in the refrigerator for 4 to 8 hours.
1 cup plain Greek yogurt	
2 tablespoons extra-virgin olive oil	
4 cloves garlic, minced	*2* Heat the grill over medium heat. Shake off any excess marinade, place the chicken on the grill skin side down, and cook for 15 minutes on each side. Flip the chicken again and finish cooking with the skin side down until the thickest part of the chicken reads 165 degrees.
1 whole lemon, chopped	
⅓ cup fresh mint, chopped	
2 teaspoons ground cumin	
½ teaspoon cayenne pepper	*3* Remove the chicken from the grill and cover with foil; allow the chicken to rest for 15 minutes before serving. Slice the chicken and serve 2 to 3 ounces per serving.
1 teaspoon coarse salt	

Per serving: Calories 261 (From Fat 83); Fat 9g (Saturated 2g); Cholesterol 113mg; Sodium 536mg; Carbohydrate 4g (Dietary Fiber 1g); Protein 40g.

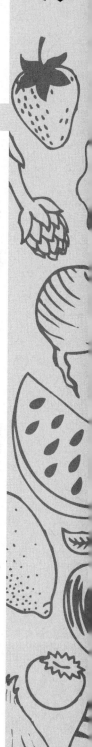

Chicken Breasts with Spinach and Feta

Prep time: 20 min • **Cook time:** 1 hr • **Yield:** 6 servings

Ingredients	*Directions*
Four 6-ounce boneless chicken breasts	*1* Preheat the oven to 350 degrees.
1 tablespoon olive oil	*2* Cut the chicken breasts lengthwise to butterfly and create a pocket for stuffing. Cut deep enough into the breast to create a large enough pocket to accommodate the stuffing, but don't cut all the way through.
4 cloves garlic, sliced	
¼ of a medium onion, chopped	
One 10-ounce package frozen spinach, defrosted	*3* In a nonstick skillet, heat the olive oil over medium heat. Add the garlic and onions and sauté for 3 minutes. Wring out the spinach to remove any excess liquid and add it, the parsley, and oregano to the pan.
½ cup parsley	
1 teaspoon dried oregano	
¼ cup feta cheese, crumbled	*4* Heat the spinach mixture for 5 minutes and remove it from the heat, straining off any additional liquid. Stir in the crumbled feta.
Nonstick cooking spray	
1 lemon, cut into wedges	
	5 Using a spoon, stuff the chicken breasts with the spinach mixture. Place the stuffed chicken breasts onto a baking sheet and spray them lightly with cooking spray.
	6 Bake the chicken for 40 to 45 minutes or until cooked completely. Slice the chicken to display the stuffing and serve with the lemon wedges.

Per serving: Calories 188 (From Fat 62); Fat 7g (Saturated 2g); Cholesterol 78mg; Sodium 240mg; Carbohydrate 5g (Dietary Fiber 2g); Protein 27g.

Adding a Touch of Morocco and Spain

You find no shortage of flavor when you begin cooking with traditional Moroccan and Spanish meals. Moroccan cuisine brings North Africa's unique flavors and regional foods; it's very flavorful because Moroccan cooks are famous for abundantly using spices and dried fruits in their cooking. Of course, you also see the use of fresh vegetables, typical of the entire Mediterranean region. To sample Moroccan food at home, try these recipes from this section:

- ✔ Moroccan Chicken with Tomatoes and Zucchini
- ✔ Chicken Curry

Traditional Spanish cooking relies heavily on olive oil and garlic — the perfect pair. Spanish cuisine is also full of smoky flavors, which sometimes come from salty smoked meats such as chorizo. Chicken is another common ingredient. Cooks in Spain use lots of spices, such as paprika and saffron, as well as herbs such as parsley, oregano, rosemary, and thyme. In this section, you can find these Spanish-inspired recipes:

- ✔ Chicken in Paprika Sauce
- ✔ Spanish Kabobs
- ✔ Breaded Chicken with Caper Mayonnaise

Moroccan Chicken with Tomatoes and Zucchini

Prep time: 5 min • **Cook time:** 25 min • **Yield:** 4 servings

Ingredients	Directions
Three 6-ounce boneless, skinless chicken breasts	**1** Cut the chicken breasts into bite-sized pieces (about 2 inches).
2 tablespoons olive oil	
6 cloves garlic, minced	**2** Heat a nonstick skillet over medium-high heat; add the olive oil, garlic, ginger, and chicken pieces and cook for 5 minutes or until the chicken is browned on all sides.
1 teaspoon grated fresh ginger, or 1 teaspoon ground ginger	
2 zucchinis	**3** Meanwhile, cut the zucchinis lengthwise into quarters and chop it into ½-inch moon shapes.
¼ teaspoon pepper	
½ cup plus ½ cup cilantro, chopped	**4** Add the zucchini, ½ cup of the cilantro, and the canned tomatoes to the skillet; stir and cover for 15 minutes or until the chicken is cooked completely. Add the remaining cilantro and serve.
One 14.8-ounce can tomatoes, chopped	

Per serving: Calories 249 (From Fat 95); Fat 11g (Saturated 2g); Cholesterol 82mg; Sodium 313mg; Carbohydrate 9g (Dietary Fiber 2g); Protein 30g.

Tip: Try serving this dish over quick-cooking couscous or with curried rice.

Note: Flip to the color insert for a photo of this recipe.

Chicken in Paprika Sauce

Prep time: 10 min • **Cook time:** 20 min • **Yield:** 6 servings

Ingredients	Directions
Three 6-ounce boneless, skinless chicken breasts	*1* Cut the chicken breasts into 1-inch pieces. Combine the flour, salt, and 1 tablespoon of the paprika in a bowl and toss the chicken pieces with the flour to coat.
¼ **cup flour**	
1 teaspoon salt	
1 tablespoon plus 1 tablespoon paprika	*2* Heat the olive oil in a nonstick skillet over medium heat. Add the chicken pieces, stirring to cook for about 4 minutes or until they're lightly browned and cooked through. Remove the chicken from the skillet and set aside.
2 tablespoons olive oil	
1 large red bell pepper, chopped	*3* Add the peppers and onions to the skillet and sauté for 5 minutes. Add the stock and remaining paprika and bring the mixture to a boil.
1 small onion, chopped	
2 cups chicken stock	*4* Turn off the heat. Using a stick blender or food processor, blend the sauce until it's smooth or your desired consistency.
¼ **cup sour cream**	
	5 Return the chicken and sauce to the pan and simmer over medium-low heat for 5 minutes, until the chicken is cooked through. Remove from the heat, stir in the sour cream, and serve.

Per serving: Calories 216 (From Fat 89); Fat 10g (Saturated 3g); Cholesterol 62mg; Sodium 610mg; Carbohydrate 10g (Dietary Fiber 1g); Protein 21g.

Tip: Serve over one of our quick-cooking couscous recipes, polenta, or the Golden Pilaf (see Chapter 13 for these sides).

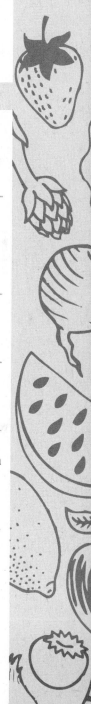

Breaded Chicken with Caper Mayonnaise

Prep time: 12 min • **Cook time:** 24 min • **Yield:** 8 servings

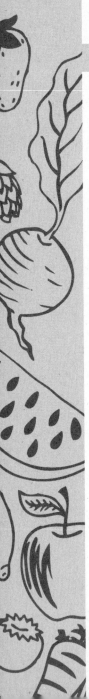

Ingredients	Directions
Four 6-ounce boneless, skinless chicken breasts	**1** Preheat the oven to 300 degrees. Cut each chicken breast piece in half lengthwise to create thin fillets.
¼ **cup flour**	
¼ **teaspoon salt**	**2** In a shallow bowl, combine the flour, salt, and pepper. In another bowl, combine the eggs and water. Mix the breadcrumbs, paprika, and thyme in a third bowl.
¼ **teaspoon pepper**	
2 eggs, lightly beaten	
2 tablespoons water	**3** Dredge the chicken in the flour mixture and shake off any excess. Dip the chicken into the egg mixture and then coat the chicken with the breadcrumbs and place onto a baking sheet.
1 cup breadcrumbs	
½ **teaspoon paprika**	
¼ **teaspoon ground thyme**	
1 tablespoon olive oil	**4** Heat the olive oil in a heavy skillet over medium-high heat. Add the chicken in batches and brown on each side (6 to 8 minutes per side). Keep the chicken warm in the oven on an ovenproof serving platter until you cook all the pieces.
Zest of 1 lemon	
¼ **cup mayonnaise**	
2 tablespoons capers, drained and rinsed	**5** Meanwhile, prepare the mayonnaise by combining the lemon zest, mayonnaise, capers, and parsley. Serve the mayonnaise with the cooked chicken.
¼ **cup parsley, chopped**	

Per serving: Calories 213 (From Fat 64); Fat 7g (Saturated 1g); Cholesterol 56mg; Sodium 401mg; Carbohydrate 15g (Dietary Fiber 1g); Protein 21g.

Spanish Kabobs

Prep time: 20 min, plus marinating time • **Cook time:** 16 min • **Yield:** 4 servings

Ingredients	Directions
Three 6-ounce boneless, skinless chicken breasts	*1* Cut the chicken into bite-sized pieces (about 2 inches).
¼ cup almonds	
1 teaspoon ground cumin	*2* In a food processor, pulse the almonds, cumin, coriander, paprika, and garlic for 3 minutes. Add the red wine vinegar and olive oil and mix for 1 minute. Season the mixture with salt to taste.
½ teaspoon coriander	
1 teaspoon paprika	
4 cloves garlic, minced	
2 tablespoons red wine vinegar	*3* Pour the mixture over chicken pieces and coat. Marinate in the refrigerator for at least 30 minutes.
2 tablespoons olive oil	*4* Lightly grease grill grates with oil and then heat the grill over medium-high heat. Skewer the chicken pieces and grill for 6 to 8 minutes on each side or until cooked thoroughly. Place on a serving dish and top with the cilantro.
Salt to taste	
½ cup cilantro, chopped	

Per serving: Calories 262 (From Fat 132); Fat 15g (Saturated 2g); Cholesterol 82mg; Sodium 155mg; Carbohydrate 2g (Dietary Fiber 1g); Protein 29g.

Tip: If you use wooden skewers, be sure to soak them in water ahead of time so they don't burn.

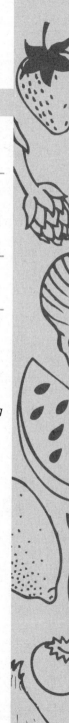

Chicken Curry

Prep time: 10 min • **Cook time:** 30 min • **Yield:** 6 servings

Ingredients	*Directions*
Four 6-ounce boneless, skinless chicken breasts	**1** Cut the chicken breasts into 1-inch pieces. Toss the chicken pieces with the flour to coat. Dust off the excess flour from the pieces.
2 tablespoons flour	
1 tablespoon olive oil	**2** In a Dutch oven, heat the olive oil over medium-high heat. Add the chicken pieces and brown on all sides, about 6 minutes. Add the onion, garlic, carrots, celery, and ginger and sauté for 4 minutes.
1 onion, chopped	
2 cloves garlic, chopped	
2 carrots, sliced	
2 stalks celery, sliced	**3** Add the spices (paprika through turmeric), broth, tomatoes, chickpeas, zucchini, and raisins; cover, lower the heat to low, and simmer for 25 minutes. Sprinkle with the cilantro and serve.
1 tablespoon minced fresh ginger	
1 teaspoon paprika	
½ teaspoon coriander	
1 teaspoon ground cumin	
1 teaspoon dried oregano	
¼ teaspoon cayenne pepper	
½ teaspoon turmeric	
1½ cups chicken broth	
One 14.8-ounce can diced tomatoes	
One 14.8-ounce can chickpeas, drained and rinsed	
1 zucchini, sliced	
¼ cup golden raisins	
½ cup cilantro, chopped	

Per serving: Calories 372 (From Fat 97); Fat 11g (Saturated 2g); Cholesterol 73mg; Sodium 613mg; Carbohydrate 36g (Dietary Fiber 9g); Protein 35g.

Tip: If you're feeling overwhelmed by the spice list, you can always substitute 1 tablespoon of a pre-made curry blend in place of the paprika, coriander, cumin, oregano, cayenne, and turmeric.

Chapter 18

Going Under the Sea with Seafood Options

In This Chapter

▶ Diving into delicious, light fish recipes

▶ Creating savory shellfish specialties

▶ Making quick and easy standby seafood recipes for busy days

Coastal living brings a rich variety of delicious, fresh seafood. The people who live on the Mediterranean coast utilize all the food bounties that nature has provided them, so you see no shortage of fish and shellfish entrees and sides in the Mediterranean diet. We encourage you to embrace seafood (figuratively speaking; you don't have to go hug a fish).

If you struggle with cooking fish, you aren't alone! It's one of the most common challenges we hear about. This chapter shows you simple steps to cook flavorful fish to perfection, even if you're short on time. And if you already consider yourself a pretty good seafood cook, you can enjoy diving into the classics in this chapter.

Although we provide some delicious recipes in this chapter, feel free to substitute the fresh fish or seafood unique to your area. For example, if lakes and streams are closer to you than the ocean, swap some local trout into one of this chapter's recipes. Use the following table to see what types of fish you can substitute into the recipes in this chapter.

Calls for	*Substitute with*
Cod	Snapper, mahi-mahi, walleye, or perch
Halibut	Grouper, cod, salmon, tilapia, or snapper
Tuna	Wahoo, halibut, salmon, or trout
Salmon	Trout, whitefish, or striped bass
Sea bass	Tuna, halibut, or trout

Making Light and Healthy Fish Entrees

Eating fish is an important part of a healthy diet; fish provides a lean source of protein and is rich in omega-3 fatty acids, which are important for heart health and mental health. Consuming fish several times a week is one of the Mediterranean population's healthy habits.

This section demonstrates some delicious ways to serve up omega-3-rich foods such as halibut, salmon, sea bass, and tuna. Make sure to check out the table earlier in the chapter if you want to substitute a different type of fish in the following recipes.

Shoring up seafood safety

Consuming seafood regularly is a good strategy for overall health and wellness, but all seafood contains traces of *mercury*, a neurotoxin that accumulates in streams and oceans from industrial pollution. Babies and small children are at the highest risk because mercury levels may exceed the safety limits for their small weight.

For the average healthy adult, limiting your intake of the high-mercury fish listed here can keep you pretty safe. Pregnant women, nursing moms, women who may become pregnant, and small children should use the following tips for seafood safety from the Environmental Protection Agency:

✔ Avoid shark, swordfish, king mackerel (kingfish), and tilefish because they contain high levels of mercury.

✔ Choose light canned tuna as opposed to albacore canned tuna because the former has less mercury.

✔ Consume up to 12 ounces per week of lower-mercury seafood, including shrimp, salmon, pollock, and catfish.

✔ Check your local advisories on any local fish caught in lakes and streams. If no advisories are available, eat up to 6 ounces per week of such local fish with no additional fish (of any kind) that week.

Halibut with Olives and Capers

Prep time: 8 min • **Cook time:** 30 min • **Yield:** 8 servings

Ingredients	Directions
2 pounds halibut, cut into approximately 1½-inch pieces	*1* Preheat the oven to 400 degrees.
Salt and pepper to taste	*2* Place the fish into a baking pan and season with the salt and pepper. Combine the tomatoes, onions, olives, parsley, capers, garlic, bell peppers, white wine, and olive oil.
Two 15-ounce cans crushed tomatoes, drained	
1 large onion, coarsely chopped	*3* Pour the sauce over the fish. Bake the fish for 30 minutes or until it flakes easily with a fork. Sprinkle with the feta and serve.
1 cup kalamata olives, pitted and halved	
½ cup fresh parsley, chopped	
2 tablespoons capers, drained	
6 cloves garlic, thinly sliced	
1 red bell pepper, seeded and diced	
1 yellow bell pepper, seeded and diced	
½ cup white wine	
¼ cup olive oil	
½ cup crumbled feta cheese	

Per serving: Calories 288 (From Fat 120); Fat 13g (Saturated 3g); Cholesterol 45mg; Sodium 538mg; Carbohydrate 13g (Dietary Fiber 3g); Protein 27g.

Vary It! In Step 2, blend the sauce until smooth and put aside. Bake the fish without the sauce and then pour the blended sauce over the cooked fish and top with the feta.

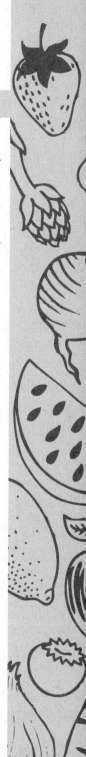

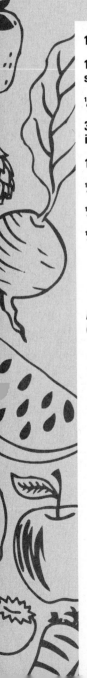

Baked Salmon with Fresh Vegetables

Prep time: 5 min • **Cook time:** 35 min • **Yield:** 4 servings

Ingredients	Directions
1 lemon, cut into ¼-inch slices	*1* Preheat the oven to 400 degrees.
1½ pounds skin-on salmon fillets	*2* Place a large piece of foil onto a baking sheet. Lay half of the lemon slices in the center of the foil and center the salmon (skin side down) on top. Sprinkle the surface of the salmon with sea salt.
½ teaspoon sea salt	
3 Roma or plum tomatoes, cut into ¼-inch slices	
1 medium onion, ¼-inch slices	*3* Layer the tomatoes, onions, mushrooms, parsley, and remaining lemon slices on top of the fish. Drizzle with the wine and fold over the edges of the foil to seal the salmon in a packet.
½ pound mushrooms, sliced	
½ cup parsley, chopped	
¼ cup white wine	
	3 Bake the salmon for 45 minutes. Remove from oven, discard the top layer of lemons and serve, watching out for steam as you open the packet.

Per serving: Calories 271 (From Fat 57); Fat 6g (Saturated 1g); Cholesterol 88mg; Sodium 422mg; Carbohydrate 11g (Dietary Fiber 2g); Protein 37g.

Sea Bass with Caper and Almond-Lemon Sauce

Prep time: 10 min • **Cook time:** 8 min • **Yield:** 4 servings

Ingredients	Directions
¼ cup breadcrumbs	*1* Pulse the breadcrumbs, almonds, garlic, lemon juice, and water in a food processor for 1 minute, scraping down the sides as needed. Gradually stream in the extra-virgin olive oil just until the sauce is creamy. Season with salt to taste. Set aside.
½ cup almonds	
2 cloves garlic	
¼ cup lemon juice	
¼ cup water	*2* Lightly season the sea bass with the salt. In a heavy skillet, heat the olive oil and butter over medium heat. Add the capers and sea bass and cook for 4 minutes on each side. Remove from the pan and place on a serving platter; drizzle with the pan drippings.
¼ cup extra-virgin olive oil	
Four 4- to 6-ounce sea bass fillets	
¼ teaspoon salt, plus more to taste	*3* Pour half the almond and lemon sauce over the sea bass to serve, leaving the remaining sauce to be added as desired.
1 tablespoon olive oil	
2 tablespoons butter	
2 tablespoons capers, drained and rinsed	

Per serving: Calories 431 (From Fat 287); Fat 32g (Saturated 6g); Cholesterol 60mg; Sodium 435mg; Carbohydrate 9g (Dietary Fiber 2g); Protein 29g.

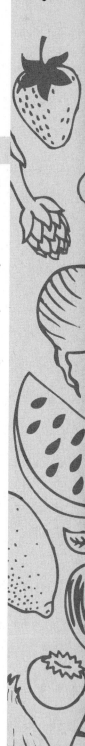

Grilled Tuna with Braised Fennel

Prep time: 8 min • **Cook time:** 16 min • **Yield:** 4 servings

Ingredients	*Directions*
¼ cup plus 1 tablespoon olive oil	*1* Preheat the grill over medium-high heat.
2 fennel bulbs, sliced ¼-inch thick	*2* In a heavy skillet, heat ¼ cup of the olive oil over medium heat. Add the fennel, onions, and garlic and sauté for 8 minutes, stirring frequently. Add the olives and capers and cook over low heat for 5 minutes.
1 onion, sliced in ¼-inch slices	
3 cloves garlic, chopped	
¼ cup kalamata olives, pitted and chopped	*3* Brush the fish with the remaining olive oil and season lightly with salt and pepper. Grill the fish for 3 minutes on each side or until slightly rare in the center.
¼ cup capers, drained and rinsed	
Four 6-ounce yellowtail tuna fillets	*4* Add the parsley and lemon juice to the fennel mixture, season with salt, stir, and serve over the fish.
¼ cup parsley, chopped	
Juice of 2 lemons	
Salt and pepper to taste	

Per serving: Calories 345 (From Fat 172); Fat 19g (Saturated 3g); Cholesterol 51mg; Sodium 439mg; Carbohydrate 16g (Dietary Fiber 5g); Protein 29g.

Note: Check out Chapter 12 for an illustration on how to slice fennel.

Crafting Some Shellfish Specialties

If you love seafood, shellfish is probably at the top of your list. Sizzling hot shrimp or the perfect tender scallop may make you want to run to the nearest seafood restaurant. The good news is you don't have to eat out. This section gives you those perfect recipes you can make any night of the week from the comfort of your own home.

Despite health scares about the high cholesterol levels found in shellfish, shrimp and the like can be part of a healthy diet. The American Heart Association recommends limiting your daily cholesterol intake to less than 300 milligrams per day (less than 200 milligrams if you have heart disease). Shrimp, mussels, and scallops all come in under these thresholds, so you can rest assured that shellfish can fit into your heart-healthy diet. Plus, shrimp and crab are both excellent sources of omega-3 fatty acids that promote heart health. Look at it this way: The folks in the Mediterranean have been eating like this for hundreds of years.

Keeping safe with shellfish

Shellfish is rich and delicious and contains healthy omega-3 fatty acids, but keep in mind that shellfish, especially oysters, clams, mussels, and scallops, can carry bacteria called Vibrio Vulnificus, which can multiply in numbers when refrigerated and can cause diarrhea, vomiting, and blistering skin, and can even lead to death. Most healthy people destroy the bacteria in the intestinal tract or with the immune system, but there are cases where that doesn't happen.

Because you can't know for sure if the shellfish you've purchased contains Vibrio Vulnificus, you can easily avoid putting yourself at risk by making sure you cook your shellfish thoroughly to destroy the bacteria. Cook scallops until they're white and firm and mollusks until the shells open. Make sure to discard any that don't open.

Sautéed Shrimp with White Wine and Feta

Prep time: 5 min • **Cook time:** 12 min • **Yield:** 6 servings

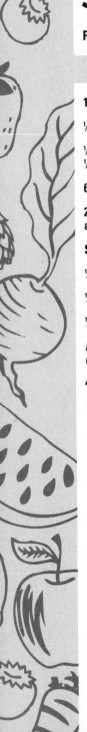

Ingredients	*Directions*
1 tablespoon olive oil	*1* Heat the olive oil in a large nonstick skillet over medium heat. Add the red pepper flakes and onion and sauté for 3 minutes. Add the garlic and cook for 3 minutes.
½ teaspoon red pepper flakes	
½ medium onion, cut into ¼-inch slices	
6 cloves garlic, sliced	*2* Season the shrimp with salt and pepper; add them to the skillet and sauté for 2 minutes per side. Add the wine and parsley and cook for 1 minute or until the shrimp is cooked. Crumble the feta over the top and serve.
2 pounds shrimp, peeled and deveined	
Salt and pepper to taste	
½ cup white wine	
¼ cup parsley, chopped	
¼ cup feta, crumbled	

Per serving: Calories 222 (From Fat 56); Fat 6g (Saturated 2g); Cholesterol 235mg; Sodium 297mg; Carbohydrate 4g (Dietary Fiber 0g); Protein 32g.

Note: Refer to Chapter 8 for an illustration on how to peel and devein shrimp.

Mussels with Tomatoes and Basil

Prep time: 5 min • **Cook time:** 15 min • **Yield:** 6 servings

Ingredients	*Directions*
1 tablespoon olive oil 1 onion, chopped 2 celery stalks, chopped 6 cloves garlic, chopped ½ teaspoon dried oregano One 14.8-ounce can tomatoes, chopped 1 teaspoon red pepper flakes 1 teaspoon honey 2 cups white wine 2 pounds mussels, cleaned Salt and pepper to taste ¼ cup basil, thinly sliced 6 slices crusty French bread	*1* In a medium saucepan, heat the olive oil over medium heat. Add the onions, celery, and garlic and cook for 5 minutes. Add the oregano, tomatoes, crushed red peppers, and honey. Simmer for 10 minutes.
	2 Meanwhile, bring the mussels and wine to a boil in a large skillet; cover and simmer for 10 minutes or until the mussels open.
	3 Pour the wine and mussels into the tomato sauce and stir. Season with salt and pepper to taste. Top with the basil and serve with the crusty French bread.

Per serving: *Calories 343 (From Fat 58); Fat 6g (Saturated 1g); Cholesterol 42mg; Sodium 767mg; Carbohydrate 34g (Dietary Fiber 2g); Protein 23g.*

Note: Discard any mussels that don't open for food safety. See the sidebar "Keeping safe with shellfish" in this chapter for more on why.

Tip: Figure 18-1 shows gives you mussel-cleaning guidance.

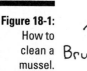

Figure 18-1:
How to clean a mussel.

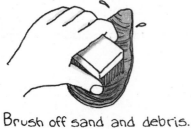

Brush off sand and debris.

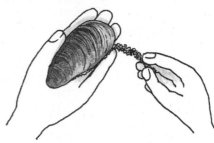

Remove the beard by pulling gently toward the hinged shell to loosen.

Marsala Scallops

Prep time: 5 min • **Cook time:** 8 min • **Yield:** 4 servings

Ingredients	*Directions*
24 sea scallops	*1* Pat the scallops dry with a paper towel. Combine the flour, salt, and pepper and dust the scallops lightly with the mixture.
⅓ cup flour	
½ teaspoon salt	
¼ teaspoon pepper	*2* Heat the olive oil in a nonstick skillet over medium-high heat. Sear the scallops for 1 to 3 minutes on each side or until cooked. Remove the scallops and deglaze the pan with the wine.
¼ cup olive oil	
⅓ cup Marsala wine or vermouth	
	3 Bring the wine to a simmer and allow the mixture to reduce, about 3 minutes. Return the scallops to the pan, toss to coat with the sauce, and serve.

Per serving: Calories 274 (From Fat 129); Fat 14g (Saturated 2g); Cholesterol 30mg; Sodium 438mg; Carbohydrate 13g (Dietary Fiber 0g); Protein 16g.

Getting a little sunshine

The Mediterranean coast is so beautiful, who wouldn't want to enjoy time outside? Everybody's body needs sunshine so that the body can produce healthy levels of vitamin D, which is associated with bone health, increased immune function, and lower cholesterol. Not to mention the fact that a warm sunny day can go a long way to lift your spirits.

Note: Don't ignore the fact that too much exposure to sunlight is associated with skin cancer and wrinkles. You can still enjoy sunshine in a healthy way. If you don't have personal history or family history of skin cancer, spending 15 to 20 minutes in the sun without sunscreen to produce some vitamin D is okay. If you're spending longer amounts of time in the sun, enjoy yourself with proper sunscreen and use hats and sunglasses for protection.

Cioppino

Prep time: 20 min • **Cook time:** 1 hr • **Yield:** 10 servings

Ingredients	*Directions*

3 tablespoons olive oil

6 cloves garlic, sliced

2 onions, chopped

1 stalk celery, chopped

1 bay leaf

½ teaspoon dried oregano

1 teaspoon red pepper flakes

1 teaspoon salt, plus more for soaking

½ teaspoon pepper

2 tablespoons tomato paste

1½ cups hearty red wine (Burgundy, Zinfandel, or Cabernet)

One 28-ounce can diced tomatoes

1¼ cups bottled clam juice

2 cups chicken stock

1 pound littleneck clams, scrubbed

1 pound halibut fillets, cut into 2-inch pieces

2 pounds large shrimp, shelled and deveined

1 pound scallops

½ cup parsley, chopped

10 slices French baguette

1 Heat the olive oil in a large Dutch oven over medium-high heat. Add the garlic, onions, celery, bay leaf, oregano, red pepper flakes, salt, and pepper and cook for 8 minutes, stirring frequently.

2 Stir in the tomato paste and cook for 2 minutes, continuing to stir. Add the wine, tomatoes, clam juice, and stock; cover and simmer for 30 minutes. Taste the base to check the seasonings and add additional salt and pepper as needed.

3 Meanwhile, soak the clams in cold, salted water and drain. When the base is ready, add the clams, halibut, shrimp, and scallops; cook for 10 minutes. Stir in the parsley and serve with the French baguette.

Per serving: Calories 223 (From Fat 49); Fat 5g (Saturated 1g); Cholesterol 4mg; Sodium 772mg; Carbohydrate 30g (Dietary Fiber 2g); Protein 8g.

Note: For food safety, discard any clamshells that don't open. See the "Keeping safe with shellfish" sidebar in this chapter for details.

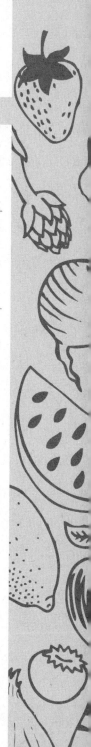

Paella

Prep time: 30 min • **Cook time:** 35 min • **Yield:** 8 servings

Ingredients	*Directions*
1 tablespoon plus 2 tablespoons olive oil	**1** Combine 1 tablespoon of the olive oil, the smoked paprika, oregano, and turmeric. Coat the chicken breasts with the oil-spice mixture and set aside.
1 tablespoon smoked paprika	
2 teaspoons dried oregano	**2** Heat 1 tablespoon of the olive oil in a large skillet over medium heat. Add the rice, garlic, and cook for 2 to 3 minutes to toast the rice.
¼ teaspoon plus ¼ teaspoon turmeric	
1 pound boneless, skinless chicken breasts, cut into 2-inch pieces	**3** Add the chicken stock, saffron, turmeric, bay leaf, and ¼ cup of the parsley. Bring the mixture to a boil, cover, and reduce the heat to a simmer for 20 to 30 minutes or until the rice is cooked. Remove bay leaf.
2 cups short-grain white rice	
4 cups chicken stock	
1 pinch saffron	**4** Heat the remaining olive oil in a large skillet over medium heat. Add the chicken, onions, bell pepper, and chorizo and cook for 5 minutes.
1 bay leaf	
¼ cup plus ¼ cup parsley, chopped	**5** Add chicken mixture to cooked rice and toss. Add the seafood over the top of the rice mixture, cover and cook until mussels and clams open, about 10 minutes.
1 onion, chopped	
1 red bell pepper, chopped	
8 ounces Spanish chorizo, cut into ½-inch slices	**6** Top with the remaining parsley and the lemon zest before serving.
1 pound shrimp, mussels, and/or littleneck clams	
Zest of 1 lemon	

Per serving: *Calories 536 (From Fat 183); Fat 20g (Saturated 5g); Cholesterol 151mg; Sodium 677mg; Carbohydrate 47g (Dietary Fiber 2g); Protein 37g*

Note: For food safety, discard any clamshells and mussels that don't open. See the "Keeping safe with shellfish" sidebar in this chapter for details. Check out the color insert for a photo of this recipe.

Vary It! You can make paella exactly the way you enjoy it. If you prefer just mussels, double them and omit the clams, or vice versa. If you don't love shellfish, use chicken, chorizo, and a fish such as halibut.

Putting Together Easy Seafood for Busy People on the Run

Although our goal in this book is to get you to slow down and enjoy cooking and eating, we know that doing so all the time can be a challenge. We also understand that your life is busy, what with running children to this rehearsal and that practice, working and commuting, and keeping your household in order. For that reason, we want to give you some quick seafood recipes that you can prepare and take with you as you run from errand to errand.

The most important piece is to get you eating fish a couple of times a week if you aren't already doing so. Having some easy and tasty recipes like the ones in this section on hand can help you enjoy fish more often. You'll find that cooking fish is actually much easier than cooking a steak.

Seeing sardines in a new light

Sardines get no respect. They're healthy for you, but many people aren't so sure about eating those little fish. Just ask the folks on the Mediterranean coast how to do it; they've been eating them regularly for hundreds of years.

Believe it or not, sardines are loaded in nutrients. They're a great source of lean protein, vitamin B-12, omega-3 fatty acids, and calcium. You can also find that they're one of the few food sources concentrated in vitamin D. This combination of nutrients is great for your heart health.

Because sardines are at the bottom of the food chain, they don't contain high levels of mercury or other contaminants. You won't find a shortage of them either, because they're found in abundance in the Atlantic and Pacific Oceans and the Mediterranean Sea.

You can find canned sardines in any major grocery store right by the canned tuna. Squirt them with lemon juice and serve them on crackers as a snack; add them to salads; or mix them with lemon juice, dill, and onions for a nice spread. If you enjoy fish, give sardines a try! Your heart will thank you for it.

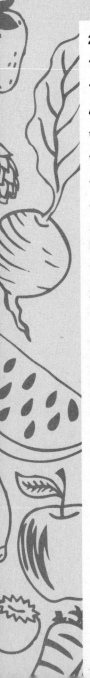

Clams in Chile-Wine Sauce

Prep time: 5 min • **Cook time:** 15 min • **Yield:** 4 servings

Ingredients	Directions
2 tablespoons olive oil	*1* In a large skillet, heat the olive oil over medium-high heat. Add the onions, celery, and garlic and sauté for 3 minutes.
1 onion, chopped	
1 celery stalk, chopped	
4 cloves garlic, chopped	*2* Add the spices to the pan and cook for 2 minutes. Add the clams and chile and cook for 3 minutes. Add the wine and cover for 5 minutes, shaking the pan to coat. Top with the parsley and serve.
½ teaspoon ground ginger	
¼ teaspoon paprika	
1 teaspoon turmeric	
1½ pounds clams	
1 red chile, sliced in half lengthwise	
¼ cup dry white wine	
2 tablespoons parsley, chopped	

Per serving: Calories 231 (From Fat 77); Fat 9g (Saturated 1g); Cholesterol 58mg; Sodium 116mg; Carbohydrate 12g (Dietary Fiber 1g); Protein 23g.

Note: For food safety, discard any clamshells that don't open. See the "Keeping safe with shellfish" sidebar in this chapter for details.

Grilled Scallops

Prep time: 15 min, plus marinating time • **Cook time:** 8 min • **Yield:** 4 servings

Ingredients	Directions
2 pounds sea scallops	*1* Rinse the scallops under water and pat dry. Toss scallops with the garlic, olive oil, butter, and parsley. Allow the scallops to marinate for 10 minutes. Spray the grill with nonstick cooking spray and heat the grill over medium-high heat.
4 cloves garlic, chopped	
2 tablespoons olive oil	
1 tablespoon butter, melted	
2 tablespoons parsley, finely chopped	*2* Skewer the scallops and grill them for 1 to 3 minutes on each side or until slightly firm to the touch and opaque. Drizzle with the lemon juice and top with the lemon zest and sea salt just before serving.
Nonstick cooking spray	
Zest and juice of 1 lemon	
¼ teaspoon sea salt	

Per serving: Calories 285 (From Fat 102); Fat 11g (Saturated 3g); Cholesterol 82mg; Sodium 531mg; Carbohydrate 5g (Dietary Fiber 0g); Protein 38g.

Tip: Soak wooden skewers in water before grilling so they don't burn on the grill.

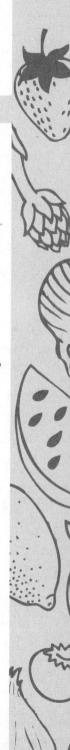

Shrimp Kabobs

Prep time: 10 min • **Cook time:** 8 min • **Yield:** 4 servings

Ingredients	*Directions*
3 small zucchinis, cut into 1-inch rounds	*1* In a large saucepan, heat 3 cups water to a boil. Add the zucchini and cook for 1 minute. Immediately place the zucchini in an ice bath to halt cooking.
1 pound large raw shrimp, peeled and deveined	
2 tablespoons olive oil	*2* Alternate pieces of the shrimp and zucchini on skewers. Combine the olive oil, garlic, lemon zest, paprika, and salt. Brush the kabobs with the lemon mixture and set aside for 10 minutes.
4 cloves garlic, chopped	
1 lemon, zested and cut into wedges	
2 teaspoons paprika	*3* Spray the grill with nonstick cooking spray and heat the grill over medium-high heat. Combine the cilantro, almonds, and olives and set aside.
½ teaspoon salt	
Nonstick cooking spray	*4* Grill the kabobs for 3 to 4 minutes per side until the shrimp is pink and opaque. Serve with the cilantro mixture and lemon wedges.
¼ cup cilantro, chopped	
¼ cup almonds, chopped	
4 green olives, chopped	

Per serving: Calories 264 (From Fat 130); Fat 14g (Saturated 2g); Cholesterol 172mg; Sodium 539mg; Carbohydrate 8g (Dietary Fiber 3g); Protein 27g.

Tip: Soak wooden skewers in water before grilling so they don't burn on the grill.

Chapter 19

Making One-of-a-Kind Meat and Pork Entrees

In This Chapter

▶ Making the perfect steak

▶ Surveying special Mediterranean beef dishes

▶ Finding some new favorite pork recipes

*O*n the Mediterranean coast, beef and pork were originally used most often for special occasions by people who could afford them. Today, people consume both meats on a more-regular basis. However, to fully realize the health benefits associated with the traditional Mediterranean diet philosophy, we encourage going old-school and eating these items no more than two to three times a month.

When you do eat beef or pork, use the following strategies to help reap the benefits of the Mediterranean style of eating:

✔ **Watch the type of cut you consume.** Although beef and pork are great sources of protein, some cuts can be higher in saturated fat, which is shown to be linked to heart disease and certain cancers. Check out the "Getting the skinny on the leanest cuts of beef" sidebar in this chapter for info on which beef cuts to choose and which ones to avoid.

✔ **Eat smaller portions.** As with poultry and fish, people in the Mediterranean consume smaller portions of beef and pork than are typical in the United States and Canada. Stick with 2- to 3-ounce servings and incorporate those smaller meat portions with lots of vegetables, fruits, and legumes.

Getting the skinny on the leanest cuts of beef

If you eat beef infrequently, enjoy it and don't worry too much about what cuts you're eating. On the flip side, if you enjoy eating beef several times a week, choosing a few leaner cuts means you can have your steak and eat it, too. The saturated fats found in animal proteins such as beef may increase inflammation in your body (leaving you at a greater risk for heart disease, type 2 diabetes, and certain cancers) and usually translate to more calories, which can contribute to weight gain. Meanwhile, stay away from T-bone, rib-eye, ribs, and porterhouse steaks, which have the most grams of saturated fat.

Here are the leanest cuts of beef:

Cut of Beef	Grams of Saturated Fat (3-ounce serving)	Grams of Total Fat
Top round	1.4	4.2
Eye round	1.5	4.2
Round tip	2.0	6.0
Top sirloin	2.4	6.0
Bottom round	2.0	6.3
Top loin	3.0	8.0
Tenderloin	3.2	8.5

In this chapter, we show you how to put together creative, delicious beef and pork recipes to serve on a weeknight, as well as some classic specialties for your next celebration.

Enjoying a Great Steak

No matter what country you live in, nothing tastes as good as a perfectly cooked steak. In this section, we challenge you to eat steak the Mediterranean way: smaller portion sizes and amazing fresh flavors and ingredients. Although the serving may be smaller, the taste quotient is just as high. You can make up for the smaller size with one of our amazing legume (Chapter 14) or vegetable (Chapter 12) recipes.

As you slow down and enjoy your steak, you see how living the Mediterranean lifestyle offers better health and more flavor than you may have experienced with your old recipes.

Zesty Mediterranean Flank Steak

Prep time: 30 min, plus marinating time • **Cook time:** 20 min • **Yield:** 6 servings

Ingredients	*Directions*
Zest and juice of 1 lemon, plus 1 tablespoon juice	*1* Whisk together the lemon juice (minus 1 tablespoon) and zest, rosemary, garlic, ¼ cup of the olive oil, and the sea salt in a small bowl.
1 tablespoon fresh rosemary, minced	
4 cloves garlic, minced	*2* Pour the mixture over the meat in a glass dish and flip the meat to coat; cover and marinate in the refrigerator for 2 to 12 hours.
¼ cup plus 1 tablespoon olive oil	
¼ teaspoon sea salt	*3* Heat the grill over medium-high heat. Combine the avocados, tomatoes, parsley, and remaining lemon juice and olive oil. Allow the flavors to blend at room temperature while the meat cooks.
2 pounds flank steak, trimmed of excess fat	
2 avocados, cubed	
2 tomatoes, cubed	*4* Grill the meat for 6 to 8 minutes until it reaches the desired doneness (3 to 4 minutes on one side and 2 minutes on the other). Remove the meat from the heat and cover with foil for at least 5 minutes before slicing.
¼ cup parsley, chopped	
Salt and pepper to taste	
	5 Slice the meat on the bias for serving. Season the tomato and avocado mixture with salt and pepper and divide evenly over each flank steak serving.

Note: Check out the color insert for a photo of this dish.

Per serving: Calories 350 (From Fat 192); Fat 21g (Saturated 7g); Cholesterol 92mg; Sodium 191mg; Carbohydrate 8g (Dietary Fiber 4g); Protein 32g.

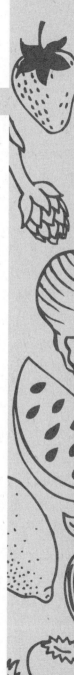

Spanish Spiced Rib-eye

Prep time: 5 min plus marinating time • **Cook time:** 20 min • **Yield:** 6 servings

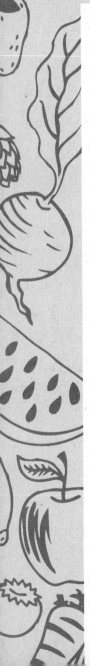

Ingredients	Directions
1 teaspoon smoked paprika	**1** Combine the paprika, sea salt, lemon zest, and pepper in a small bowl. Rub the meat on both sides. Set aside and allow the meat to marinate at room temperature for 30 to 45 minutes.
¼ teaspoon sea salt	
Zest of 1 lemon	
½ teaspoon pepper	
Two ¾-pound rib-eye steaks	**2** Meanwhile, combine the olive oil, olives, garlic, lemon juice, and parsley.
2 tablespoons olive oil	
½ cup green olives	**3** Heat the grill to medium high heat. Cook the meat for 7 to 10 minutes on each side, depending on thickness and desired doneness.
1 clove garlic, minced	
2 tablespoons lemon juice	
2 tablespoons parsley, chopped	**4** Remove the meat from the heat and cover with foil. Allow the meat to rest for 5 minutes. Thinly slice the meat and evenly divide the olive mixture on top of each serving.

Per serving: Calories 321 (From Fat 209); Fat 23g (Saturated 8g); Cholesterol 61mg; Sodium 359mg; Carbohydrate 0g (Dietary Fiber 0g); Protein 26g.

Filet with Gremolata

Prep time: 15 min • **Cook time:** 16 min • **Yield:** 4 servings

Ingredients	Directions
Four 5-ounce filets of steak	*1* Season the meat with the salt and pepper and allow the meat to come to room temperature.
½ teaspoon sea salt	
½ teaspoon pepper	*2* Heat the grill over medium heat. Cook the filets for 4 to 6 minutes on each side or until they reach the desired doneness.
⅓ cup gremolata	
	3 Remove the meat from the heat and cover with foil for 5 minutes. Spoon the gremolata evenly over the top of each serving and serve.

Per serving: Calories 361 (From Fat 234); Fat 26g (Saturated 7g); Cholesterol 88mg; Sodium 368mg; Carbohydrate 1g (Dietary Fiber 0g); Protein 29g.

Tip: You can find gremolatas with a variety of fresh herbs. Thyme, rosemary, oregano, and mint make great additions to this recipe. Or try the Gremolata recipe in Chapter 9.

Mary had a little lamb, goose, and rabbit

Game meats such as goose, rabbit, and lamb are popular choices in Mediterranean cuisine. We recognize that you can't always walk into a local grocery store in the United States and pick up these types of meats easily (and that the thought of doing so may make you a little squeamish), so we don't include any recipes for them in this book. That said, these meats are an important part of the cooking culture in both Italy and Greece, so we want to at least share a little information about them:

✔ Goose meat is similar to duck; it's darker than a lot of poultry and has a rich flavor. Folks in the Mediterranean hunt and clean goose and then cook it into many wonderful dishes, such as goose breast with mandarins and cinnamon.

✔ Lamb is a very tender, flavorful cut of meat used widely on the Mediterranean coast. You may even be able to find some in your local grocery store. Greece is known for its delicious lamb dishes, including skewered kabobs and ribs.

✔ Rabbit has the texture of chicken with a slightly more gamey, often sweet flavor. Italians are known for amazing rabbit dishes such as rabbit amandine (a rabbit and almond recipe).

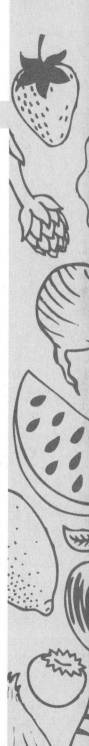

Pomegranate Steak

Prep time: 30 min plus marinating time • **Cook time:** 16 min • **Yield:** 4 servings

Ingredients	*Directions*
Two ½-pound sirloin steaks	*1* Season the meat with the salt, pepper, and rosemary. Set aside and allow the meat to marinate for 15 to 30 minutes at room temperature.
¼ teaspoon sea salt	
½ teaspoon pepper	
1 tablespoon fresh rosemary, minced	*2* Heat the grill to medium-high heat. Cook the steaks for 4 to 8 minutes on each side or until they reach the desired doneness.
¼ cup walnuts, chopped	
1 shallot, minced	*3* Combine the walnuts, shallot, and parsley in a small bowl. Top the steaks with 1 to 2 tablespoons of the pomegranate syrup and the walnut mixture to serve, reserving the remaining to be added as desired.
2 tablespoons parsley, chopped	
½ cup pomegranate reduction	

Per serving: Calories 251 (From Fat 143); Fat 16g (Saturated 3g); Cholesterol 42mg; Sodium 194mg; Carbohydrate 3g (Dietary Fiber 1g); Protein 23g.

Vary It! This recipe also works well with pork chops.

Tip: Use the pomegranate reduction in Chapter 10.

Exploring Beef Specialties

Historically, only the affluent Mediterranean-coast residents used beef; it was too expensive for common folks and would only show up on their tables during special occasions and holidays. Even though beef is now more common throughout the region, it remains a supporting player in a meal instead of being the main focus. Because of the smaller portion size, beef specialties in the Mediterranean region focus on flavor — quality over quantity. This section presents some of the unique beef classics of the Mediterranean region.

With any beef recipe, let your beef rest for 2 to 3 minutes off the heat before slicing for quality and to ensure you don't burn your fingers.

Safety first when handling beef

Beef can be a delicious part of a healthy diet, but you want to be certain that you handle beef carefully to avoid contamination from Escherichia coli (commonly known as E. coli), bacteria that can cause food poisoning leading to severe diarrhea. Here are some tips for handling your beef safely from the supermarket to the table.

✔ **When you pick up beef at the store, make sure to use an extra bag to separate it from your other groceries.** Even if the package is sealed, having extra protection from any leakage that may seep out is smart. Many stores bag beef separately anyway.

✔ **As soon as you arrive home, immediately refrigerate your beef and use within 3 to 5 days.** You can also safely put it in the freezer and use within 9 to 12 months. If you are storing in the freezer for more than 2 months, double wrap your meat in heavy foil or freezer bags to help decrease the chance of *freezer burn*, or gray spots that occur when air reaches the surface of the meat and affect the beef quality and taste.

✔ **When defrosting, slowly defrost over a day or two in the refrigerator.** Your second best option is to submerge the beef (still in its package) in cold water and run under cold water.

✔ **Choose a work surface such as a cutting board when preparing your beef for cooking.** Using a cutting board helps to prevent spillage onto your countertop, where other foods may be prepped. The debate on whether wood or plastic cutting boards are best for working with meat still rages, but no matter which one you choose, keeping one cutting board special for meats to avoid any cross-contamination is a good idea. Make sure to wash your hands and work surface with antibacterial soap when you're done to destroy any of the bacteria that may be present in the raw meat.

✔ **Cook beef to an internal temperature of 145 degrees as measured with a food thermometer.** Doing so ensures that you destroy any bacteria found in the meat.

Greek Meatballs with Tomato and Red Pepper Puree

Prep time: 17 min • **Cook time:** 50 min • **Yield:** 4 servings

Ingredients	Directions
1 tablespoon plus 1 tablespoon olive oil	**1** In a Dutch oven, heat 1 tablespoon of the olive oil over medium-high heat; add the bell peppers and sauté for 5 minutes. Reduce the heat to medium and add half the garlic; sauté for 2 minutes.
2 red bell peppers, seeded and chopped	
1 clove plus 1 clove garlic, minced	**2** Add the canned tomatoes, stock, cumin, coriander, and oregano and simmer while you prepare the meatballs.
Two 14.5-ounce cans diced tomatoes	
2 cups beef stock	**3** Meanwhile, combine the ground beef, rice, onion, and remaining olive oil and garlic in a medium bowl. Knead the mixture with your hands and roll into 1-inch balls.
1 teaspoon ground cumin	
1 teaspoon coriander	
1 teaspoon dried oregano	**4** Using a stick blender, blender, or food processor, blend the sauce until it's the desired consistency. Season the sauce with salt and pepper to taste and then return it to the Dutch oven.
Salt and pepper to taste	
1 pound lean ground beef	
½ cup uncooked basmati rice	**5** Add the meatballs to the sauce and simmer for 55 minutes or until the rice is no longer crunchy, stirring occasionally to coat the meatballs with the sauce. Transfer the meatballs and sauce to a large platter to serve.
1 onion, minced	

Per serving: Calories 450 (From Fat 171); Fat 19g (Saturated 6g); Cholesterol 40mg; Sodium 627mg; Carbohydrate 40g (Dietary Fiber 5g); Protein 30g.

Tip: To reduce cooking time, use prepared rice in the meatballs and cook them for only 20 minutes in the sauce, making sure they're cooked through.

Tip: This recipe is great doubled and enjoyed the next day or frozen to enjoy at a later time. Freeze up to 1 month.

Pastitsio

Prep time: 1 hour • **Cook time:** 45 min • **Yield:** 16 servings

Ingredients	*Directions*
1 tablespoon olive oil	*1* Preheat the oven to 400 degrees. Heat the olive oil in a large saucepan over medium-high heat. Sauté the onions for 5 minutes. Add the ground beef and sauté until the meat is completely cooked, about 10 minutes.
1 medium onion, chopped	
2 pounds lean ground beef	
One 6-ounce can tomato paste	*2* Dilute the tomato paste with the water and add it to the pan. Add the nutmeg, allspice, cinnamon, salt, and pepper; cover and simmer for about 5 minutes. Uncover and simmer for another 5 minutes to reduce the liquid.
¾ cup water	
1 teaspoon nutmeg	
1 teaspoon allspice	
1 teaspoon cinnamon	*3* Remove the beef mixture from the heat. Chill the mixture in the refrigerator while you begin the rest of the layers.
¼ teaspoon salt	
½ teaspoon pepper	
2 eggs, lightly beaten	*4* Cook the macaroni according to package directions (about 12 to 14 minutes) or until al dente. Drain the macaroni well and spread half of it into a 9-x-13-inch baking pan. Sprinkle with ¼ cup of the cheese.
1½ pounds elbow macaroni	
½ cup plus 1 cup Parmesan cheese, freshly grated	
2 cups Béchamel	*5* Combine the eggs with the meat mixture and spread the entire mixture over the macaroni. Add the remaining macaroni and sprinkle with another ¼ cup of the cheese.
	6 Prepare the Béchamel according to the recipe in Chapter 9 and add the remaining cheese to the white sauce. Pour the sauce over the dish, cover with foil and bake for about 30 minutes. Remove the foil and bake 15 minutes longer or until golden brown.
	7 Remove the pastitsio from oven and let stand approximately 15 minutes before cutting into serving portions.

Per serving: Calories 346 (From Fat 92); Fat 10g (Saturated 5g); Cholesterol 53mg; Sodium 346mg; Carbohydrate 39g (Dietary Fiber 2g); Protein 24g.

Note: This dish is commonly served at large Greek family gatherings or holidays.

Vary It! You can substitute cooked lentils for the ground beef, making this meal vegetarian.

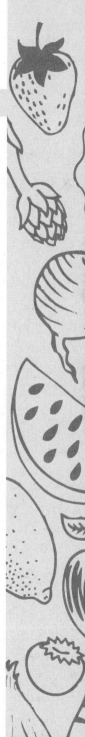

Mediterranean Beef Kabobs

Prep time: 30 min, plus marinating time • **Cook time:** 15 min • **Yield:** 8 servings

Ingredients	*Directions*
½ cup olive oil	*1* Combine the olive oil, vinegar, mustard, garlic, oregano, and sugar. Season the dressing with salt and pepper to taste.
½ cup balsamic vinegar	
2 teaspoons prepared yellow mustard	
3 cloves garlic, minced	*2* Toss the meat and vegetables with the dressing in a large bowl to coat evenly. Marinate the mixture in the refrigerator for 2 to 12 hours, stirring every hour or so to coat.
1 tablespoon dried oregano	
2 teaspoons sugar	
Salt and pepper to taste	*3* Drain and discard the marinade. Skewer the kabobs, alternating meat pieces with vegetables.
2 pounds sirloin steak, cut into 1-inch cubes	
2 red bell peppers, cut into 1-inch wedges	*4* Heat the grill over medium-high heat. Cook the kabobs for 5 to 6 minutes on each side or until the meat is cooked well done. Serve.
3 zucchinis, cut into 1-inch rounds	
1 onion, cut into 1-inch pieces	

Per serving: Calories 293 (From Fat 138); Fat 15g (Saturated 3g); Cholesterol 60mg; Sodium 92mg; Carbohydrate 12g (Dietary Fiber 2g); Protein 26g.

Tip: If you're using wooden skewers, soak them in water before grilling so that they don't burn.

Tip: If you prefer your veggies softer, skewer them on their own and get them on the grill about 10 minutes prior to your meat.

Meaty Eggplant Casserole

Prep time: 30 min • **Cook time:** 1 hr, 10 min • **Yield:** 6 servings

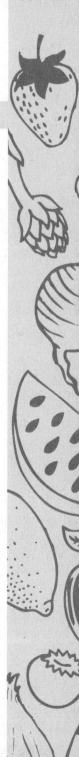

Ingredients	*Directions*
2 eggplants, sliced diagonally 2 teaspoons salt ¼ cup plus 1 tablespoon olive oil 1 pound lean ground beef 2 large or 3 medium onions, thinly sliced 3 tomatoes, peeled and chopped, or one 14.5-ounce can chopped tomatoes 2 tablespoons tomato paste 2 cloves garlic, crushed 1 teaspoon allspice 1 teaspoon sugar Salt to taste Nonstick cooking spray ½ cup feta cheese	*1* Sprinkle both sides of the eggplant slices with the salt. Pile the slices in colander, cover them with a small plate and a weight, and leave for 20 minutes. Rinse with water and press dry with a towel. *2* Heat a griddle or nonstick skillet over medium-high heat. Brush both sides of each eggplant slice with olive oil (¼ cup total) and cook for about 4 minutes per side. *3* In a nonstick skillet (can be the eggplant skillet), cook the ground beef over medium heat until browned, about 10 minutes. Drain off the excess fat and set the beef aside. Cook the onions in the remaining olive oil until soft and pale yellow, about 6 minutes. *4* Add the tomatoes, tomato paste, and garlic; season with the allspice and sugar, and salt to taste. Cook the sauce for 5 minutes. Return the ground beef to the pan and stir. *5* Preheat the oven to 350 degrees. Spray a large glass casserole dish with nonstick cooking spray. Layer the eggplant and sauce in the casserole dish, starting with eggplant and finishing with sauce. Bake for 20 minutes. *6* Crumble the cheese on top of the casserole and bake for 5 minutes. Allow the casserole to rest for 5 minutes before serving.

Per serving: *Calories 413 (From Fat 235); Fat 26g (Saturated 8g); Cholesterol 58mg; Sodium 922mg; Carbohydrate 28g (Dietary Fiber 9g); Protein 19g.*

Note: This Turkish inspired dish highlights how meat can accent a main dish without being the star.

Perfecting Pork

In the old days, roasting an entire pig was the centerpiece of many Mediterranean celebrations. Because pigs were small enough to raise, pork became more common for the everyday person.

As they do with many meats, people in the Mediterranean use smaller portion sizes of pork as a side dish or one component of a meal, such as adding sausage in a lasagne or ham in a soup or salad. In this section, we focus on pork as a stand-alone entree.

Considering cured meats

Cured meats are popular in Mediterranean cooking. The curing process helps preserve meat by aging, drying, or canning to prevent spoiling and the growth of microorganisms. Salt is used in nearly all curing processes, either added dry as a rub or in the brining solution.

Here are a few popular cured meats used in Mediterranean cuisine:

✔ **Pancetta** is a style of bacon seasoned with spices like fennel, peppercorns, hot peppers, and garlic before curing. This meat has a bite of spice to it and will crisp in cooking much like regular bacon does.

✔ **Prosciutto** is a delicate, thin ham with a mild albeit salty flavor perfect for adding that punch of savory to any dish. Pair the salty flavor with fruit, such as honeydew or cantaloupe, for a winning combination.

✔ **Salami** is popular for sandwiches and as a snack with crackers. The flavor is a combination of salty, sweet, and spicy all at the same time.

Cured meats have a big punch of flavor in a small serving, providing big flavor to sandwiches, pizzas, soups, stews, vegetable dishes, and other side dishes. They're definitely higher in sodium, and in some cases fat than regular meats, so in true Mediterranean fashion, you want to use small amounts of cured meats to enhance the flavors of other foods instead of making them the star. Recipes throughout this book use cured meats in small portions.

Pork Chops with Tomatoes and Bell Peppers

Prep time: 8 min • **Cook time:** 1 hr, 10 min • **Yield:** 6 servings

Ingredients	Directions
Six 6- to 8-ounce bone-in, 1-inch thick pork chops	*1* Season the chops on each side with the pepper. In a heavy skillet, heat the olive oil over medium-high heat. Brown the chops for 2 minutes on each side and remove them from the pan.
½ teaspoon pepper	
2 tablespoons olive oil	
2 cloves garlic, sliced	*2* Add the garlic and rosemary to the skillet and sauté for 2 minutes. Deglaze the pan with the stock, scraping the bottom to release the browned bits. Bring to a boil and turn off the heat.
1 teaspoon rosemary, minced	
2 cups low-sodium chicken stock	
2 cups parboiled rice, white or brown	*3* Preheat the oven to 350 degrees. Spread the rice along the bottom of a glass casserole dish and top with the pork chops. Layer the onions, tomatoes, and bell peppers over the chops and secure with toothpicks.
1 large tomato, cut into 6 slices	
1 large onion, cut into 6 slices	
1 green bell pepper, cut into 6 slices	*4* Pour the stock mixture over the dish, cover with foil, and bake for 1 hour. Serve each chop with a lemon wedge.
1 lemon, cut into 6 wedges	

Per serving: Calories 484 (From Fat 84); Fat 9g (Saturated 2g); Cholesterol 74mg; Sodium 492mg; Carbohydrate 57g (Dietary Fiber 3g); Protein 42g.

Tip: Parboiled refers to partially cooking the rice. We recommend boiling white rice for 10 minutes and brown rice for 15 minutes prior to preparing. Drain off any excess water prior to putting the rice into baking pan.

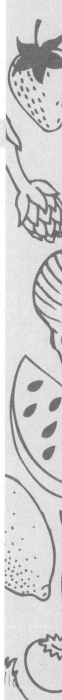

Lemon Pork Chops

Prep time: 5 min, plus marinating time • **Cook time:** 20 min • **Yield:** 4 servings

Ingredients	Directions
½ cup parsley, chopped	*1* Combine the parsley, garlic, olive oil, lemon juice, and salt. Place the chops in a glass dish and pour the marinade over top, coating on each side.
4 cloves garlic, chopped	
¼ cup olive oil	
½ cup lemon juice	*2* Marinate the chops for 30 minutes to 4 hours in the refrigerator. Remove the chops from the refrigerator at least 30 minutes before grilling to return them to room temperature.
¼ teaspoon salt	
Four 4-ounce, ½-inch-thick pork chops	
	3 Heat the grill over medium-high heat. Grill each chop for 4 to 15 minutes on each side or until the internal temperature reaches 145 degrees. Remove the chops from the grill and allow the meat to rest for 3 minutes before serving.

Per serving: Calories 247 (From Fat 148); Fat 16g (Saturated 3g); Cholesterol 53mg; Sodium 413mg; Carbohydrate 0g (Dietary Fiber 0g); Protein 25g.

Roasted Pork Loin with Apricots

Prep time: 8 min • **Cook time:** 48 min • **Yield:** 6 servings

Ingredients	*Directions*
1 tablespoon olive oil	*1* Preheat the oven to 350 degrees.
One 1- to 1.5-pound pork tenderloin	*2* Rub the olive oil over the tenderloin. Combine the cumin, coriander, orange zest, and ginger in a small bowl and rub the spice mixture onto the meat.
½ teaspoon ground cumin	
½ teaspoon ground coriander	
1 tablespoon freshly grated orange zest	*3* Spray a 9-x-13-inch casserole dish with nonstick cooking spray and layer the onion slices on the bottom. Top with the tenderloin and add the chicken broth and apricots.
1 teaspoon ground ginger	
Nonstick cooking spray	
1 small onion, cut into thin slices	*4* Bake for 40 minutes or until the internal temperature reaches 145 degrees. Remove the tenderloin from the pan and place on a serving platter. Set the pan with the apricots aside.
1 cup chicken broth	
½ cup thinly sliced dried apricots	*5* In a small saucepan, heat the butter over medium heat. Add the flour and whisk for 2 minutes. Add the pork pan drippings, apricots, and onions to the pan along with the wine and bring the mixture to a boil.
1 tablespoon butter	
1 tablespoon flour	
⅓ cup dry white wine	*6* Remove the mixture from the heat and season with salt to taste. Pour the apricot sauce over the tenderloin and top with the cilantro to serve.
Salt to taste	
¼ cup cilantro, chopped	

Per serving: Calories 177 (From Fat 54); Fat 6g (Saturated 2g); Cholesterol 54mg; Sodium 215mg; Carbohydrate 12g (Dietary Fiber 1g); Protein 17g.

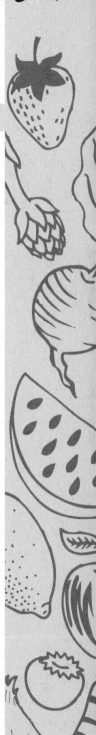

Pork Sausage with White Beans and Tomatoes

Prep time: 5 min • **Cook time:** 40 min • **Yield:** 6 servings

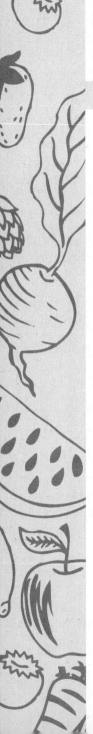

Ingredients	Directions
1 pound fresh Italian sausage	**1** Preheat the oven to 450 degrees. Remove the sausage from the casing and cut into 1-inch pieces. Toss the sausage and tomatoes with 2 tablespoons olive oil, the balsamic vinegar, and the garlic. Pour the mixture into a shallow roasting pan.
8 Roma or plum tomatoes, quartered lengthwise	
2 tablespoons plus 1 tablespoon olive oil	
2 tablespoons balsamic vinegar	**2** Place the pan into oven, reduce the heat to 400 degrees, and cook for 30 minutes.
4 cloves garlic, sliced	
One 14.5-ounce can cannellini or navy beans	**3** Meanwhile, combine the beans, remaining olive oil, and thyme. Add the beans to the sausage and tomatoes, stir to mix, and return to the oven for 10 minutes. Season with the lemon juice and salt to taste and serve.
1 teaspoon fresh thyme, chopped	
2 tablespoons lemon juice	
Salt to taste	

Per serving: Calories 426 (From Fat 278); Fat 31g (Saturated 10g); Cholesterol 57mg; Sodium 876mg; Carbohydrate 21g (Dietary Fiber 5g); Protein 17g.

Note: Check out the color insert for a photo of this recipe.

Chapter 20

Don't Forget Dessert!

In This Chapter

▶ Eating desserts the Mediterranean way

▶ Making some classic desserts from the Mediterranean coast

▶ Creating amazing fruit-based desserts

▶ Baking wonderful cookies for all occasions

Serving up a variety of great desserts is common practice on the Mediterranean coast. So how do the people who live there stay heart healthy and manage their weights? Moderation is the secret.

For weekly dessert treats, Mediterranean residents often eat just plain fruit or a small cookie such as biscotti. You also see fruit desserts lightly sweetened with a little sugar or honey. The more-robust desserts the region is famous for, such as baklava, are reserved for special occasions like holidays and festivals. Some desserts are served for a specific symbolic meaning, such as desserts made with eggs at Easter.

As with all Mediterranean-style cooking, the dessert menu often includes an abundance of the region's commonly grown foods, such as nuts, apricots, dates, lemons, and oranges. Even though the desserts you're used to probably contain stuff that isn't so good for you, many Mediterranean dessert recipes have healthy ingredients.

Enjoying a delicious treat once in a while without worrying about sugar, fat, and calories is the trick. That way, you never feel deprived, but you don't overdo it to the point that you gain weight or put yourself at increased risk for diet-related diseases, such as cardiovascular disease or diabetes.

In this chapter you can find a variety of desserts for all occasions. Many of these recipes certainly make the cut for a weekly treat because they're lower in fat, calories, and sugar than many store-bought desserts. Consider treating yourself to Rice Pudding, Baked Farina, Crepes with Berries, Baked Apples with Raisins and Walnuts, Pucker Up Lemon Cookies, and the biscotti recipes on a fairly regular basis. We recommend serving recipes such as Walnut Baklava or Ricotta Cake once in awhile for special occasions.

Devouring Quintessential Mediterranean Desserts

People of the Mediterranean are masters at creating amazing desserts, many of which take painstaking hours to prepare. But your busy life may not allow you to spend that much time toiling in the kitchen, so this section focuses on a few easier-to-make classics. Walnut Baklava and Ricotta Cake are beautiful presentations for your next celebration or holiday, and Rice Pudding and Baked Farina are great for conquering your sweet tooth on a more weekly basis.

Nutty for nuts

A bowl of nuts with a nutcracker is a common appearance on countertops across the Mediterranean region, especially during the holidays. The early Romans considered the walnut food for the gods and also commonly used its oil. Italians mastered the art of roasting chestnuts at Christmastime, bringing a tradition that's told in songs and stories around the world.

Having a bowl of walnuts or roasted chestnuts on your counter is a wonderful snack any time of year for visitors and family coming and going. Nuts provide healthy fats to your diet, helping you reduce your risk of heart disease. But remember: Everything in moderation; nuts also have a lot of calories, which can add up quickly. Enjoy an ounce or two of nuts each day to help keep your heart healthy. Here are a few ways to enjoy nuts:

✔ Sprinkle some walnuts, almonds, or pistachios on your salads.

✔ Have an ounce of your favorite nuts as a snack with a piece of fruit.

✔ Set out some nuts with a nutcracker for family and friends at parties, celebrations, or holidays.

✔ Add toasted almonds to green beans and toasted walnuts to asparagus.

✔ Add toasted almonds or walnuts to your oatmeal.

✔ Make your own salad dressings, using peanut or walnut oil as the base.

✔ Enjoy the added benefit of nuts in your desserts; try the recipes in this chapter!

If you have allergies to nuts, you can certainly still use some of the recipes in this chapter by omitting the nuts. Just stay away from the Baklava. We suggest you keep the baklava recipe the same because the nuts are important in the end product.

Ricotta Cake

Prep time: 35 min • **Cook time:** 45 min, plus cooling time • **Yield:** 12 servings

Ingredients	Directions
1 tablespoon plus ½ cup butter	*1* Preheat the oven to 325 degrees. Coat a springform cake pan with 1 tablespoon butter and dust evenly with 1 tablespoon of the flour.
1 tablespoon plus ⅔ cup flour	
¼ cup olive oil	
¾ cup sugar	*2* In a mixing bowl, beat the butter, olive oil, and sugar until smooth and fluffy. In a separate mixing bowl, combine the remaining flour, the baking powder, and the salt and set aside.
2 teaspoons baking powder	
⅛ teaspoon salt	
4 eggs, separated	*3* In a third mixing bowl, beat the egg whites until stiff peaks form. Add the egg yolks, ricotta, and orange zest to the butter mixture and stir. Mix in the flour mixture until a smooth batter forms.
1 cup lowfat ricotta cheese	
3 tablespoons orange zest	
¼ cup apricot preserves or jam	*4* Fold the egg whites into the cake batter and pour it into prepared pan. Bake the cake for 45 minutes or until done in the center.
½ cup walnuts, chopped	
	5 Cool for 25 minutes. Use a knife to separate the cake from edges and then release spring form.
	6 In a small saucepan or microwave-safe dish, heat the apricot preserves until liquefied; add the walnuts and drizzle over the cake before serving.

Per serving: Calories 266 (From Fat 158); Fat 18g (Saturated 7g); Cholesterol 29mg; Sodium 192mg; Carbohydrate 24g (Dietary Fiber 0g); Protein 5g.

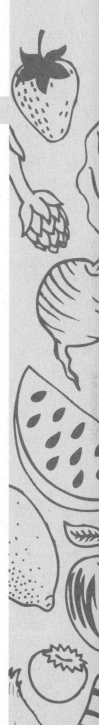

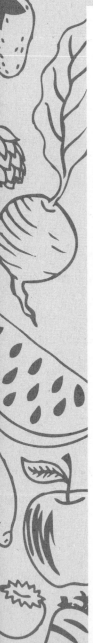

Walnut Baklava

Prep time: 45 min • **Cook time:** 1 hr, plus resting time • **Yield:** 32 servings

Ingredients	Directions
1½ cups water	**1** Preheat the oven to 325 degrees. In a heavy saucepan, combine the water, 1½ cups sugar, honey, lemon juice, and cinnamon sticks. Bring to a boil over medium-high heat and cook for 20 minutes. Remove from the heat, cover, and cool in the fridge. Remove cinnamon stick.
½ cup honey	
1½ cups plus ¼ cup sugar	
2 tablespoons lemon juice	
2 cinnamon sticks	**2** Pulse the nuts, the remaining sugar, the cinnamon, cardamom, and zests in a food processor until coarsely chopped (about 20 pulses). Combine the butter and olive oil and brush the mixture on the sides of a 9-x-13-inch pan with a pastry brush.
3 cups walnuts	
2 cups pistachios, shelled	
2 teaspoons cinnamon	
1 teaspoon cardamom	**3** Unroll the phyllo dough and cut the entire stack in half.
2 teaspoon orange zest	
1 teaspoon lemon zest	**4** Place 1 sheet of phyllo on the bottom of the pan and brush it with the butter mixture. Repeat with 7 more sheets. Place half the nut mixture on the phyllo dough.
½ cup butter, melted	
½ cup olive oil	
½ pound phyllo dough (about 20 sheets)	**5** Layer 4 more sheets of phyllo over the nuts, brushing each layer with the butter mixture. Top with the remaining nut mixture and an additional 8 layers of butter-brushed phyllo.
	6 Using a sharp knife, score the top layer of eight sheets of phyllo to make 8 cuts across and 4 cuts lengthwise, making sure not to cut beyond the top nut layer.
	7 Bake the baklava for 1 hour or until it's golden and crisp. Remove from the oven and ladle the honey mixture over the baklava. Allow it to set and absorb the sauce for at least 30 minutes before serving.

Per serving: Calories 254 (From Fat 149); Fat 17g (Saturated 3g); Cholesterol 8mg; Sodium 78mg; Carbohydrate 25g (Dietary Fiber 2g); Protein 4g.

Note: If you have a nut allergy or sensitivity, we recommend skipping this recipe rather than omitting the nuts, because they're an important part of the final product.

Rice Pudding

Prep time: 15 min • **Cook time:** 45 min • **Yield:** 6 servings

Ingredients	Directions
½ cup basmati rice	**1** Soak the rice in water for 10 minutes and drain.
4 cups milk	
3 tablespoons sugar	**2** In a heavy saucepan, bring the milk and sugar to a low boil over medium-high heat. Add the rice, raisins, cardamom, and cinnamon and simmer over low heat until thickened (about 45 minutes), stirring frequently.
¼ cup raisins	
½ teaspoon cardamom	
¼ teaspoon cinnamon	
½ teaspoon rose water (optional)	**3** Remove from the heat and add the rose water (if desired). Combine the almonds and orange zest. Ladle the pudding into serving bowls and garnish with the almond mixture. Serve hot or cold.
¼ almonds, chopped	
1 tablespoon orange zest	

Per serving: Calories 207 (From Fat 43); Fat 5g (Saturated 1g); Cholesterol 8mg; Sodium 75mg; Carbohydrate 34g (Dietary Fiber 1g); Protein 8g.

How many nuts are enough?

Nuts are widely used in Mediterranean cuisine making a healthy satisfying snack and adding wonderful flavor to many recipes. You want to be careful though with how much you eat. Although they contain healthy fats, they still can add up in calories, which means potential for weight gain. A serving size of nuts is typically about one ounce, which breaks down to the following for the specific type of nut:

- ✔ Almonds: 20 to 24
- ✔ Brazil nuts: 6 to 8
- ✔ Cashews: 16 to 18
- ✔ Hazelnuts: 18 to 20
- ✔ Macadamias: 10 to 12

- ✔ Peanuts (really a legume): 28
- ✔ Pecans: 15 halves
- ✔ Pine nuts: 150 to 157
- ✔ Pistachios: 45 to 47
- ✔ Walnuts: 14 halves

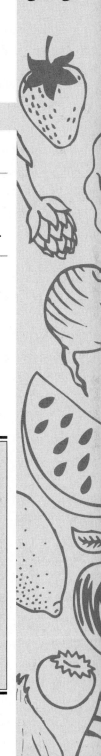

Baked Farina

Prep time: 25 min • **Cook time:** 1 hr, plus cooling time • **Yield:** 24 servings

Ingredients	*Directions*
Nonstick cooking spray 8 cups milk	*1* Preheat the oven to 350 degrees. Spray a 9-x-13-inch pan with nonstick cooking spray.
¼ cup butter 1 cup sugar 2 eggs 1¼ cup farina	*2* In a large saucepan, heat the milk, butter, and sugar over medium-high heat until almost boiling. Stir frequently to avoid scalding or burning the milk. Meanwhile, in a medium mixing bowl, beat the eggs until fluffy.
1 teaspoon orange blossom water or vanilla extract ¼ cup honey 1 tablespoon water	*3* Remove the milk from the heat and add the farina, whisking constantly for 1 minute. Add the orange blossom water. Temper the eggs by slowly drizzling 1 cup of the hot milk mixture while beating.
	4 Add the tempered egg mixture back into the milk mixture and whisk to blend. Pour the batter into the prepared pan and bake for 1 hour or until set and slightly golden on top.
	5 In a microwave-safe bowl, heat the honey and water for 30 seconds or until thin and liquefied. Poke holes in the surface of the cake and drizzle the honey mixture over the surface. Cool the cake for 30 minutes before cutting and serving.

Per serving: *Calories 129 (From Fat 25); Fat 3g (Saturated 2g); Cholesterol 9mg; Sodium 54mg; Carbohydrate 22g (Dietary Fiber 0g); Protein 4g.*

Note: Farina is a cereal grain made from wheat. You may know it better by its brand names, Cream of Wheat or Malt-o-Meal.

Adding a Touch of Fruit to Sweeten Your Meal

Using fruit in desserts (from cakes to cookies) is common practice in the Mediterranean. Actually, fruit itself is often a simple dessert, which is another key to the health benefits found in the Mediterranean lifestyle.

Getting in the habit of eating a little fruit when you have a sweet tooth is a great wellness strategy. Eating abundant amounts of fruit means consuming more healthy nutrients such as vitamins, antioxidants, and fiber, which help you lower your risk of certain diseases.

This section shows you some great ways to incorporate fruit in your dessert. These desserts are more satisfying; lower in calories, fat, and sugar; and richer in healthy nutrients than the processed sweets you can pick up at the store.

Berry delicious and healthy

Berries, such as strawberries, blueberries, and blackberries, are sweet, make the perfect quick dessert, and provide powerful health benefits. They're loaded in different nutrients including antioxidants, vitamins, minerals, and phytochemicals, which can all help lower your risk of diseases such as heart disease and certain cancers.

The only downside to berries is they can spoil quickly. The best way to get berries is to pick them or to buy them at a local farmers' market. When buying berries at your grocery store, make sure the berries have no soft spots or mold for best quality.

Use the berry-featuring recipes in this chapter (such as the Greek-Style Nesting Berries) for delicious desserts, or try some of these ideas for some quick treats:

- Dip fresh strawberries in chocolate sauce.

- Add a dollop of whipped cream to a bowl of your favorite berries. Top with some pistachios, slivered almonds, or shaved dark chocolate.

- Add fresh berries to vanilla or chocolate frozen yogurt.

- Mix your favorite berries with chocolate pudding.

- Blend berries, banana, and yogurt to make a fruit smoothie. Freeze your fruit smoothie with popsicle sticks to make a delicious frozen treat!

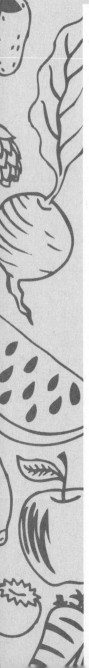

Panna Cotta

Prep time: 15 min, plus chilling time • **Cook time:** 7 min • **Yield:** 4 servings

Ingredients	Directions
1 teaspoon unflavored gelatin	*1* In a small bowl, sprinkle the gelatin over ¼ cup of the cream. Allow the mixture to stand for 1 minute to soften the gelatin.
¾ cup plus 2 tablespoons heavy whipping cream	
3 tablespoons whole milk	*2* In a heavy saucepan, combine the remaining cream, milk, and sugar. Bring the mixture to a boil over medium heat while continuously stirring. Remove the mixture from the heat and whisk in the gelatin mixture until the gelatin dissolves.
2 tablespoons sugar	
2 tablespoons honey	
1 cup blackberries, strawberries, or raspberries	*3* Pour the mixture into 4 small custard cups and chill for at least 4 hours.
	4 To serve, unmold the panna cotta onto serving plates. Drizzle honey over each panna cotta and serve with the berries.

Per serving: Calories 260 (From Fat 179); Fat 20g (Saturated 12g); Cholesterol 73mg; Sodium 32mg; Carbohydrate 21g (Dietary Fiber 2g); Protein 2g.

Greek-Style Nesting Berries

Prep time: 35 min • **Cook time:** 1 hr • **Yield:** 8 servings

Ingredients	Directions
4 egg whites, room temperature **1 cup plus 2 tablespoons sugar** **2 teaspoons cornstarch** **1 teaspoon white vinegar** **½ teaspoon plus ½ teaspoon orange blossom water** **2 cups blackberries, strawberries, and blueberries** **½ cup heavy whipping cream**	*1* Preheat the oven to 250 degrees. Place a piece of parchment paper on a baking sheet. With a pen, trace a 9-inch circle on the parchment paper.
	2 Beat the egg whites in a stainless steel bowl on medium speed for 2 minutes. Increase the speed and slowly add 1 cup of the sugar in a slow, steady stream, beating until stiff peaks form (about 3 to 4 minutes) to form the meringue.
	3 Whisk together the cornstarch, vinegar, and ½ teaspoon of the orange blossom water. Fold the mixture into the meringue, being careful not to overstir and deflate the batter.
	4 Spoon the meringue into the 9-inch circle and spread the batter out to the edges, creating an even disk shape (it doesn't need to be flat on the surface).
	5 Bake the meringue for 1 hour or until it's firm to the touch yet slightly soft in the center. Remove from the oven and cool on a wire cooling rack for at least 30 minutes.
	6 In a separate bowl, gently combine the berries, orange blossom water, and sugar and set aside.
	7 In a clean, cold stainless steel bowl, whip the cream on medium-high speed until soft peaks form. Cut the meringue into 8 slices and top with the berry mixture and a dollop of whipped cream.

Per serving: Calories 196 (From Fat 51); Fat 6g (Saturated 3g); Cholesterol 20mg; Sodium 34mg; Carbohydrate 36g (Dietary Fiber 1g); Protein 2g.

Tip: You can substitute 2 teaspoons of orange zest for the orange blossom water in the berry mixture. You can also buy whipped cream and omit Step 7.

Tip: This recipe is best when enjoyed the day you prepare it. You can also make smaller "nests" and store them in a sealed container at room temperature for a week.

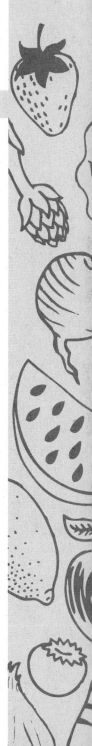

Crepes with Berries

Prep time: 5 min, plus chilling time • **Cook time:** 12 min • **Yield:** 8 servings

Ingredients	*Directions*
2 eggs	**1** Combine the eggs, milk, flour, salt, and butter in a blender until smooth, about 2 minutes. Cover and refrigerate the batter for 1 hour.
1 cup milk	
⅔ cup flour	
⅛ teaspoon salt	**2** In a small bowl, gently combine the berries and sugar. Cover and set aside at room temperature. Spray a nonstick skillet with nonstick cooking spray and heat over medium heat.
1 tablespoon butter, melted	
1½ cups strawberries, blackberries, raspberries, and/ or blueberries	**3** Ladle ¼ cup of the batter into the skillet and quickly rotate and coat the pan with the batter to make a thin crepe as shown in Figure 20-1.
2 tablespoons sugar	
Nonstick cooking spray	**4** Cook for 1 minute (look for golden brown edges) and then flip and cook for 30 seconds or until golden. Remove from the pan, place on a plate, and cover with a warm towel.
Powdered sugar for dusting	
	5 Repeat Steps 3 and 4 with the remaining batter. Fold each crepe in half and then in half again. Top each crepe with berries and dust with powdered sugar to serve.

Per serving: *Calories 108 (From Fat 17); Fat 2g (Saturated 1g); Cholesterol 5mg; Sodium 73mg; Carbohydrate 19g (Dietary Fiber 1g); Protein 3g.*

POURING CREPE BATTER INTO A PAN

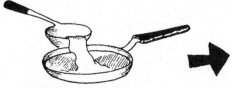

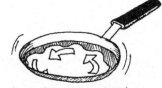

Figure 20-1: Making crepes is easy.

Pour the batter into the crepe pan with a ladle or measuring cup.

Swirl the pan around so the batter runs to the edges and covers the bottom of the pan.

Baked Apples with Raisins and Walnuts

Prep time: 35 min • **Cook time:** 45 min • **Yield:** 8 servings

Ingredients	*Directions*
8 Braeburn or Golden Delicious apples	*1* Preheat the oven to 350 degrees. Core the apples whole (as shown in Figure 20-2) and peel off 1 inch of the skin from the top of the apple.
¾ cup walnuts, chopped	
1 tablespoon orange zest	*2* Combine the walnuts, orange zest, raisins, cinnamon, and cloves. Stuff each apple evenly with 2 tablespoons of nut filling and top with 1 teaspoon of butter. Bake the stuffed apples in a 9-x-13-inch baking dish for 10 minutes.
¼ cup raisins or golden raisins, chopped	
½ teaspoon cinnamon	
¼ teaspoon cloves	
8 teaspoons plus 2 tablespoons butter	*3* Meanwhile, bring the sugar, water, and cinnamon stick to a boil in a heavy saucepan over medium-high heat for 5 minutes. Whisk in the remaining butter and remove from the heat. Discard the cinnamon stick.
½ cup sugar	
½ cup water	*4* Remove the apples from the oven and douse with the sauce. Continue baking for 35 minutes. Serve hot or at room temperature.
1 cinnamon stick	

Per serving: Calories 245 (From Fat 107); Fat 12g (Saturated 3g); Cholesterol 11mg; Sodium 33mg; Carbohydrate 37g (Dietary Fiber 4g); Protein 2g.

HOW TO CORE AN APPLE

Figure 20-2:
How to core
an apple.

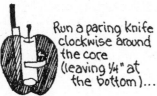 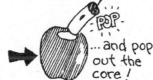

Run a paring knife clockwise around the core (leaving ¼" at the bottom)... POP ...and pop out the core!

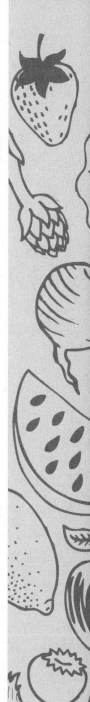

Lemon Ices

Prep time: 5 min, plus freezing time 2 hours • **Yield:** 6 servings

Ingredients	*Directions*
2 cups water	**1** Heat the sugar and water in a heavy saucepan over medium heat until the sugar has dissolved. Add the lemon zest and juice and stir to combine.
¾ cup sugar	
Zest and juice of 5 lemons	
	2 Pour the mixture into a 9-x-13-inch glass baking dish. Freeze the mixture until all the liquid is gone, scraping every 20 minutes. During the last hour of freezing, scrape every 10 minutes to create a finer ice. Spoon into cups and serve.

Per serving: Calories 107 (From Fat 0); Fat 0g (Saturated 0g); Cholesterol 0mg; Sodium 1mg; Carbohydrate 28g (Dietary Fiber 0g); Protein 0g.

Tip: For a smoother consistency, you can chill the lemon mixture in an ice-cream maker. Both methods are considered traditional depending on the area of the Mediterranean.

Note: The color insert in this book shows a photo of this recipe.

Date and Walnut Drops

Prep time: 10 min • **Yield:** 24 servings

Ingredients	Directions
24 dates	**1** Cut each date lengthwise and remove and discard the seed. Stuff each date with 1 almond or walnut.
24 almonds or walnut halves	
½ cup sugar	**2** In a small bowl, combine the sugar and orange zest. Gently roll the stuffed dates in the sugar and serve.
Zest of 1 orange	

Per serving: Calories 109 (From Fat 24); Fat 3g (Saturated 0g); Cholesterol 0mg; Sodium 0mg; Carbohydrate 23g (Dietary Fiber 2g); Protein 1g.

Note: The color insert in this book shows a photo of this recipe.

Make room for walnuts

You may hear a lot of buzz in the media about including omega-3 fatty acids in your diet. *Omega-3 fatty acids* are basically poly-unsaturated fats that have been found to help thin blood and prevent blood platelets from clotting and sticking to artery walls. Consuming these fatty acids is so important because your body doesn't produce them, which means you have to get them through the foods you eat. Unfortunately, most people don't eat enough omega-3s, and this deficiency can lead to an improper balance of fats that contributes to inflammation in your body. (The recommended intake for omega-3 fatty acids is about 1.1 grams per day.) Omega-3s have been shown to reduce inflammation, lowering your risk of heart disease and other chronic diseases. (Head to Chapter 2 for more on the health benefits of omega-3s.)

Walnuts are an omega-3 source that's so simple to add to your weekly food routine. A serving of 1.5 ounces of walnuts provides 3.8 grams of omega-3. Mix them into oatmeal or yogurt for a nutty crunch, toss them into a salad, or just eat them plain as a snack. You can even add them to hot pasta dishes for a nutty flavor and some texture. They can also give a healthy kick to baked treats like cookies or brownies.

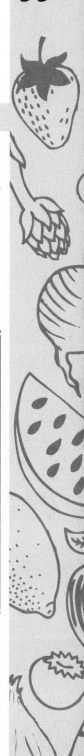

Going Cuckoo for Cookies

People in the Mediterranean use decadent cookies for all kinds of occasions, such as holidays and weddings, like American culture does. However, one difference is that people on the Mediterranean coast traditionally use certain light cookies, primarily biscotti, for breakfast.

If you like this concept, eating a biscotti cookie that includes nuts with your morning coffee, some yogurt or milk, and some fruit isn't necessarily a horrible way to start your day because biscotti aren't terribly high in sugar, fat, or calories. The heart-healthy nuts contain protein and healthy fats to help you feel satisfied. In this section, we show you how to make biscotti, as well as a variety of unique and beautiful cookies that are perfect for your next celebration.

You may be thinking, "Cookies for breakfast? Sign me up!" But beware; not all cookies are created equal. Don't replace the breakfast biscotti with something like creamy sandwich cookies, or the whole concept will backfire. We still recommend having a healthy breakfast that includes whole grains, protein, and healthy fats.

If you're allergic to nuts, you can certainly try many of these recipes and omit the nuts. See how you like the taste!

A spoonful of honey makes the cold symptoms go away

Honey is a popular ingredient in Mediterranean cooking and also has some interesting health benefits along with its sweet, satisfying flavor. In a small study, researchers from Penn State College of Medicine found that a single night-time dose of buckwheat honey helped to alleviate cough in kids age 2 to 18 with upper respiratory tract infections. A spoonful of honey beats cough medicine any day!

Another study from the University of Ottawa found that two specific types of honey called manuka and sidr were effective at killing off bacteria associated with sinusitis. Chronic sinusitis occurs when the nasal membranes become inflamed leading to stuffy nose, headaches, and difficulty breathing.

More research is needed in this area, but the good news is that a little honey is certainly not bad for you. If you're battling a cold or have sinusitis, give honey a try.

Pucker Up Lemon Polenta Cookies

Prep time: 15 min, plus chilling time 30 • **Cook time:** 14 minutes • **Yield:** 36 servings

Ingredients	Directions
½ cup room-temperature butter ¼ cup sugar ¼ cup brown sugar, packed 1 tablespoon honey Zest and juice of 1 lemon, plus 1 tablespoon juice 1 egg 1 teaspoon vanilla ¼ cup pistachios 1⅓ cups flour ½ cup cornmeal ½ teaspoon cardamom ¼ teaspoon salt 1 tablespoon half and half ½ cup powdered sugar	*1* With an electric mixer, cream the butter, sugar, brown sugar, honey, and lemon zest until fluffy, approximately 5 minutes. Add the egg, vanilla, and lemon juice (minus 1 tablespoon) and mix until incorporated. *2* In a food processor, grind the pistachios to a flour consistency. In a small bowl, combine the ground nuts, flour, cornmeal, cardamom, and salt. *3* Add the dry mixture to the wet ingredients and mix until combined. Chill the dough for 30 minutes in refrigerator. *4* Preheat the oven to 350 degrees. Roll the dough into balls 1 tablespoon at a time, place the balls 2 inches apart on a cookie sheet, and flatten gently. Repeat with remaining dough. *5* Bake for 10 to 14 minutes or until the edges brown. Remove from the oven and cool completely on a wire rack. *6* Whisk together the remaining lemon juice, the half and half, and the powdered sugar in a small bowl. Drizzle the cooled cookies with the glaze and cool until the glaze hardens. Serve.

Per serving: Calories 77 (From Fat 28); Fat 3g (Saturated 2g); Cholesterol 7mg; Sodium 65mg; Carbohydrate 12g (Dietary Fiber 0g); Protein 1g.

Tip: You can store the cookies at room temperature in a covered container for a week or freeze them for a month.

Note: Check out the color insert for a photo of this recipe.

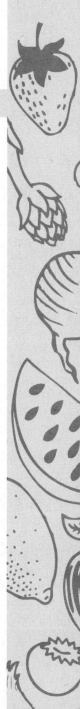

Orange Cardamom Cookies

Prep time: 15 min, plus chilling time • **Cook time:** 30 min • **Yield:** 48 servings

Ingredients	*Directions*
3 cups flour	*1* In a large mixing bowl, whisk together the flour, baking soda, cream of tartar, ½ teaspoon of the cardamom, and the salt. Set aside.
¾ teaspoon baking soda	
1 teaspoon cream of tartar	
½ teaspoon plus 1 teaspoon cardamom	*2* Using a stand mixer, cream the butter and 1½ cups of the sugar until creamy, about 4 minutes. Add the eggs and mix for 1 minute. Add the orange blossom water, orange zest, and milk and gently mix for 1 minute.
½ teaspoon salt	
1 stick room-temperature butter	
1½ cups plus ¾ cup sugar	*3* Mix the flour mixture into the batter just until combined. Chill the dough in the refrigerator for at least 1 hour.
2 eggs	
½ teaspoon orange blossom water or vanilla extract	*4* Combine the remaining sugar and cardamom. Roll the chilled dough into 1-inch balls. Roll the dough in the cardamom sugar and place each ball about 2 inches apart on a baking sheet.
1 tablespoon orange zest	
¼ cup milk	
	5 Bake the cookies for 10 to 12 minutes or until the edges are slightly golden brown. Allow the cookies to cool on the baking sheet for 3 minutes and then transfer to a cooling rack. Serve.

Per serving: Calories 83 (From Fat 18); Fat 2g (Saturated 1g); Cholesterol 5mg; Sodium 61mg; Carbohydrate 15g (Dietary Fiber 0g); Protein 1g.

Orange, Chocolate, and Pistachio Biscotti

Prep time: 25 min • **Cook Time:** 35 min, plus cooling time • **Yield:** 36 servings

Ingredients	Directions
¾ cup pistachios, shelled	*1* Preheat the oven to 350 degrees. Place parchment paper on two baking sheets.
¼ cup semisweet chocolate chips, lightly chopped	
2 cups plus ¼ cup flour	*2* In a large bowl, combine 2 cups flour, the sugar, salt, baking powder, and baking soda. Cut in the butter and mix with a spoon. Add the pistachios and chocolate chips.
1 cup sugar	
⅛ teaspoon salt	
1 teaspoon baking powder	*3* In a small bowl, combine the eggs, egg yolk, and orange blossom water. Using a stand mixer, mix the egg mixture into the flour mixture, forming the dough.
¼ teaspoon baking soda	
3 tablespoons room temperature butter	*4* Lightly dust your hands with the remaining flour and form the dough into a ball. Dust your work surface with the remaining flour and knead the dough 5 times, no more than 1 minute. Divide the dough in half.
2 whole eggs plus 1 egg yolk	
1 teaspoon orange blossom water	*5* Roll each piece of dough into a log 8 inches long, 3 inches wide, and 1 inch thick. Place each log onto the parchment paper about 5 inches apart. Bake the logs for 20 minutes.
	6 Remove the logs from the oven and cool for 10 minutes. Gently transfer to a cutting board and use a sharp knife to cut biscotti pieces horizontally every ½ inch.
	7 Place the cookies cut side down onto two baking sheets lined with parchment paper. Bake the cookies for 5 minutes; turn each cookie over and bake for an additional 10 minutes. Let the cookies cool completely on baking sheets before storing.

Per serving: Calories 80 (From Fat 23); Fat 3g (Saturated 1g); Cholesterol 3mg; Sodium 42mg; Carbohydrate 13g (Dietary Fiber 1g); Protein 2g.

Tip: You can replace the orange blossom water with 1 tablespoon of orange zest.

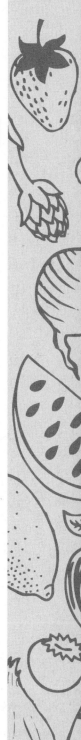

Classic Biscotti

Prep time: 25 minutes • **Cook time:** 35 minutes, plus cooling time • **Yield:** 36 servings

Ingredients	Directions
½ **cup toasted hazelnuts, skins removed**	**1** Preheat the oven to 350 degrees. Place a piece of parchment paper on a baking sheet.
½ **cup toasted almonds**	
2 **cups plus** ¼ **cup flour**	**2** In a large bowl, mix 2 cups of the flour, the sugar, salt, baking powder, baking soda, and orange zest. Cut in the butter and mix with a spoon. Add the hazelnuts and the almonds and stir to combine.
1 **cup sugar**	
1 **teaspoon baking powder**	
¼ **teaspoon baking soda**	**3** In a small bowl, combine the eggs, egg yolk, and vanilla extract. Using a stand mixer, mix the egg mixture into the flour mixture, forming the dough.
1 **teaspoon orange zest**	
⅛ **teaspoon salt**	
3 **tablespoons room temperature butter**	**4** Lightly dust your hands with some of the remaining flour and form the dough into a ball. Dust your work surface with the remaining flour and knead the dough 5 times, no longer than 1 minute. Divide the dough in half.
2 **whole eggs plus 1 egg yolk**	
1 **teaspoon vanilla extract**	
	5 Roll each piece of dough into a log 8 inches long, 3 inches wide, and 1 inch thick. Place each log onto the parchment paper about 5 inches apart. Bake the logs for 20 minutes.
	6 Remove the logs from the oven and cool for 10 minutes. Gently transfer the logs to a cutting board and use a sharp knife to cut biscotti pieces horizontally every ½ inch.
	7 Place the cookies cut side down onto two baking sheets lined with parchment paper. Bake the cookies for 5 minutes; turn each cookie over and bake for an additional 10 minutes. Let the cookies cool completely on baking sheets before storing.

Per serving: Calories 84 (From Fat 29); Fat 3g (Saturated 1g); Cholesterol 3mg; Sodium 42mg; Carbohydrate 12g (Dietary Fiber 1g); Protein 2g.

Tip: Keep the cookies in a tightly covered container; you can store them at room temperature for 2 weeks.

Part V
The Part of Tens

The 5th Wave — By Rich Tennant

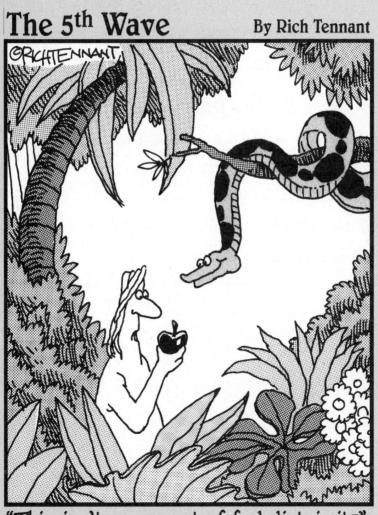

"This isn't some sort of fad diet, is it?"

In this part . . .

This part explains how you can get more plant-based foods into your diet and shoots down some common misconceptions about the Mediterranean way of life. (You probably already guessed that you can't healthily stuff yourself with pasta, wine, and cheese.)

The appendix in this part contains some useful information for converting the temperatures and measurements in this book to their metric equivalents.

Chapter 21

Ten Tips for Getting More Plant-Based Foods in Your Diet

In This Chapter

▶ Upping your intake of fruits, veggies, and herbs

▶ Finding simple ways to get whole grains and legumes into your daily meals

*T*he biggest concept behind a Mediterranean style diet is adding more plant-based foods, such as fruits, vegetables, herbs, legumes, and even whole grains, to every meal. Fruits and vegetables are the main components of this push; you want to have five to nine servings of fruits and vegetables each day. Hitting that number may be a simple change for some people, but it may be a bigger challenge for others. Similarly, you may be at a loss as to how legumes, herbs, and whole grains can fit into your lifestyle. When you aren't used to eating many fruits, vegetables, and the like, knowing how to add them to your diet may be quite difficult. Fortunately, adding plant-based foods to your diet isn't rocket science. This chapter is here to help make the shift effortless and tasty.

Increasing the variety of the plant-based foods you eat each day means you also get a good variety of the nutrients your body needs.

Keeping Sliced Vegetables on Hand

One of the easiest ways to consume more veggies is to eat them raw as snacks. The key to making it simple is to pre-slice a bunch of different vegetables, such as bell peppers, broccoli, carrots, and any other favorites, for the week at one time. Then you can grab some of the veggies and your favorite dip — such as the Hummus or the Roasted Eggplant Dip from Chapter 8 — while sitting at your desk or watching a movie for an instant healthy snack. In addition, you can throw whatever cut veggies you don't use as snacks into a soup, pasta dish, or salad or some scrambled eggs.

Including a Fruit or Vegetable with Every Meal

Always planning to have a fruit or vegetable with every meal is a good mindset to get you into the Mediterranean spirit. After you have this little mental guideline in your head, you can find all sorts of creative ways to make it happen. For example, you can spruce up your sandwich with dark leafy greens and tomatoes, add some fruit to your yogurt, or slice up some raw veggies to have on hand as a snack. You can make this habit work for you in all kinds of ways. By focusing on this guideline, you'll naturally start incorporating five to nine servings of fruits and vegetables during the day.

Keeping a Fruit Bowl on Your Counter

Rather than the old mantra "out of sight, out of mind," you want to go for "in sight, in mind." Keep a fruit bowl on your counter to remind you to eat some fruit during the day with your meal or snacks. If you have kids, you may be surprised how much more fruit they eat when it's in plain sight. Having a bowl of fresh fruit also looks beautiful and sets the stage for your kitchen to be a healthy, nutritious spot.

Don't just settle for a few bananas; fill the bowl up with all kinds of fresh, seasonal fruit so that you have choices and aren't left with the same type of fruit all day.

Adding Fruit to Your Cereals

Adding fruit to your cereals is a great strategy that gives your meal more flavor and makes it more satisfying. Slice up any sort of fresh fruit, such as bananas, nectarines, or peaches, or sprinkle some fresh berries on your cereal or oatmeal. Dried fruit is also a wonderful choice and is easy to store in your pantry. Just choose dried fruits with no added sugars.

You can add fresh fruit to your cereal year-round. Just keep frozen fruits and berries in your freezer so you can thaw them in the microwave in a few seconds. Their warm, juicy texture is perfect on top of oatmeal or low-fat granola.

Dressing Up Your Salad with Fresh Fruits and Vegetables

Don't settle for a boring old leafy green salad. You can create a savory or sweet masterpiece by incorporating some fruits and veggies. For example, add sliced bell peppers, tomatoes, and fresh herbs, such as dill, for a savory experience. Sweeten up another salad by adding mandarin orange slices along with some walnuts.

Salads in general are a great way to up your plant food intake. Use salads frequently as an additional vegetable side or as your entree with some kind of protein (such as chicken or egg).

Sneaking Veggies and Herbs into Your Egg Dishes

You can use vegetables to add tons of flavor and texture to the most basic egg dishes, such as scrambled eggs. Chop up fresh tomatoes (okay, those are technically a fruit), fresh spinach, onions, or even zucchini. If you have leftover steamed veggies, they're perfect to throw into an egg dish the next morning.

You can also add fresh herbs to the mix to add significant flavor. Basil, parsley, and oregano are all great flavors with eggs. Fresh salsa is also an excellent addition to egg dishes. For some recipe ideas, check out the egg dishes in Chapter 7. Remember, though, that egg dishes don't just have to be for breakfast; they can be great, quick meal ideas for lunch and dinner, too.

Punching Up Your Pasta with Fresh Produce

Pasta dishes are the perfect food to add fresh vegetables and herbs to. Even if you already use a vegetable-based sauce such as marinara, you can up the vegetable quotient by adding blanched broccoli, carrots, and bell peppers. Doing so adds more variety and helps you eat less pasta than you may otherwise.

And don't forget about herbs! Fresh herbs can turn your pasta dish into something spectacular. Experiment yourself and see what types of blends work well for you. One idea: Next time you're eating a pasta salad, try adding some fresh basil leaves.

Starting Off with a Little Vegetable Soup

Beginning a meal with a cup of vegetable soup is an easy strategy for adding more vegetables and helping with weight management. Use low-calorie vegetable or tomato soup as a starter for your meals. The soup can help you feel full and satisfied so that you eat less of the main meal.

Supercharging Soups and Stews with Whole Grains

You can add some flavor and texture to soups and stews by incorporating whole grains such as whole-wheat pasta or pearl barley into them. Adding whole grains to plain vegetable soup can recreate a side dish as a complete meal. Whole grains provide fiber and other healthful nutrients and add to the variety of plant-based foods you take in during your day. Check out Chapter 5 for more information about the health benefits of whole grains.

Adding Beans to, Well, Everything

Beans are versatile, flavorful, and easy to use with many different dishes. Look for ways to include them every day.

Always keep some dried and canned beans on hand in your pantry. You can rinse canned beans and add them to soups, stews, salads, pasta dishes, or grain dishes.

Chapter 22

Ten Myths about the Mediterranean Diet

In This Chapter

▶ Uncovering some common misconceptions about the Mediterranean diet

▶ Discovering the right balance to make a Mediterranean lifestyle healthy

*F*ollowing a Mediterranean lifestyle definitely offers many benefits, such as better health, flavorful food, and lots of fun, without depriving you. However, not everything you've heard about this way of life is necessarily true. Proclamations that you can eat huge, rich meals and drink tons of wine are a little misleading. This chapter debunks some of the myths you may have heard so that you make sure you stay on the right track.

People Who Live in the Mediterranean Are All Healthy

The Mediterranean coast covers a large region including parts of Africa, Morocco, Greece, Turkey, France, and Italy, just to name a few. Not all countries or all regions practice the same healthy habits. For instance, people in northern Italy more commonly use lard and butter in cooking, which tips their diet's balance toward more saturated fats than you see in southern Italy, where people primarily use olive oil.

In general, however, the Mediterranean lifestyle we tout in this book is inspired by the Greek island of Crete and other areas of Greece, plus Spain, Morocco, and southern Italy.

You Can Eat as Much Cheese as You Want

One misconception about the Mediterranean diet is that you can eat as much cheese as your heart (or stomach) desires. Unfortunately, this myth isn't true. Eating too much cheese can add up in unwanted calories and saturated fats. People in certain regions of the Mediterranean do consume large amounts of cheese, but these regions don't share in the same health benefits that the more rural areas this diet is centered on do. (See the preceding section for specifics on what those areas are.)

Consuming cheese is a common Mediterranean practice, but you want to do so in a moderate way. Using strong-flavored cheeses such as feta or goat cheese helps you get a lot of flavor while using much less cheese.

Drinking as Much Wine as You Want Is Heart Healthy

Wine certainly does have unique health benefits for your heart (head to Chapter 2 for details on what these are). However, drinking in moderation is the key. Residents on the Mediterranean coast don't actually drink as much alcohol as you may think. Enjoying a glass of wine with dinner is common, but downing two to three glasses is not. Frequently drinking more than one to two glasses of wine can actually be bad for your heart (not to mention your decision-making). To stay on the healthy side of the fence, enjoy a glass of wine with your meal a few times a week — and maybe hide the karaoke machine.

You Can Eat Desserts Regularly and Manage Your Weight

Eating too many desserts isn't good for your midsection or your overall weight. People of the Mediterranean coast primarily eat a diet full of vegetables, fruits, whole grains, and legumes, and not every meal includes a luxurious dessert. The region does offer some of the most delicious traditional desserts, such as baklava, but these dishes are served for special occasions (such as holidays or weddings) maybe once or twice a year. For the most part, Mediterranean folks eat fruit for dessert or enjoy low-calorie cookies such as biscotti. Portion sizes of these desserts are also smaller than you may be used to; one to two biscotti is plenty.

Eating Large Bowls of Pasta with Bread Is Totally Fine

The Mediterranean diet conjures up thoughts of Italian cooking and pasta, pasta, pasta! And what's pasta without bread to soak up all that sauce? Eating big bowls of pasta with garlic bread is one of those myths where the truth isn't always what it may seem on the surface.

Yes, Italians in particular eat a lot of pasta, but not in the type of portion sizes that Americans are accustomed to. In the Mediterranean, pasta is typically a side dish with about a ½-cup to 1-cup serving size. Pasta isn't the stand-alone dish; instead, people have salads, meat sides, and vegetable sides to fill their plates. A slice of bread (as in one slice) often joins the meal, for a total of two to three starch servings for that meal. Chapter 15 provides delicious pasta recipes with the right portion sizes.

You Don't Have to Go to the Gym

This one is technically true, but part of the mindset behind it needs debunking. People who lived on the Mediterranean coast 60 years ago likely weren't hitting the gym for exercise, so no, you don't specifically have to drag yourself to the gym every day to model their lifestyle. That's a relief, right?

However, you're not off the hook on physical activity entirely. These people didn't need a workout because they were much more active in daily life, performing manual work and walking where they needed to go rather than driving everywhere in a car. A more convenient life means you have to seek out ways to get exercise each and every day.

The Diet Can't Be Healthy Because It Contains So Much Fat

People on the Mediterranean coast do eat more fat than is recommended in the United States, but that doesn't mean their diet is considered high-fat. The average fat intake in the Mediterranean is about 35 percent of daily calories, and the average U.S. intake is 36 percent.

The key to Mediterranean diet is the *type* of fat consumed. Folks in the Mediterranean region eat more heart-healthy monounsaturated fats, such as those in olive oil and avocados, than they do saturated fats found in meats, butter, and dairy.

The Health Benefits are All about the Diet

Diet (that is, a way of eating) is a key contributor to the health benefits prominent in certain regions of the Mediterranean coast, but it isn't the only contributor. Physical activity (see the earlier section "You Don't Have to Go to the Gym"), stress management, rest and play, and proper vitamin D levels from ample sunshine are also important components. A combination of all these factors is likely what results in the health benefits seen by researchers. After all, eating a healthy diet, getting physical activity, and managing your stress are still the most common recommendations for engaging in any healthy lifestyle.

People from the Mediterranean Eat Huge Meals and Never Gain Weight

Maintaining weight in spite of eating large meals *is* sometimes possible for the people of this region, but the catch is that they eat many small servings of low-calorie foods rather than large servings of high-calorie foods — that is, loads of vegetables (both raw and cooked) and small portions of meats, grains, and legumes. The important point is the make-up of the meal, not the size. You can't eat just anything at a large meal, even on the Mediterranean diet. The meal has to have the right balance of foods and still come in at a relatively low calorie level.

You Can Continue a Busy Life and Fully Adopt a Mediterranean Diet

Everything about the Mediterranean lifestyle is about slowing down: taking time to choose your foods, cook them, and have a hearty meal with your family; spending time with your loved ones; and giving yourself plenty of time for rest and play. You only get 24 hours in a day, so to provide all this time for food, activity, community, and rest, you may have to sacrifice a busy work life. If that is impossible, don't fret! Make a goal to adopt a few Mediterranean lifestyle choices. Even a few small changes can still make a big impact on your overall health and well-being.

Appendix

Metric Conversion Guide

ote: The recipes in this book weren't developed or tested using metric measurements. There may be some variation in quality when converting to metric units.

Common Abbreviations

Abbreviation(s)	What It Stands For
cm	Centimeter
C., c.	Cup
G, g	Gram
kg	Kilogram
L, l	Liter
lb.	Pound
mL, ml	Milliliter
oz.	Ounce
pt.	Pint
t., tsp.	Teaspoon
T., Tb., Tbsp.	Tablespoon

Volume

U.S. Units	Canadian Metric	Australian Metric
¼ teaspoon	1 milliliter	1 milliliter
½ teaspoon	2 milliliters	2 milliliters
1 teaspoon	5 milliliters	5 milliliters
1 tablespoon	15 milliliters	20 milliliters
¼ cup	50 milliliters	60 milliliters
⅓ cup	75 milliliters	80 milliliters
½ cup	125 milliliters	125 milliliters
⅔ cup	150 milliliters	170 milliliters
¾ cup	175 milliliters	190 milliliters
1 cup	250 milliliters	250 milliliters
1 quart	1 liter	1 liter
1½ quarts	1.5 liters	1.5 liters
2 quarts	2 liters	2 liters
2½ quarts	2.5 liters	2.5 liters
3 quarts	3 liters	3 liters
4 quarts (1 gallon)	4 liters	4 liters

Weight

U.S. Units	Canadian Metric	Australian Metric
1 ounce	30 grams	30 grams
2 ounces	55 grams	60 grams
3 ounces	85 grams	90 grams
4 ounces (¼ pound)	115 grams	125 grams
8 ounces (½ pound)	225 grams	225 grams
16 ounces (1 pound)	455 grams	500 grams (½ kilogram)

Length

Inches	Centimeters
0.5	1.5
1	2.5
2	5.0
3	7.5
4	10.0
5	12.5
6	15.0
7	17.5
8	20.5
9	23.0
10	25.5
11	28.0
12	30.5

Temperature (Degrees)

Fahrenheit	Celsius
32	0
212	100
250	120
275	140
300	150
325	160
350	180
375	190
400	200
425	220
450	230
475	240
500	260

Index

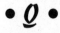

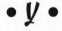